P9-CJW-235

ADVANCE PRAISE FOR

The Gluten-Free Edge

"If you want to learn more about how to optimize your performance and body composition, then read this book. Seriously."
—RYAN D. ANDREWS, MS, MA, RD, CSCS, coach with Precision Nutrition

"Insights from history, science, and nutrition, combined with striking personal accounts from elite athletes, make it an engaging read all the way through. The NFCA is proud to find our Athletes for Awareness among these pages, and we expect this book will inspire more to come!"—ALICE BAST, and the team at the National Foundation for Celiac Awareness

"Finally! A book that validates the science behind everything I've observed with our athletes: Gluten-free equals improved performance. If you want to go faster, get leaner, and have the energy to go the distance, get the facts from *The Gluten-Free Edge*. You will be blown away by this book—and once you read it you'll never want to go back to eating, feeling, and underperforming the way you did before. A must-read for all athletes!"—MIRIAM G. ZACHARIAS, PhD, MS, Vice President of the National Association of Nutrition Professionals

"Nutritional needs are forefront in the minds of athletes, including trail runners. This well-written and thoroughly researched book demystifies gluten and provides a realistic approach to food as it relates to and assists with performance."
—NANCY HOBBS, Executive Director, American Trail Running Association

"*The Gluten-Free Edge* is a great book for both the weekend warrior and the professional. Even as an ultra-endurance swimmer and 50-year-old competitive athlete, I found much to learn. The authors help you navigate a complicated subject with simple and personal stories that everyone can understand."
—BRUCE GORDON, marathon swimmer

"*The Gluten-Free Edge* provides very powerful personal stories and lessons for anyone contemplating the shift toward a gluten-free lifestyle. Great insights for athletes and non-athletes alike, especially those suffering from celiac disease or undiagnosed gluten intolerance." —SETH BRONHEIM, MS, RD, CDN, Director of Nutrition and Fitness, Generation UCAN, www.generationucan.com

HILLSBORO   RARIES
WITHDRAWN   IDEAS
COOPERATIVE LIBRARY SERVICES

ALSO BY PETER BRONSKI

At the Mercy of the Mountains: True Stories of Survival and Tragedy in New York's Adirondacks

Hunting Nature's Fury: A Storm Chaser's Obsession with Tornadoes, Hurricanes, and Other Natural Disasters

Powder Ghost Towns: Epic Backcountry Runs in Colorado's Lost Ski Resorts

WITH KELLI BRONSKI

Artisanal Gluten-Free Cooking: 275 Great-Tasting, From-Scratch Recipes from Around the World, Perfect for Every Meal and Anyone on a Gluten-Free Diet— and Even Those Who Aren't

Artisanal Gluten-Free Cupcakes: 50 From-Scratch Recipes to Delight Every Cupcake Devotee—Gluten-Free and Otherwise

THE
Gluten-Free
EDGE

A NUTRITION AND
TRAINING GUIDE FOR PEAK
ATHLETIC PERFORMANCE
AND AN ACTIVE
GLUTEN-FREE LIFE

Peter Bronski and
Melissa McLean Jory, MNT

FOREWORD BY AMY YODER BEGLEY

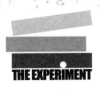

THE EXPERIMENT

NEW YORK

HILLSBORO PUBLIC LIBRARIES
Hillsboro, OR
Member of Washington County
COOPERATIVE LIBRARY SERVICES

THE GLUTEN-FREE EDGE: *A Nutrition and Training Guide for Peak Athletic Performance and an Active Gluten-Free Life*
Copyright © Peter Bronski and Melissa McLean Jory, 2012
Foreword copyright © Amy Yoder Begley, 2012
The photo credits on page 358 are a continuation of this copyright page.

All rights reserved. Except for brief passages quoted in newspaper, magazine, radio, television, or online reviews, no portion of this book may be reproduced, distributed, or transmitted in any form or by any means, electronic or mechanical, including photocopying, recording, or information storage or retrieval system, without the prior written permission of the publisher.

The Experiment, LLC
260 Fifth Avenue
New York, NY 10001–6408
www.theexperimentpublishing.com

The Experiment's books are available at special discounts when purchased in bulk for premiums and sales promotions as well as for fundraising or educational use. For details, contact us at info@theexperimentpublishing.com.

Many of the designations used by manufacturers and sellers to distinguish their products are claimed as trademarks. Where those designations appear in this book and The Experiment was aware of a trademark claim, the designations have been capitalized.

This book is not intended as a substitute for the medical advice of physicians or other clinicians. Readers should consult with a physician, dietitian, or other health-care professional before beginning or making any changes to a diet, exercise, or health program. The authors and publisher expressly disclaim responsibility for any liability, loss, or risk—personal or otherwise—which is incurred, directly or indirectly, as a consequence of the use and application of any of the contents of this book.

Library of Congress Cataloging-in-Publication Data
Bronski, Peter.
The gluten-free edge : a nutrition and training guide for peak athletic performance and an active gluten-free life / Peter Bronski and Melissa McLean Jory ; foreword by Amy Yoder Begley.
p. cm.
Includes bibliographical references and index.
ISBN 978-1-61519-052-2 (pbk.)—ISBN 978-1-61519-149-9 (ebook) 1. Gluten-free diet—Popular works. 2. Gluten-free diet—Recipes. I. Jory, Melissa McLean. II. Title.
RM237.86.B753 2012
615.8'54—dc23
2012005134

ISBN 978-1-61519-052-2
Ebook ISBN 978-1-61519-149-9

4965 0319 8/12

Cover design by Howard Grossman | 12edesign.com
Cover photograph of tennis player © Thomas M. Barwick INC | Getty Images
Cover photograph of jogger © Maridav | 123RF
Text design by Pauline Neuwirth, Neuwirth & Associates, Inc.

Manufactured in the United States of America
Distributed by Workman Publishing Company, Inc.
Distributed simultaneously in Canada by Thomas Allen and Son Ltd.
First published July 2012

10 9 8 7 6 5 4 3 2 1

To Kelli, Marin, and Charlotte, my constant "support crew" . . .
in racing and in life
—Peter

For my mom and my family, for their love and support, and to the memory
of my dad, who, by example, taught me to love the mountains
—Melissa

CONTENTS

Foreword by Amy Yoder Begley   ix

Introduction   1

   Pete's Story   8

   Melissa's Story   13

1. G IS FOR GLUTEN   19

2. WHY ALL ATHLETES SHOULD CARE ABOUT GLUTEN   35

3. GET YOUR MOTOR RUNNING: HOW THE BODY STORES AND USES ENERGY   69

4. FUELING THE ENGINE: THE FOOD FOUNDATION   79

5. SPECIAL CONSIDERATIONS   116

6. HIGH OCTANE: GLUTEN-FREE FOR MAXIMUM PERFORMANCE   134

7. CHANNEL YOUR INNER CAMEL: THE IMPORTANCE OF PROPER HYDRATION   163

8. GETTING PERSONAL: SPORT-, GENDER-, AND AGE-SPECIFIC ADVICE   183

9. TIME FOR A TUNE-UP   218

10. NO TRAIN, NO GAIN: TRAINING AND EXERCISE STRATEGIES TO COMPLEMENT NUTRITION   228

11. ON YOUR MARK, GET SET, COOK! FLAVORFUL, NUTRIENT-DENSE RECIPES   247

   Breakfasts   253

   Smoothies   261

   On the Go: Snacks and Trail Food   264

   Salads and Savory Dips   272

   Lunches and Dinners   279

   Desserts   307

Metric Conversion Charts 311

Glossary 313

Notes 325

Photo Acknowledgments 358

Acknowledgments 359

Index 362

About the Authors 372

FOREWORD

by Amy Yoder Begley

WHEN I WAS diagnosed with celiac disease in 2006, it was a relief to have an answer, but overwhelming to learn how to live a gluten-free life while training for distance races. I spent hours in the bookstore trying to find a book with all the answers. I spent even longer reading labels. Learning to cook gluten-free and to eat safely while traveling was a trial-and-error process. My perseverance ultimately paid off, and I made the 2008 Beijing Olympic Team in the 10,000 meters two years after my diagnosis. That diagnosis was a doorway to a healthier life that allowed me to reach my potential and accomplish my dreams.

Now, I get weekly emails from athletes with questions about eating and training gluten-free, and I am excited to be able to point them to one resource, *The Gluten-Free Edge*. It is an informative book that covers everything a newly diagnosed celiac or a veteran gluten-free athlete could want to know. If you don't have a medical reason to go gluten-free but are wondering whether it will boost your performance, *The Gluten-Free Edge* will leave you convinced. I have a degree in exercise science and I still learned new things from these pages.

The Gluten-Free Edge is the first book for all athletes that explains what gluten is and how it affects digestion and the body in an easy-to-read yet scientific manner. Pete and Melissa also break down the complicated aspects of energy systems, nutrition, hydration, and training programs so that you can easily apply them to your gluten-free life. And they conclude with a great mix of nutrient-dense, gluten-free recipes specifically tailored for athletes.

They also include examples of athletes from many sports who have benefited from going gluten-free, whether they have celiac or gluten intolerance or just switched for improved performance. Each athlete took a different route to becoming gluten-free, but all of them will inspire you with their accomplishments. They prove that it's possible to reach your goals while being 100 percent gluten-free.

I enjoyed reading *The Gluten-Free Edge*, and I am excited to recommend this book to athletes everywhere. It will encourage the newly diagnosed and prove a valuable resource to those already experiencing the gluten-free edge.

AMY YODER BEGLEY is an Olympian and six-time national champion American middle and long distance runner. Gluten-free since her diagnosis with celiac disease in 2006, she represented the United States in the 10,000-meter track event at the 2008 Summer Olympics in Beijing. She lives in Oregon with her husband.

INTRODUCTION

W HEN THE ANCIENT Greeks held the world's first Olympics in 776
BC, they did more than give us the forerunner to today's modern
Olympics. They also gave us the fields of sports medicine, athletic training, and nutrition. Ancient Greece was one of the first cultures to embrace sports and fitness, one of the first in which athletes adhered to
sport-specific training regimens, and perhaps *the* first where athletes
adopted particular diets to maximize their performance. Athletes then,
as now, were looking to gain an edge.

Diet has long proven central to the equation. The diet in ancient
Greece—a predecessor to today's heralded Mediterranean diet—focused
heavily on fresh fruits and vegetables. Figs and grapes were especially
popular fruits, alongside apples, pears, and dates. Beans, peas, onions,
radishes, squash, beets, garlic, and wild greens were the vegetables of
choice. Cereal grains, especially gluten-containing wheat and barley,
provided complex carbohydrates. Fat came chiefly from olive oil. Fish
was a popular source of protein, as was feta cheese, but meat consumption was rare among the general population. Honey was used for sweetening foods, and wine—often diluted with water—was the drink of
choice.[1]

Athletes of the day looking to gain a competitive advantage over their
opponents adopted different eating habits, however. Some of those athletic diets were notable for recommending what athletes *should* eat.

Charmis of Sparta—who trained on a diet of dried figs—won the 200-yard sprint at the Olympic Games in 668 BC, touching off a dried fig fad. Soon, dried figs, cheese, and wheat became the diet of choice for athletes.

In the sixth century BC, Eurymenes of Samos became an Olympic victor as the first recorded athlete to train with a diet heavily reliant upon meat, very unusual for an ancient Greek. In the early fifth century BC, long-distance runner Dromeus of Stymphalus continued the meat-heavy diet craze among athletes. The most famous athlete to proclaim the benefits of eating meat, however, was the legendary wrestler Milo of Croton, who won six consecutive Olympic games. (He was said to consume 20 pounds of meat, another 20 pounds of bread, and 18 pints of wine *per day.*)[2]

On the other hand, Xenophon—writing in the fifth century BC—was unique for recommending what athletes *shouldn't* eat, in particular bread.[3] Bread and porridge—made with wheat and/or barley—were ubiquitous staples of the ancient Greek diet. (Plato called them "good and beneficial food."[4]) Yet, an important subset of the era's elite athletes voluntarily abstained, following Xenophon's advice. Although they wouldn't have called it by the name, they had, in essence, gone gluten-free.

With the benefit of 2,500 years of hindsight, there's a certain poetry to this juxtaposition. Not only did these early athletes forgo bread in a culture whose cuisine was built upon gluten-containing wheat and barley, but ancient Greece also gave us what is widely considered to be the first description of gluten intolerance. During the late first and early second centuries AD, Greek physician and writer Aretaeus of Cappadocia observed patients with a digestive disorder that gave them a distended stomach and symptoms that included diarrhea. He labeled their condition *koiliakos,* from which the name for celiac disease is derived.[5] (Archaeologists have since unearthed another case, also from the first century AD, of ancient celiac disease. In Cosa, an archaeological site in the Tuscany region of Italy, a young wealthy woman—living in an area of widespread wheat cultivation—died with signs of severe malnutrition, anemia, and osteoporosis, classic symptoms of celiac disease.[6])

This book strikes at the heart of the ancient Greek dichotomy—that athletes, through diet and training, were striving to look, feel, and perform their best (some of them doing so through a rudimentary gluten-free diet), while some members of that same population were struggling with a gluten-induced condition we'd later know as celiac disease. Herodicus, who lived during the fifth century BC and is considered the father of sports medicine, offers valuable perspective: He believed that poor health was the result of an imbalance between diet and physical activity.[7]

This book also strikes a tone of brutal honesty. No matter what we *think* you should eat and how we believe going gluten-free may benefit you, we've grounded *The Gluten-Free Edge* in the best of what established and cutting-edge science tells us today, and illustrated the science with examples from athletes. If the truth is cloudy and not black-and-white, or if researchers have yet to get to the bottom of a particular issue, we won't make more out of something than is actually there. But if the evidence is convincing—and in many cases it is—we'll tell you.

We're aware that—as gluten-free athletes with celiac disease ourselves, as gluten-free bloggers, as a gluten-free cookbook author and gluten-free nutritionist—we bring a certain perspective to the table. And we know that when you're a hammer, every problem can begin to look like a nail. We're not here to tell you that going gluten-free is the holy grail for every person, or every athlete. But there's very good reason for any person to read this book, and especially for athletes to pay attention to our message, to digest the information, so to speak, and make an important personal decision. Is the gluten-free edge for you?

Today, the influence of diet and an active lifestyle on our health is more important than ever. Rapidly rising rates of gluten intolerance, obesity, and other health problems—the result, in part, of a gluten-laden diet and sedentary lifestyle—is making many of us sick, even killing some of us. Consider this alone: Celiac disease, a severe autoimmune response to gluten in the diet, affecting an estimated one in one hundred people, is 4.5 times as common today as it was just fifty short years ago.[8] Under the broader umbrella of gluten intolerance, diverse and varied symptoms ranging from chronic severe diarrhea to crippling headaches to much worse can have devastating effects on health and can negatively impact quality of life.

The Gluten-Free Edge is about fighting back against that reversible trend. It is about regaining health and vitality; about not just improving quality of life, but about thriving in an active gluten-free life. For athletes, it is about excelling in sport to your maximum potential; about gaining an edge that you may not have even realized was missing.

Athletes, in many ways, are aptly suited to discovering the gluten-free edge. Like the ancient Greeks, they are finely attuned to their body and mindful of the food they eat to fuel their performance. And as many are discovering, going gluten-free can offer great benefits.

No athlete has brought awareness to the issue more than Serbian tennis star Novak Djokovic. After being diagnosed with gluten intolerance, he switched to a gluten-free diet, and almost overnight, his 2011 season became one for the ages. Of the four Grand Slam tournaments, Djokovic won three: the Australian Open, Wimbledon, and the U.S. Open. He went on an incredible forty-three-match winning streak and ended the year with a 70–6 record. He went from being *one* of the top tennis players in the world to officially solidifying his spot as *the* top-ranked tennis player on Earth. The performance had many calling it the "best year ever" in men's tennis.[9]

But you don't have to be a superstar to benefit from the gluten-free edge. Some of the best athletes on the planet happen to live simple lifestyles—no elaborate gyms and fitness centers, no high-tech training tools or heart rate monitors, no expensive running shoes or other sports equipment, no personal athletic trainers or sports psychologists or on-call nutritionists or team chefs or physiologists. They do share one thing in common with Djokovic and a growing list of other athletes, however: They're gluten-free. Frequently, they're referred to simply as *superathletes.*

For example, the Tarahumara tribe of Mexico's Copper Canyons, known as the Rarámuri (the Running People) in their native tongue, are renowned for their incredible endurance on ultradistance trail runs through notoriously unforgiving terrain. The Tarahumara might run for twenty-four, forty-eight, or even seventy-two hours at a stretch, covering 50 to 100 miles, or much more. It's the kind of extreme physical exertion where, if you don't have the right fuel in the tank, at some point you're going to self-destruct. But the Tarahumara don't, and their diet is an important part of why.

Corn, a naturally gluten-free cereal grain, is central to their diet, both as *pinole* (coarsely ground cornmeal used in myriad ways as a base for other dishes) and as corn beer. Much of the balance of the diet is similarly plant based: chia seeds (often consumed as *iskiate*—ground chia seeds in water with a touch of sugar and lime), pinto beans, chile peppers, squash, and wild greens. What little meat the Tarahumara eat usually comes from mice, fish, or goats. As simple as the diet appears at first blush, it turns out to be surprisingly rich in complex carbohydrates, amino acids, omega-3 and omega-6 fatty acids, calcium, iron, fiber, and more.[10]

What their diet *doesn't* have is gluten.

Neither does the diet of the Kalenjin tribe in Kenya.

Like the Tarahumara, the Kalenjin are known as great runners. Although they shine at several distances, they are best known for producing many of the world's best marathoners. Just one example: Between 1991 and 2011, eighteen of twenty-one winners of the Boston Marathon were Kenyan. The Kalenjin tribe—which makes up roughly 10 percent of Kenya's population—accounts for more than 75 percent of Kenya's elite distance runners at the international level of competition.[11]

Also like the Tarahumara, the Kalenjin diet is naturally gluten-free. *Ugali*—a slurry made with ground corn flour (or sometimes millet or sorghum), water, and salt—is used as a base for many dishes. It is to the Kalenjin what *pinole* is to the Tarahumara. Kidney beans, cooked greens and vegetables, fruit, eggs, milk, and a small amount of roasted meat round out the diet. The Kalenjin accomplish their incredible athletic achievements without wheat, barley, or rye.[12]

We're not saying that being gluten-free is the sole secret behind their seeming superpowers. Many factors help to explain why the Tarahumara and the Kalenjin have become superathletes, of which diet is just one. But as any serious athlete will tell you, diet matters.

In fact, as some of the Tarahumara have adopted a more Western diet—filled with gluten and refined wheat flour—they've begun to lose some of the elite physical prowess for which they're so famous.[13] A similar story is being told elsewhere around the world.

Researchers are increasingly finding that gluten and gluten intolerance, once thought to primarily affect populations of European descent, are causing a global health crisis. Places such as Mexico, parts of Africa, and East Asia, cultures with historically gluten-free cuisines—where gluten-related disease has been almost unheard of—have seen disease rates spike as gluten has been introduced to the diet. Likewise, high rates of celiac disease are being found throughout the Middle Eastern countries in wheat- and barley-based food cultures once thought to be immune to gluten intolerance problems.[14]

A simple conclusion has emerged: Eating gluten is making people sick, and the more of it that we eat, the sicker we get as a society.

For some, the health consequences are devastating. For others, they're more subtle. Either way, though, they're hardly inevitable. Each of us has the power to decide what foods we put into our body. Each of us can embrace the gluten-free edge. And as we've seen with Novak Djokovic, the benefits can be tremendous.

Whether you're male or female, young of age or young at heart, this book is for you. If you want to live a healthy, active, gluten-free lifestyle, it begins here and now. It doesn't matter where you sit along the athletic spectrum: novice, recreational athlete, serious weekend warrior, elite amateur, or professional. In fact, throughout the book you'll find interviews with and profiles of many athletes. They're inspiring examples of people living and benefiting from the gluten-free edge *today*. They put a face and a name and personal story to all the gluten-free nutrition and athletic science.

You'll find distance runner (and foreword author) Amy Yoder Begley (six-time U.S. national champion), mountain biker Brian Lopes (world champion), swimmer and nutritionist Anita Nall Richesson (Olympic gold medalist), triathlete Heather Wurtele (Ironman champion), and mountaineer Dave Hahn (thirteen Mount Everest summits). You'll find collegiate athletes such as lacrosse player Kristen Taylor, cross country runner Andie Cozzarelli, soccer player Kelsey Holbert, and basketball player Diana Rolniak. And you'll read about recreational athletes such as runner Michael Danke, cyclist Ashley DiVeronica, Pilates instructor Liana Mauro, yoga expert Amy Ippoliti, and many more.

MLB. NFL. NHL. NBA. If you poke around, you'll find gluten-free athletes in most any major professional sporting league. They're proof positive that, whether you're gluten-free for medical reasons or voluntarily, as a gluten-free athlete you can perform at the very highest levels of sport.

For every athlete we profile, for every athlete we mention by name, there are ten more standing in the wings. Gluten-free athletes are everywhere. We wish we could give each of them a place in this book, but the beauty of the situation is that we can't, because there are simply too many of them.

If you're gluten-free for medical reasons *and* an athlete, welcome home. You're one of us. We'll guide you through the nutritional requirements and unique concerns of gluten-free athletes.

If you're a "conventional" athlete curious about the benefits of adopting a gluten-free diet, you're in the right place.* We explain how going gluten-free can potentially improve your performance, even if you think you feel fine eating gluten now.

This book is for you, whether you practice a lifestyle sport such as yoga, running, or cycling; enjoy outdoor adventure sports such as hiking, mountain biking, or rock and ice climbing; focus on competitive sports such as triathlon or tennis; or play team sports such as lacrosse, football, basketball, or soccer. No matter what sport you play and at what level, you can apply the information contained within these pages *now*, to help you look, feel, and perform your best.

Learn what to eat and what not to eat, why gluten causes problems, and how to take full advantage of the gluten-free edge, from avoiding common pitfalls to principles for fitness and training. And enjoy nutrient-dense, power-packed recipes to fuel your active lifestyle.

Don't hesitate. Turn the page and start experiencing the gluten-free edge. An active, gluten-free life is just around the corner.

---

*Throughout this book, we use the terms "healthy athlete" and "conventional athlete" interchangeably to refer to athletes who do *not* have an overt form of gluten intolerance.

Pete's Story

IT WAS MID-APRIL 2007. Winter was officially over but still held its cold, snowy grip on the high country of Colorado's Rocky Mountains. My wife, Kelli, and I had planned a winter-conditions ascent of 14,196-foot Mount Yale, in the Collegiate Peaks range.

The day dawned beautiful—crisp, cold, sunny, not a cloud in the sky. Locals called days like those "Colorado Bluebird" days. Except, for me, a black cloud hung over the otherwise gorgeous mountain landscape. I was sick, and had been for several years.

I woke that morning feeling heavily fatigued, as usual. Worse, on the drive to the trailhead from our then-home in Boulder, I had to make emergency bathroom stops at gas stations at least three times. The chronic severe diarrhea that had become a fixture of my life was rearing its ugly head. Again. That morning in April 2007 it left me malnourished, weak, and dehydrated. It was no way to start the climb of a 14,000-foot mountain peak.

At the third gas station—in the town of Buena Vista in the Arkansas River valley at the foot of the Collegiate Peaks—I bought a travel pack of antidiarrheal caplets, washed them down with a swig of water, and hoped for the best.

Back in our Jeep for the final leg of our drive to the trailhead, Kelli spoke up.

"Maybe we should turn around. Are you sure this a good idea? Do you feel up to it?"

My male ego was too proud. I was too stubborn and reluctant to make the smart choice and back down. Instead I insisted we give it a try.

We worked our way up Avalanche Gulch to a saddle between Mount Yale and an adjacent peak. From there, we began ascending Yale's rocky, snowy, icy East Ridge. But somewhere above 12,500 feet, I slumped onto a boulder. I could go no higher. Then I began to cry.

I was young. I was fit. I was an athlete. This wasn't supposed to happen. Not to me. I had climbed bigger mountains than this. What was wrong with me? Why was I so sick? Answers to those questions had been elusive.

My self-destruction on Mount Yale was one of many low points over a two-year period. Going jogging in my neighborhood, a flat out-and-back on pavement—a modest 1.5-mile round-trip—was a challenge. I could seldom complete longer runs through the neighborhood without ducking into the community recreation center to use the restroom (if it was open) or into the trees in the adjacent open space park (if it wasn't). Hiking and climbing in the mountains, I always carried paper napkins or toilet paper in my backpack for the sudden and inevitable calls of nature that sent me scurrying off trail into the forest or behind a boulder. I developed anxiety riding in cars and airplanes: What if I needed to use the facilities? I spent a not insignificant part of each day—including after each meal, it seemed—in the bathroom.

I was a long way gone from the athlete I'd been just a few years before.

As a child, I was always active—playing team sports such as soccer and baseball, hiking, swimming and surfing in the ocean. Later, I wrestled, played varsity lacrosse in high school, and became co-captain of the varsity soccer team. In college, I embraced outdoor adventure sports, especially mountaineering. Climbing trips and larger expeditions took me to the Alps, the Andes, the Cascades, and beyond. Eventually, I blended my background in competitive sports with my passion for the outdoors as an adventure racer.

Meanwhile, I'd been lactose intolerant for as long as I could remember. I came from a family of sensitive stomachs, with many of us prone to symptoms like those of irritable bowel syndrome. At the time, it was nothing I considered abnormal.

Then, sometime in early 2005, things changed in a big way. I can't say exactly what flipped the switch. Looking back, I don't recall a particular defining moment when I went from being healthy to being sick.

Nevertheless, my health fell off the rails; my quality of life diminished. The good health that I had largely taken for granted was no longer. I struggled with activities that previously had come easily to me athletically. The change drastically impacted my lifestyle, which was defined by being active and fit and in the mountains.

Earlier searches for answers hadn't yielded much. But as I grew sicker, my desperation—and urgency—grew, too. And so in January 2007 I began seeing a new doctor, a holistic practitioner who combined Eastern and Western medicine philosophies. I sat on the edge of the table in an examining room and rattled off a long list of symptoms and the progression of my problems. No sooner had I finished that he looked me in the eye.

"Your problem is gluten."

My problem was what? For me, *gluten* may as well have been a word from an unfamiliar foreign language. I'm not sure I'd ever consciously heard it before. He explained that gluten is a family of proteins found in wheat, barley, and rye, not to mention ancient varieties of wheat such as spelt, emmer, and einkorn, as well as hybrids such as triticale (wheat crossed with rye), and any foods made from them: traditional forms of bread, bagels, pizza, pasta, cake, and cookies.

I couldn't believe it. Ironically, in an attempt to eat healthier, I'd somewhat recently started incorporating more whole grains and whole-grain foods into my diet, versus more refined starches. At that time, *whole grains* to me meant *whole wheat*; but whole wheat meant more protein, and meant more gluten—and more gluten meant that I was unknowingly poisoning myself. Plato may have called wheat and company "good and beneficial foods," but for me they were anything but.

Going gluten-free, I soon learned, had a steep learning curve. At least it did for me in early 2007. I didn't realize all the places where gluten might hide in foods. I also didn't realize the severity of my own condition: that healing and recovery would require strict lifelong adherence to a gluten-free diet. Just trying to go low gluten, as I initially attempted to do, wasn't going to cut it.

Which is why—three months after a doctor told me to go gluten-free—I crumpled onto that rock high on the side of a mountain in Colorado. I was defeated. But only temporarily. I resolved then and there to make the necessary changes to regain my health, to regain my lifestyle, to simply regain my life.

Sitting in the doctor's office one morning days later, I looked at him.

"Tell me what I need to do," I said.

At last fully educated, I made the switch to a genuine gluten-free diet and pretty much haven't looked back since.

Weeks later, sitting with Kelli in the living room of our home, I had a sudden realization. My symptoms were gone—the chronic severe diarrhea, the stomach pain, the fatigue, the muscle trembles. It was a deafening silence. Mine was a body so quiet of symptoms that I couldn't do anything but notice the difference. I felt better than I had in perhaps a decade.

It was a sign of continued good things to come. Today, I feel so healthy and so good, I can't imagine ever going back to eating gluten. (A few rare instances of cross-contamination have unfortunately reminded me of just how bad I felt once—including getting "glutened" the night before a ski mountaineering race near Aspen, Colorado, which left me fatigued and dehydrated before I even started the race after a long night of diarrhea, abdominal pain, and muscle trembles—a strong motivator for staying gluten-free today.)

In the end, my doctor made a de facto celiac disease diagnosis, based primarily on a supervised elimination diet, my constellation of symptoms, my incredibly positive response to the gluten-free diet, and a few other curious changes (for example, my lifelong lactose intolerance "miraculously" resolved once I was gluten-free). I never did get a blood test, or an intestinal biopsy, often described as the gold standard of celiac diagnosis. For those tests to be accurate, you need to be eating gluten, and there was no way I was going back to that just for the sake of a piece of paper that said, "Yes, you officially have celiac disease." My body had already told me everything I needed to know.

In the years since, I not only recovered to where I'd been physically, athletically, before I got sick; I surpassed any previous athletic accomplishment. I now weigh in my thirties what I did as a varsity athlete in high school. I began ski mountaineering racing during the winter. My adventure racing transitioned into Xterra off-road triathlons, and in 2009 I went to the U.S. National Championship as a competitor. I returned to high-altitude mountaineering, summiting my first 6,000-meter peak. A friend and I became one of a just a handful of groups to successfully repeat the Trooper Traverse, a four-day ski mountaineering route through Colorado's Rockies from Leadville to Aspen, first pioneered by a group of elite 10th Mountain Division ski troopers in 1944.

Most recently, I've been competing in trail running races as an ultramarathoner. Once challenged by running 1.5 miles on flat pavement, I now run 50-plus miles on trails with 10,000 vertical feet of elevation gain. That's the equivalent of running back-to-back marathons, off-road, while climbing to the top of the Empire State Building eight times.

I don't say this to boast. I say it from a perspective of joy, gratitude, and contentment. I'm convinced that none of these accomplishments would have happened, none of them would have been possible, without the gluten-free edge. For me, it was more than an edge. It was everything, because it gave me back my life.

Having regained my own life, I now try to help others regain theirs. I've coauthored gluten-free cookbooks, cofounded a popular gluten-free blog, and serve as an Athlete for Awareness for the National Foundation for Celiac Awareness. At the end of the day, those efforts—and this book—are about sharing my knowledge and experience with others, to help them—and you—live a healthy, active, joyous gluten-free life.

For me, going gluten-free—though born of medical necessity, rather than of choice—has been a blessing with rich rewards. I hope it can be for you, too.

—PETER BRONSKI, 2012

Melissa's Story

BARNEY MCLEAN WAS born in 1917 and grew up in the small mountain town of Hot Sulphur Springs, Colorado, home to the first winter sports carnival held west of the Mississippi. He strapped on his first pair of homemade skis at age four and the sport of skiing was never the same.

By 1950, he had won every major ski race in North America, including nine national championships—in ski jumping, as well as the downhill, slalom, and combined alpine events. He was named to three U.S. Olympic teams, serving as captain of the team for the 1948 games. At the age of thirty-three, he was named coach of the U.S. FIS team. Among ski racers, the Fédération Internationale de Ski championships—now known as the Alpine World Ski Championships—rate almost as important as the Olympics.

Ski Illustrated magazine named him Skier of the Year in 1942. Five years later, the National Ski Association awarded him its All-American Ski Trophy. And in 1952, *Ski Magazine* called him "America's best known skier."

I called him Dad.

He was a hardy man with a rugged spirit and an unshakable inner strength. Scattered throughout our modest Colorado home were reminders of his commitment to good health: a chin-up bar installed in the kitchen doorjamb (which my mother loathed), outdoor gear stowed in every corner of the house, a trampoline in the backyard, and a makeshift utility bench in the carport where he could build, work on, and wax skis. He jumped rope, did sit-ups and push-ups, rode a bike, and played tennis. Being active was in his DNA.

I was an only child—my dad's special girl—but I was also the son he never had. I grew up skiing, backpacking, hiking, camping, and flying around the mountains in small airplanes. (Dad had been a flight instructor and Arctic survival specialist for the Air Force.)

Like my father, I started skiing at a young age. We'd ride up the chairlift together, my dad challenging me to hold my legs straight out, ski tips to the sky. I'd moan and wiggle, thighs burning, hoping he'd give up before I did. He had legs of steel, so that was unlikely, but to a little girl the challenge was fun. If I could keep my legs straight the whole way up the lift, the reward was often part of a candy bar he had stashed in his jacket pocket. I still do this "chairlift challenge" on occasion, all these years later.

I also remember us "sitting" together, knees bent at 90-degree angles, with our backs pressed against the living room wall, as if we were on straight-backed chairs, but with no seats beneath us. "This'll help keep your legs strong," he'd say as the minutes went by.

Dad went on to be named to the U.S. Ski Hall of Fame, the Colorado Ski Hall of Fame, and the Colorado Sports Hall of Fame. In 1996, *Ski Magazine* called him an "American skiing legend," and four years later, *Sports Illustrated* called him one of Colorado's fifty greatest athletes of the twentieth century.

Most important, he was a good guy. Generous, quiet, humble, he was never one to mention his considerable achievements. In fact, he's probably protesting from above as I write this, but I wanted to paint this picture of who my dad was—strong, hardworking, athletically gifted, a determined man with an unflappable constitution.

Because then, his story—and my story—changed. There was a chink in his armor, though no one knew it for years. It was, I'm convinced, a weakness to gluten—the Trojan horse in his otherwise healthy diet. A man who was once a strong athlete ended up malnourished, suffering from a serious "failure to thrive," the victim of a devastating collapse of health that for him didn't become evident until later in life.

His last ten years were the most difficult, and then came the end.

It was July 18, 2005. I came home from a yoga class to find a phone message from my dad. He was sick. At my parent's house, I found him throwing up what looked like coffee grinds. Although I didn't know exactly what was wrong, I'd had EMT training and knew it probably meant that he was bleeding internally. I took him to the hospital. After an agonizing night in the emergency room, he died early the next morning.

Although elderly when he died, those final years were more difficult than they should have been. His osteoporosis was so bad that his pelvic X-ray looked like Swiss cheese. His spine was an arthritic mess; the pain difficult to manage. He had severe anemia, chronic intestinal problems, and nutrient deficiencies—all despite a seemingly healthy diet. At the time of his death, he weighed just 118 pounds. A testimony to his strength, love of the sport, and sheer determination, he skied every year from age four onward, taking his last run at age eighty-seven, just a few months before he died.

His death certificate says he died of natural causes. I'm not so sure. In fact, I'm convinced otherwise.

Despite good medical care, somewhere along the way something was missed. Armed with the knowledge I have now, looking back I believe that undiagnosed and unmanaged celiac disease contributed to his death. I should know, because I have celiac disease, too, though the road to diagnosis was hardly straightforward.

It started with my daughter. For years she suffered from skin rashes, asthma, intestinal problems, and headaches. While spending a semester of study abroad in London with a daily diet of fresh baguettes, her symptoms grew worse. Shortly thereafter, my daughter was diagnosed with multiple food allergies. Wheat—and thus, gluten—was high on the list.

Around the same time, a dermatologist suggested that wheat might be the cause of an inflamed, itchy rash I had on my elbows. I also developed a strange autoimmune condition called Dupuytren's contracture that affects the connective tissue in my hands and feet. Slowly, pieces of our family puzzle started to fall into place.

I spent the year and a half after my dad's death buried in research with a focus on gluten intolerance. I already had a degree in exercise science and a background in medicine and health, but I felt that I needed in-depth nutrition knowledge to add to the mix. Although my father's death prompted me to explore nutrition further, it was an interest I inherited from my mother. She was a gourmet cook who made real food from scratch. As a child, I ate her beets, broccoli, and spinach with no complaints, along with nourishing stews and soups accompanied by homemade biscuits, breads, and desserts.

In 2007, I became a master graduate of the Nutrition Therapy Institute in Denver. Shortly after, I completed a two-hundred-hour course in yoga teacher training, which had been on my to-do list for years. My life of sports and nutrition, exercise and food, was falling into place. More and more, I learned—and experienced—how body, mind, and spirit health are intimately connected. I had found my calling.

Meanwhile, I had found more—namely, diagnoses for my daughter and me. We both had celiac disease. Once she was gluten-free, my daughter's asthma and headaches went away and her stomach problems improved. My chronic joint pain, which I had attributed to years of gymnastics, a few nasty mountain bike misadventures, hundreds of miles of hard-core backpacking, and the occasional high-impact ski crash—slowly disappeared. Within a year or so, I was pain-free.

The rashes on my elbows were later diagnosed as dermatitis herpetiformis, the skin manifestation of celiac disease. It took a long time for the rashes to subside, and if I am unintentionally zapped by gluten, they come back in a day or two with a vengeance. So do the canker sores I've suffered with since childhood.

The common thread between my dad, me, and my daughter, boils down to one thing: gluten. If one person in the family has an intolerance, it's likely others will as well. My story is an example of how gluten intolerance generally, and celiac disease specifically, can manifest through generations. For my dad, it was probably triggered later in life; I developed it in midlife; and for my daughter, it was activated as a teenager.

I, of course, am a genetic carrier for celiac disease. Genetic and antibody testing revealed that my husband carries one of the genetic markers as well. Thanks to us, our kids all have two copies of the genes for celiac disease, though my daughter and I are the only ones with elevated antibodies to gluten—so far. I'm keeping my eye on everyone else. Celiac disease can be triggered at any time of life.

But it doesn't have to be. Celiac disease is the only autoimmune disease for which we know the trigger: gluten. How lucky that a condition so potentially devastating can be controlled with little more than diet. For this I am grateful.

I'm grateful, too, for my dad and the gift he unknowingly gave me. Because of his experience with this disease, I can look to the future—for my children, as well as myself—with a positive outlook, blessed with the knowledge we need to chart a path of health that avoids what he went through in his last years.

That knowledge has also become my mission: to increase awareness of celiac disease, and to help people heal and thrive. Not just to get by, but to climb mountains, ski, run marathons, compete, endure. My father did once, as I do now, and so can you.

—MELISSA McLEAN JORY, 2012

1

G Is for Gluten

EVER SINCE SHE was sixteen years old, Ashley DiVeronica—a thirty-year-old marketing professional and successful competitive amateur cyclist from south Florida—had stomach trouble. Serious stomach trouble. So bad that at age seventeen she was hospitalized. "I couldn't keep food in me," she recalls. "My days were planned around how close I could be to a bathroom."

Doctors initially suspected Crohn's disease, which runs in her family. For years, medical professionals told her she had a severe form of irritable bowel syndrome. Misdiagnosed, it took a full decade for DiVeronica to finally find an answer to her health woes. At age twenty-seven, she switched gastroenterologists. "The first thing he said to me was, 'Have you ever been tested for celiac disease?'" she remembers.

Tests came back positive. It was time, he explained, for her to switch to a gluten-free diet. "I had no idea what gluten was!" she says today.

Ashley, meet gluten. Gluten, meet Ashley.

It's time for you to formally meet gluten, too. This may be a book about the gluten-free lifestyle and how athletes can perform at their best following a gluten-free diet, but we'd be remiss if we didn't start out talking at least a little bit about what's *not* in this book: gluten. Otherwise, we'd be guilty of ignoring the 800-pound gorilla in the room.

There are compelling reasons to go gluten-free—especially if you're an athlete—and we're about to explain them. Those reasons start not with the benefits of the gluten-free diet (which we address as well), but with the problems inherent to gluten. It's like a case of "Keep your friends close, and your enemies closer." Know gluten, and you'll appreciate that much more the power behind the gluten-free edge.

WHAT IS GLUTEN?

Gluten is the common word used to describe a group of plant-based storage proteins.* All cereal grains have storage proteins, but *gluten* typically refers specifically to the proteins in wheat, barley, and rye that cause problems for people with gluten intolerance. They're also known as *prolamins*, because they're rich in the amino acid proline. In wheat, the prolamins are gliadin and glutenin; in barley, hordein; and in rye, secalin. And it's not the whole protein that's the problem. It's a piece of the larger protein, which researchers call a fraction, and some gluten fractions are more problematic than others.

As in other proteins, amino acids serve as the building blocks of gluten. And also like other proteins, gluten has levels of structure. *Primary structure* refers to the actual sequence of amino acids that comprise a given protein. *Secondary* and *tertiary structure* refer to how that string of amino acids twists, turns, and folds to create a three-dimensional molecule. And *quarternary structure* (not all proteins have this) refers to multiple three-dimensional protein subunits that bond to one another.

All but the primary structure are held together with relatively weak bonds. Breaking down a protein's secondary, tertiary, or quarternary structure is known as *denaturing*, and we do it all the time. If you've ever beaten an egg white into soft or stiff peaks, you've denatured its proteins. This type of denaturing is reversible. On the other hand, when you're cooking an egg and the color turns from clear to white, you've also denatured the proteins. This type of denaturing is decidedly *not* reversible (unless you're a magician who knows how to uncook an egg).

At the level of a protein's primary structure—its sequence of amino acids—it's up to enzymes to do the work of breaking down the protein. This is important work. For protein to be useful to your body, it first

---

*Please refer to the Glossary on page 311 for the definitions of many terms in this book.

ATHLETE INSIGHT

Ashley DiVeronica

AMATEUR COMPETITIVE CYCLIST

Born: 1981 • Lives: Florida • Gluten-Free Since: 2008

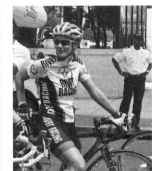

IN 2005, A friend casually suggested to Ashley DiVeronica that she "had good legs, that I would make a really good cyclist," DiVeronica explains today. She'd never really considered taking up the sport before. Intrigued, she and her mother signed up to do an MS 150 bike ride from Miami to Key Largo and back . . . even though neither of them owned a bicycle at the time.

DiVeronica went out, bought a bike, and did her first ride—30 miles, on a cruiser bike. "I took the bike back the next day and got a road bike," she says. Training eventually gave her the confidence to go out on group rides. There, fellow riders encouraged her to start racing. "I fell in love with the sport," she says.

It wasn't until 2008, when she went gluten-free following her celiac disease diagnosis, that her cycling really took off. "In hindsight, I see how much it definitely impacted my performance," she says.

Today she races throughout the state for the Rivet Racing women's cycling team in south Florida, where her training and her gluten-free diet have enabled her to capture a number of Top 5 finishes and to advance to become a Cat 3 rider.

FAVORITE GLUTEN-FREE FOODS: gluten-free oats with banana and peanut butter, Larabars, potatoes, brown rice, chicken, fish, lots of veggies, homemade protein bars, gluten-free baked ziti needs to be converted from larger peptides (multiple amino acids bonded together in a chain) into individual amino acids. Think of amino acids as beads in a necklace. Enzymatic digestion breaks apart the individual amino acid "beads" so that your body can reassemble them in all sorts of useful ways. Some enzymes gobble on the ends of the chain like Pac-Man. Others snip the chain somewhere in the middle, like a pair of scissors.

Once your body has individual amino acids at its disposal, it uses them in all sorts of important ways: for repairing and replacing tissue (including muscles, ligaments, and tendons); for hormone, enzyme, and antibody production; for bone growth and repair; for tooth enamel; for energy; and the list goes on.

Unfortunately, gluten isn't particularly cooperative—quite the contrary, in fact. It's a notoriously stubborn protein. Even in so-called healthy people who in theory have no problem with gluten, it resists the enzymes in the stomach and intestines and comes out the other end virtually undigested.[1] One of the only exceptions is pepsin, a stomach enzyme. Pepsin takes a crack a gluten, but with relatively little effect.[2] (As you'll read in chapter 2, the gluten fragments that pepsin *does* manage to digest cause their own negative effects on your health.) The small intestine does no better. And by the time gluten reaches your intestines, it's already starting to go to work causing a variety of problems (more on that in chapter 2).

As a matter of fact, the human gastrointestinal system is so bad at digesting gluten that an entire branch of celiac disease treatment research is aimed at trying to use nonhuman enzymes to, in essence, digest the gluten for us, to break it down sufficiently to nullify its toxicity to the human body.[3]

But here's the kicker: This problem doesn't just afflict those of us with gluten intolerance. As Dr. Martin Kagnoff of the University of California–San Diego noted in a 2007 issue of the *Journal of Clinical Investigation*, "There is no known difference between healthy individuals and those susceptible to developing [celiac disease] in their ability to digest these proteins."[4] More recently, in a 2011 Health.com article, Dr. Daniel Leffer, of the Celiac Center at Harvard Medical School's Beth Israel Deaconess Medical Center in Massachusetts, was just as blunt, stating, "Gluten is fairly indigestible in all people. There's probably some kind of gluten intolerance in all of us."[5]

If we're all intolerant of gluten to varying degrees, then why eat it at all? That's a good question.

Certainly, wheat, barley, and rye contain beneficial nutrients, but gluten isn't one of them. Gluten's singular saving grace is its network of unusual properties that creates a springy elasticity when glutenous flour is mixed with water. Gluten is what traditionally makes dough "doughy." This makes gluten good for baking, for sure. That's why you find it in conventional forms of breads, bagels, cakes, cookies, and pizzas, not to mention pastas and beer (sometimes called *liquid bread*).

In more recent years, gluten has also found favor in the food industry, where it's been used extensively as a binder and filler in processed foods. It sneaks into cereals, certain processed and deli meat products, some imitation crab meats, and a long list of other foods where your first reaction might be one of "They put gluten in that?" Yes, they do. It's seemingly everywhere and in everything.

AMINO ACIDS

THERE ARE TWENTY amino acids in the human body, used to build and repair body tissues. Of those, nine are known as *essential amino acids*. Whereas your body can synthesize the other eleven amino acids, essential amino acids can only be gained by eating foods that contain them. Leucine, important for recovery and rebuilding muscle after exercise, is one essential amino acid. A diet poor in essential amino acids can result in essential amino acid deficiency, which can cause a variety of negative health effects.

HOW HAS GLUTEN CHANGED?

The story starts ten thousand or so years ago, when our hunter-gatherer ancestors first domesticated cereal grains—notably, wheat and barley—

in the Fertile Crescent of Mesopotamia (in modern-day Syria, Iraq, and Turkey).[6] In the uplands of the Fertile Crescent, wild wheat and barley grew well. As early as 7000 BC, those grains had been domesticated in northeastern Mesopotamia. The region's climate—with a cool, wet growing season, followed by a warm, dry season during which the grain ripened leading up to harvest—was ideal.[7]

Those gluten-containing cereal grains were abundant, but they were also durable and stored well—desirable characteristics for early civilizations looking to buffer themselves from the dangers of famine and Mother Nature's sometimes fickle habits. Wheat also proved a crop with certain ecological and agricultural advantages: It was highly adaptable, not to mention drought and salt tolerant. Such traits made it popular among farmers. It would soon become popular among cooks, too, who discovered that flours high in gluten were great for baking.

From there, the story began to change. Wheat—the "staff of life" that enabled nomadic peoples to form more permanent and settled societies supported by agriculture—went through a long series of changes. So much so that the first wild versions of einkorn and emmer—ancestors of modern-day wheat—are distant cousins at best to the wheat and gluten we eat today.

The evolution of wheat flour began with the selection of wheat varieties for certain characteristics. Those first farmers, sowing einkorn and emmer in their fields, could scarcely have imagined that their early work would later give rise to more than twenty-five thousand genetic variations of wheat, many of them high-yield varieties with a pumped-up gluten content that makes them great for dough and baking.[8]

Over time, wheat became a leading source of vegetable protein and dietary energy for humans worldwide. Today, more of the Earth's surface is covered with wheat than with any other crop.[9]

Modern genetic modification, however, has accelerated the rate of change in wheat and, by extension, in gluten. To give you a sense of just how different today's wheat is from the original, ancient domesticated varieties, consider this: Einkorn has 14 chromosomes. Emmer has 28 chromosomes. By contrast, today's wheat varieties have 42 chromosomes, triple what einkorn did.[10]

This increase in chromosome number is what's known as *polyploidy*, when the chromosomes from more than one genome get added together to multiply the overall count. Humans, by way of example, are diploid (*di* meaning two, *ploid* meaning the number of sets of chromosomes). Each cell in your body (with the exception of sex cells for reproduction) contains two sets of chromosomes—one half contributed by your mother and the other half by your father. The human genome has 23 chromosomes. Thus, each cell contains 46 chromosomes (2 × 23).

Now let's consider wheat. The basic wheat genome contains 7 chromosomes. Einkorn is a diploid (remember, two sets of chromosomes), hence 14 chromosomes (2 × 7).

Here's where polyploidy starts to make things interesting. Emmer and durum (macaroni) wheat are tetraploid. They contain full sets of chromosomes from two different wheat genomes (denoted A and B in wheat genetics). And so, each cell in these varieties of wheat contains AABB chromosomes, where each letter represents a set of 7 chromosomes from the two genomes. Hence, tetraploid wheats, such as emmer, have a total of 28 chromosomes (4 × 7, or 2 × 7 + 2 × 7).

Can you see where this is going for modern wheat? Modern wheat is *Triticum aestivum*, also known as *bread wheat*. It has a very high gluten content and is the most common form of wheat grown today. In fact, modern bread wheat accounts for 95 percent of the surface area of Earth under wheat cultivation.[11] Modern wheat is hexaploid, containing six sets of chromosomes from three different genomes. It takes the A and B genomes from diploid and tetraploid wheats and adds a third genome, known as D. And so, hexaploid wheat contains 42 chromosomes (6 × 7, or 2 × 7 + 2 × 7 + 2 × 7).

This kind of polyploidy in and of itself isn't bad. Polyploidy is very common among plants. In fact, many other crops—including corn and potatoes—employ this form of genetics.

But in the case of modern wheat, polyploidy turns out to be problematic for human health. The rich gene bank it offers scientists has permitted rapid evolution of wheat, resulting in radical change to the plant and its gluten.[12]

Part of this radical change has been geared toward eking more wheat out of a given plot of land. For example, wheat's yield per acre nearly tripled from the early 1950s through the late 1990s.[13]

But much of the modern change in wheat has also been about packing more gluten into the grain. As many a baker and *pizzaiolo* (pizza maker) will tell you, as a general rule, the more gluten in a flour, the better the dough that flour makes.

The bottom line is that today's gluten—consumed in wheat, barley, and rye—was not the food of Plato or Socrates, who praised the grains. Heck, it wasn't even the food of your grandparents. The wheat, barley, and rye that we eat today—and the gluten they contain—are a different thing entirely.

WHY IS GLUTEN MAKING PEOPLE SICK?

Ever since—and probably, before—the first case of celiac disease was described some two thousand years ago, gluten has been making people sick.[14] Why?

We know certain things: that gluten can disrupt digestion; that it can cause inflammation; that, in people with celiac disease, it causes a severe autoimmune response. Truth be told, though, the mechanisms of a negative reaction to gluten are complex. This is a currently unfolding area of research, with scientists gaining new insights almost on a weekly basis. (We briefly discuss some of their findings in the next section, "The Gluten Intolerance Spectrum.")

Regardless, a disturbing trend has emerged. Gluten is not just making people sick. It's making *more* people *sicker* today than ever before.

For instance, the prevalence of celiac disease has notably increased in recent decades. It's tempting to attribute such a trend to rising rates of awareness about gluten intolerance issues. The more health-care practitioners know about it, the more patients can be successfully diagnosed. But there's more at work here, irrespective of awareness and rates of diagnosis.

An oft-cited University of Maryland Center for Celiac Research study from 2003 showed that the rate of celiac disease in the general population has *doubled every fifteen years* since 1974.[15] A more recent Mayo Clinic study from 2009 demonstrated that celiac disease is *4.5 times more prevalent* today than it was in the 1950s. As researchers note, our genetics haven't changed. A few measly decades are too short a time period for that. We haven't suddenly mutated as a population and become more susceptible to gluten as a result. What *has* changed is our diet.[16]

First of all, we're eating more wheat and more gluten, and seeing rising rates of gluten intolerance as a result. The highest rates of celiac disease tend to correspond to the highest per capita rates of wheat consumption in countries around the world. We're also seeing rising rates of gluten intolerance elsewhere across the globe, in countries and cultures with naturally gluten-free cuisines that are now introducing gluten into the diet. Finally, researchers are now finding gluten intolerance among Middle Eastern cultures that have been eating wheat the longest. Although they were once thought to be immune to gluten intolerance, we're finding these cultures are anything but.

It should come as no surprise, then, that we're seeing a spike in gluten intolerance in the United States. We're eating a lot of gluten, more than we have in half a century. Since the 1950s, per capita wheat flour consumption in the United States has steadily risen, disconcertingly aligning with the Mayo Clinic's findings about the rising prevalence of celiac disease since the same decade.[17]

A number of factors are to blame for why Americans are eating more gluten today. For one thing, the increasing popularity of fast foods and convenience foods—burgers, pizza, bagels, sandwiches—has injected more gluten into the diet. For another, when cholesterol and heart health concerns surfaced in the 1970s and '80s, people shifted their eating habits from animal sources to more grains, including gluten-containing wheat.

According to the United States Department of Agriculture's Economic Research Service, per capita annual wheat flour consumption in 2008 was 136.6 pounds. That's a lot of wheat . . . and a lot of gluten. And the number doesn't begin to capture all the nonflour gluten consumption in the Standard American Diet, such as when gluten is added to processed foods as filler and binder.

For another, as we previously noted, it's not just that we're eating more gluten, but that gluten itself has changed. When researchers compared einkorn to modern varieties of wheat, they found that einkorn caused fewer gluten intolerance problems and proved less toxic to people with celiac disease.[18]

Another study, from 2010, compared thirty-six modern wheat varieties to fifty wheat varieties commonly grown until about one century
ago. The researchers' conclusion? Wheat breeding has resulted in modern crops that have more of the gluten fractions that make people sick
and trigger the autoimmune reaction of celiac disease. The increased
prevalence of gluten intolerance and celiac disease is a direct result of
changes in the gluten we've been eating over the years.[19]

Let's revisit the issue of polyploidy and, in particular, the hexaploid
nature of modern bread wheat, which contains forty-two chromosomes,
fourteen each from the A, B, and D genomes.

First, the hexaploid nature of modern bread wheat results in a kind
of genetic redundancy, notes Dr. David Sands, professor of plant sciences and molecular biosciences at Montana State University. The
genes that code for gluten are strongly retained and copied; wheat can
tolerate genetic mutations and variations without ill effect to the plant
or its gluten content. In other words, gluten is not just persistent in your
GI tract; it's persistent genetically, too.

Second, the gluten fractions most toxic to humans—including certain alpha and gamma gliadins—arise from the D genome. This is why
the ancient diploid and tetraploid ancestors of modern wheat have been
shown in studies to be less toxic to humans. They lack the D genome
that codes for the most problematic forms of gluten. Not only that, but
when all three genomes—A, B, and D—are present, as they are in modern hexaploid wheat, gliadins from the D genome (remember, the most
toxic) are preferentially expressed.[20]

Einkorn, emmer, and their cousins aren't totally off the hook, either.
Although the ancient varieties by many measures have been shown to
be less toxic than modern wheat,[21] they cause their share of gluten intolerance problems as well.[22]

Granted, the relative expression of gluten fractions varies from
variety to variety of wheat, and breeding and other mechanisms can,
in a sense, be used to turn genes on or off, or to select for varieties
with lower toxicity.[23] A handful of researchers have been looking at
doing just that. They're tracing wheat back to its ancestral varieties,
then looking for baking-quality wheat and gluten without toxicity
problems.[24]

But we're unlikely to see gluten-free wheat or glutenous wheat free of toxic gluten fractions anytime soon . . . or ever. As long as people care more about "good" wheat flour than they do about their health, there's little incentive for change. Instead, we're left with a highly industrialized plant, bred for certain characteristics, some of which happen to be pretty bad for your health, all in the name of better baking.

Dr. Sands at Montana State says it another way: "Wheat breeding has changed greatly in the last sixty years. International cooperative breeding programs have given wheat breeders access to the world collection of wheat with a great diversity of genotypes, and it is not surprising that this included a diversity of types of gluten. There was selection for glutens that improved the mixing and baking characteristics of bread wheats, possibly causing more reactivity." Which is exactly what we've been seeing with rising rates of gluten intolerance.

The implications of these studies, and others like them, is clear:[25] The new varieties of wheat so prevalent in the food system are making people the sickest, are causing the most reactions to gluten. We've gone from a possibility to reality.

As a matter of fact, although we eat a heck of a lot of gluten these days and gluten consumption has been on the rise for nearly sixty years, it's not the highest it's ever been. Americans actually consumed *more* wheat flour per capita in the nineteenth century.[26] Yet their rates of celiac disease were almost certainly lower than we see today, for one simple reason: They were eating "the easy stuff." Their wheat had less gluten, and the gluten it did have was less toxic.

At the end of the day, the question of why gluten is making people sick boils down to a double whammy, a one-two punch. We're getting sick because we eat too much gluten, and the gluten that we're eating is more toxic to humans than it was in the past.

The solution is simple: Eat less gluten, or better, none at all. Go gluten-free.

That straightforward conclusion reminds us of a popular joke you've probably heard before. A patient walks into his doctor's office and says, "Doc, it hurts when I do this." The doctor, without missing a beat, responds, "Then don't do that." If gluten is causing a problem, don't do gluten.

The mechanisms of gluten intolerance may be complex, but the imperative for health, fitness, and athletics is becoming increasingly urgent and compelling. We're on the threshold of a gluten version of the familiar maxim "It's the economy, stupid." And as we'll explain in the next chapter, athletes—and not just gluten-free athletes—have reason to sit up and take notice.

THE GLUTEN INTOLERANCE SPECTRUM

Throughout this book, we use *gluten intolerance* as an umbrella term to describe all conditions that would warrant a gluten-free diet for serious medical reasons. This especially includes celiac disease, wheat allergy, and gluten sensitivity.

The boundary lines between these conditions are sometimes fuzzy. More and more, medical researchers are understanding how gluten is a problem. But as our knowledge of such conditions grows, it also becomes more complex. We're finding less black and white, and a lot more gray area.

"What is clear to us now [is that] there is this big family of gluten sufferers—people of all shapes and sizes and symptoms who suffer several forms of gluten intolerance, including celiac disease, wheat allergy, and gluten sensitivity," noted Dr. Alessio Fasano, one of the top celiac disease doctors in the world and director of the University of Maryland's Center for Celiac Research.[27]

Some forms of gluten intolerance appear to overlap with others. There's no convenient diagnostic flowchart, no perfect test for diagnosis, no textbook case. Every person's situation is a little different. But here are the basics.

CELIAC DISEASE

Celiac disease is a genetically predisposed autoimmune disease triggered by ingesting gluten. It's the only example of autoimmunity in which one specific environmental substance—you guessed it . . . gluten—is known to turn the disease "on" and "off." One hallmark of many cases is villous atrophy, or damage to the villi of the small intestine, which impacts enzymes for digestion, as well as absorption of nutrients.

Celiac disease can have immediate effects (such as stomach pain, diarrhea, or headaches), but also long-term side effects (such as malnutrition, osteoporosis, iron-deficiency anemia, elevated risk for certain cancers, and heightened mortality rates), especially when undiagnosed and untreated. It's serious stuff.[28]

Symptoms can be wide-ranging. As a result, celiac disease can be difficult to diagnose, because it often looks like something else. It's a digestive disease that doesn't always cause digestive problems. It can be triggered at any age. But when it does "activate," your immune system attacks your body's own tissues. Unchecked, the disease can be devastating.

Doctors may employ several tools for diagnosis—your list of symptoms, your response to a gluten-free diet, blood antibody testing, genetic testing, and/or an invasive small intestine biopsy, often considered the gold standard.

There's currently no cure for celiac disease. Treatment consists of strict lifelong adherence to the gluten-free diet.

Current estimates suggest that three million Americans, or about 1 in 133 people, have celiac disease. Recently, a 1 in 100 prevalence is becoming more commonly noted.

WHEAT ALLERGY

The Food and Drug Administration lists wheat as a "top eight" allergen in the United States. The allergic response in wheat allergy triggers a different immune response than does celiac disease. Gluten, however, remains a common denominator.

The rapid response in a wheat allergy reaction triggers the release of histamine. Symptoms may include rashes, abdominal distress, lip swelling, wheezing, and even anaphylaxis.[29] Current estimates suggest that wheat allergy affects 400,000 to 600,000 Americans.

There's also a condition known as *wheat-dependent, exercise-induced anaphylaxis*. It's a potentially life-threatening response to gluten that occurs specifically when wheat is ingested in conjunction with physical exercise.[30] Food alone is not enough to cause the reaction. It takes food plus exercise. Obviously, this is of special concern to athletes. Given how many athletes might "carb up" with gluten-containing pasta, toast, bagels, pizza, and so on before a workout, training session, race, or game, this should be on your radar.

GLUTEN SENSITIVITY

Gluten sensitivity represents the largest branch of gluten sufferers, and yet it is the least well-known of the gluten intolerance conditions. People with gluten sensitivity have a particular immune response to gluten, different from that in both celiac disease and wheat allergy. Typically, other conditions have first been ruled out, yet these people do have real and often serious symptoms triggered by gluten, which are alleviated by the gluten-free diet.[31]

"Imagine gluten ingestion on a spectrum," write Dr. Fasano and his colleagues in a recent research article. "At one end, you have people with celiac disease, who cannot tolerate one crumb of gluten in their diet. At the other end, you have the lucky people who can eat pizza, beer, pasta, and cookies—and have no ill effects whatsoever. In the middle, there is this murky area of gluten reactions, including gluten sensitivity."[32]

Current estimates suggest that over twenty million Americans are affected by gluten sensitivity. Some researchers suggest the condition affects 10 percent of the general population, which would put the number well past thirty million people in the United States.

EVERYBODY ELSE

And what about everyone else? Is gluten a problem for them, too? Is it a problem for you?

The answer is . . . maybe. As we've noted, there are reasons to believe that gluten could be a problem for everyone. For some, the effects may be subtle. For others, they'll be more serious.

For some of you, the answer is . . . probably. If you have a blood relative with gluten intolerance, there's an increased chance that gluten is a problem for you as well. Regardless, if you're an athlete, you're likely at heightened risk for gluten-related problems and more sensitive to its potential effects on your performance. We explain why in chapter 2.

POSSIBLE SIGNS AND SYMPTOMS OF GLUTEN EXPOSURE AND ASSOCIATED CONDITIONS

Diarrhea

Gas

Bloating

Abdominal pain

Lactose intolerance

Nausea and vomiting

Fatty, oily, bloody, or
    foul-smelling stools (steatorrhea)

Unexplained weight loss

Joint pain

Osteopenia or osteoporosis

Iron deficiency

Anemia

Chronic fatigue

Headaches

Brain fog

Muscle coordination and balance problems (ataxia)

Neuropathy

Depression

Malnutrition

Growth delay or failure to thrive

Skin rashes and disorders (dermatitis herpetiformis)

General or abdominal swelling

Nutrient deficiencies

Pain, numbness, or tingling in extremities
    (peripheral neuropathy)

Intestinal lymphoma and bowel cancer

Type 1 diabetes

Rheumatoid arthritis

Autoimmune thyroid disease

Irritable bowel syndrome

NEED TO KNOW |||||||||||||||||||||||||||||||||||||||||||||||||||||||||||||||||||||||||

- Gluten is a family of proteins found in cereal grains such as wheat, barley, and rye, as well as foods made from them.
- Selective breeding and genetic modification of grains such as wheat have resulted in higher concentrations of gluten, as well as gluten that is more toxic than it once was.
- Changes in our diet, and especially rising rates of heavy gluten consumption, are causing rapidly increasing rates of gluten intolerance.
- Gluten causes a wide range of gluten intolerance problems, including celiac disease, gluten sensitivity, and wheat allergy.

2

Why All Athletes Should Care About Gluten

I F YOU'RE A conventional athlete—a healthy person with no obvious or diagnosed problem with gluten—you may be thinking, *I don't have trouble eating gluten. Why should I go gluten-free?*

You may not realize it now, but there's a good chance that gluten is actually impacting your body. Once on a gluten-free diet, many athletes feel the change retrospectively. They're unaware that anything has been "off" until they go gluten-free and then realize that they feel and perform better than they did before. There may even be a "eureka" moment when they conclude that gluten was affecting their body in subtle—and sometimes not so subtle—ways.

IMPAIRED DIGESTION

For better or worse, the gut is not an athletic organ. Sure, training can improve how it handles and digests food—before, during, and after exercise—but at the end of the day, it's a finicky system that can be surprisingly sensitive to the balance of carbohydrates and protein and fat in your diet, the ratio of nutrients to fluid intake, and so on.[1] It requires careful calibration, a matching of diet to sport.

Yet, as seemingly fickle as the gut can be, the digestion and absorption of nutrients is a critical piece of the athletic equation.

As we noted in the previous chapter, gluten is extremely difficult for your body to digest. If that were all, gluten might not be so bad. It would be akin to dietary fiber, adding bulk to your meals. Alas, that's not where the story ends. Gluten disrupts your digestion and negatively affects your health, and eventually your athletic performance, too.

Jay Beagle, a professional ice hockey player for the NHL's Washington Capitals, found that out. "I don't really have problems with gluten. I can eat it and feel fine. I grew up eating it. I ate a lot of pasta before games. But if I want to perform at my best, I feel better when I'm eating gluten-free," he explains.

During the summer of 2010, Beagle was having digestive problems. He was eating more than 6,000 calories per day, trying to put on healthy weight in advance of the upcoming 2010–2011 ice hockey season. But there was a subtle problem. "I wasn't digesting food well," he says. "I was feeling bloated. I wasn't feeling right in my workouts. I didn't have as much energy, didn't feel as good."

One reason why athletes such as Beagle are normally attracted to wheat products such as breads and pastas is for the starches, the carbohydrates, which get broken down into sugars and converted into glycogen, to be stored in muscles and the liver for energy during athletics.

It's a good idea in principle. As Beagle discovered, though, gluten sometimes gets in the way. Even in healthy people, gluten causes starch malabsorption and other digestive problems.[2] In other words, if you eat a slice of whole-grain wheat bread with the idea that it will supply your body with a good source of carbs, gluten will inhibit your body from being able to digest and absorb those very carbs. (The starches in breads made from gluten-free flours, by comparison, are more readily digested and absorbed into the bloodstream.[3] For more, be sure to check out chapter 6.)

Already, we're seeing why you as a conventional athlete ought to consider going gluten-free. Not only is gluten difficult to digest, it also interferes with the absorption of the wheat carbs athletes may eat to fuel their body. Omitting the gluten can help resolve both of those issues. It certainly did for Beagle.

During the summer of 2011, Beagle—along with Capitals teammate Karl Alzner—made the switch to the gluten-free diet. It was purely experimental initially. "I decided to try the diet for two weeks at first and see how it went. Almost within the week, I could tell the difference," he

ATHLETE INSIGHT

Jay Beagle

PROFESSIONAL HOCKEY PLAYER, WASHINGTON CAPITALS (NHL)

Born: 1985 • Lives: Washington, DC, area • Gluten-Free Since: 2011

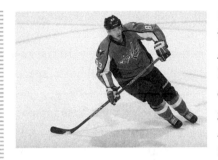

HIGHLIGHTS: STARTING AS a talented youth player in the Alberta Junior Hockey League, Beagle rose through the ranks of ice hockey, playing collegiately at the University of Alaska–Anchorage before joining professional developmental leagues such as the ECHL, and later, the AHL, considered the primary incubator for the NHL. He made his NHL debut with the New York Rangers before signing with the Washington Capitals. During the 2010–2011 season, Beagle played in a career-high thirty-one games, scoring two game-winning goals.[4]

FAVORITE GLUTEN-FREE FOODS: sweet potatoes (with some brown sugar and coconut oil); KIND bars; Go Raw Super Cookies; gluten-free corn chips with bison meat, organic cheese, and peppers for a snack; bison, wild boar, venison, and salmon, in addition to some steak, for protein

says. "I started digesting food better, started putting on better weight, because I didn't have to eat as much. I was getting the nutrients with a little less food. I no longer feel bloated. To take away that feeling of going into a workout or a practice or a game feeling full and bloated is huge. That was the main thing."

And digestion is just the tip of the iceberg. A number of factors come into play for athletes and anyone living an active lifestyle. Each factor is impacted by exercise, and in each case, gluten makes a potential problem worse. Athletes, be on alert.

LEAKY GUT AND GLUTEN TOXICITY

The gastrointestinal tract is an amazing series of organs. Take the small and large intestines, for example. The cells that make up the intestinal wall normally fit together tightly, with no spaces, like a perfect jigsaw puzzle. They form a barrier that separates the gut ecosystem from the rest of your body. When functioning properly, the intestinal wall keeps bad things in your intestines and out of your body, while letting the good things—such as nutrients—in.

Sometimes that system stops functioning properly. In the case of a leaky gut (also known as *intestinal permeability*), small holes, spaces, and gaps develop.

How does a leaky gut happen? For one, intense exercise increases the permeability of the intestine.[5] Leaky gut is also found in people with celiac disease and other autoimmune conditions. That much isn't news. But here's what is: A leaky gut is also caused by gluten, including in healthy people.[6] Although not to the same degree as that seen in athletes with celiac disease, gluten causes a leaky gut nonetheless.

Once that happens, toxins can sneak their way into your body, where they can cause inflammation and other problems. Gluten can sneak its way in, too.[7]

It's bad enough that gluten exacerbates the leaky gut problem, letting toxins into your body that can mess with how you feel and perform. But it turns out that gluten itself is also toxic. The human body just doesn't like it, including in so-called healthy people.[8] When researchers took gluten and exposed it to all sorts of different cells in a person's body—intestines, lungs, kidneys, adrenal glands—the result was always the same: "noxious effects."[9] Gluten displayed a "nonspecific cytotoxicity." It's an equal-opportunity problem maker.

Between its influence in causing leaky gut and its toxicity to human cells, gluten is like the Trojan horse *and* the army waiting inside the horse to wreak havoc. It has the key to the city and the capability to inflict harm, a dangerous combo.

And there's more. Gluten's ability to toxically invade the body doesn't stop there.

Although gluten is very resistant to digestion, the stomach enzyme pepsin does do one thing to it. Pepsin causes gluten to release bioactive peptides known as *exorphins*, chunks of gluten that remain intact and cause physiological and neurological responses.[10] In the case of gluten, those exorphins act like opioids.[11] This puts them in the same family of narcotics as opium and morphine. Opioid effects can sometimes be positive, such as their role in the runner's high, but they can also be negative, as is the case with gluten. Toxic gluten exorphins cause problems ranging from gut dysfunction to immune system changes to neurological disorders, especially when they cross the blood-brain barrier.[12] (Because of gluten's role in neurological problems, researchers are increasingly finding and understanding a curious link between gluten and schizophrenia.[13])

GASTROINTESTINAL PROBLEMS

It's no secret that sports provide plenty of health benefits. But when it comes to the GI system, those benefits only accrue up to a point. Eventually, you get diminishing returns, and then the returns start going negative.[14] It's a fact of life that some sports can cause stomach troubles.[15]

Certain types of sports are more guilty of this than are others. For example, upward of 70 percent of endurance athletes are affected by at least one GI symptom. Regardless of your chosen sport, train hard enough and it can become problematic to your digestion.[16]

Generally, the longer the duration of and the more strenuous your sport, the more likely you are to develop gastrointestinal problems, symptoms, even disorders.[17] A recent Drexel University College of Medicine study whose results were reported at the 2011 Digestive Disease Week conference gave added confirmation: If you play competitive, high-intensity sports, you're more likely to develop GI problems.[18] A subset of athletes will also wrestle with irritable bowel syndrome (IBS), a functional GI disorder that is aggravated by gluten, and which responds well to the gluten-free diet, especially among those with IBS from food hypersensitivity.[19]

Thus, as with a leaky gut, GI problems can arise strictly as a result of sport. And again, gluten is a known trigger that potentially compounds the problem.[20] Maximizing your athletic performance is all about having your body, your mind, your training, *and your diet* work together. Why add gluten to the equation, when you know it has the potential to undermine your hard-won gains?

Would you toe the starting line of an important race, swallow a few laxatives, hope for the best, and expect to perform well? We don't think so. Then why keep gluten in your diet if you are an athlete? You're just setting yourself up for what researchers call food-dependent, exercise-induced gastrointestinal distress.[21] We call it a shame, because going gluten-free is an easy way, fully within your control, to remove a known stress on your GI system, an integral part of your athletic engine.

INFLAMMATION

Inflammation is the body's natural response to injury, irritation, and toxins. It is a defensive immune response characterized by increased blood and fluid flow to the site, where you may experience swelling, pain, redness, and/or heat, and in the case of joints, loss of movement or function. Inflammation can affect a particular part of the body or the whole body.

Under normal circumstances, it's a healthy response. When you twist your ankle, or develop a blister from your running shoe or hiking boot, or get a bruise from an impact injury, your brain makes a "911 call" and various internal "first responders" are called into action. Your body is protecting itself from further injury, repairing existing injuries, and maintaining healthy tissue.

Sometimes, though, inflammation can be a bad thing. When? If the inflammatory response is misguided—if it never shuts off, if it acts against your own body and targets healthy tissue, if it is too extreme, or if it becomes chronic and ongoing. Under those circumstances, inflammation can inhibit health, performance, and recovery, and even cause damage and disease. That's why athletes stretch, and ice, and employ all sorts of anti-inflammatory tactics—including taking "vitamin I" (ibuprofen, a nonsteroidal anti-inflammatory drug).

Enhanced athletic performance and recovery are about avoiding extreme inflammation and maintaining healthy levels.

So what does gluten have to do with inflammation in conventional athletes? As it turns out, plenty. Let's look at two sides of the same coin: gluten as a cause of inflammation, and the gluten-free diet as anti-inflammatory.

Gluten can cause inflammation directly in healthy adults. If you've been reading this chapter at all, you already know why—by placing digestive stress on the GI tract, by causing a leaky gut, and through direct toxicity to the body's cells. Such inflammation can have direct and immediate effects on athletic performance and recovery.

There's a longer-term concern with that inflammation, too. While gluten-induced inflammation causes serious problems for athletes with gluten intolerance, this lower-level inflammation we're talking about among conventional athletes is nothing to scoff at, either. As we noted in chapter 1, people with gluten intolerance are at risk for heightened mortality, as compared to the general population. But the results of a study published in a 2009 issue of the *Journal of the American Medical Association* revealed some concerning findings. When researchers looked at three populations of people—those with celiac disease, those with latent celiac disease (positive blood test results, but not the intestinal damage), and a third group with mild gut inflammation—the highest mortality was found not in the celiac disease group, but in the nonceliac group of people with milder forms of chronic inflammation[22]— the type of inflammation you might find in a so-called healthy person who eats a lot of gluten regularly.

On the flip side of the coin, the gluten-free diet has been shown to have anti-inflammatory properties. This effect has been especially demonstrated in studies of gut microbiota. The gut is like a complicated ecosystem, with a delicate balance of beneficial and harmful bacteria and other microbiota. That ecosystem has proven responsive to the presence or absence of gluten in the diet.

When researchers studied healthy groups of people on either gluten-containing or gluten-free diets, the ones eating gluten had higher levels of inflammatory factors, such as certain cytokines and chemokines. This gluten-induced inflammatory response was similar to that of people with gluten intolerance,but it was found among people who supposedly don't react to gluten.[23]

Kyle Korver

PROFESSIONAL BASKETBALL PLAYER, CHICAGO BULLS (NBA)

Born: 1981 • Lives: Illinois • Gluten-Free Since: 2010

HIGHLIGHTS: KYLE KORVER comes from a basketball family—his dad and five uncles all played, as did all his brothers. Born in California but raised in Iowa, he helped lead his high school team to the state tournament for three consecutive years. Korver attended Creighton University, where he helped his team to four straight NCAA tournament appearances. He was part of the team with the best record in school history. Korver also finished his college career in the Top 10 in NCAA history for threes made (371). He joined the NBA as a second-round draft pick of the New Jersey Nets and played at the Philadelphia 76ers and Utah Jazz before joining Chicago.[24]

FAVORITE GLUTEN-FREE FOODS: gluten-free pasta with chicken or ground turkey, goat cheese, and tomatoes; quinoa and eggs with a bit of salsa the morning of big games; meat and vegetables when on the road

Those on the gluten-free diet had significant decreases in several factors known to cause inflammation. Incredibly, as with those on the gluten-containing diet, this change happened in a group of people who traditionally were told they could eat gluten without a second thought.[25] One study compared the wheat- and gluten-based European diet versus the naturally gluten-free diet in rural Burkina Faso, Africa, composed heavily of millet, sorghum, and some corn. Researchers found significant differences between the gut ecosystems of the two populations.

ATHLETE INSIGHT

Liana Mauro

PILATES INSTRUCTOR

Born: 1982 • Lives: Texas • Gluten-Free Since: 2009

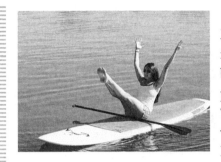

PILATES INSTRUCTOR Liana Mauro is living proof of the inflammatory problems caused by gluten, and the healing power of the gluten-free diet. "My whole life, pretty much, I was sick," she says. Her problems included bad chronic pain, especially in her joints. Mauro was eventually diagnosed with rheumatoid arthritis, a long-term autoimmune disease that leads to inflammation in the joints and surrounding tissues.

Growing up in an athletic family, facing such challenges was difficult for Mauro. One of her sisters is an Ironman triathlete; another runs marathons. Her dad is a competitive tennis player. "I would try to get involved in sports, but it wasn't comfortable for me," she says. "I always had chronic pain, headaches, fatigue. I was always sick." Her mother introduced her to Pilates when she was fifteen years old and she quickly fell in love with it. Pilates helped her manage her pain and build strength, and eventually became her career.

Meanwhile, however, some nagging health problems lingered. After years of frustration working with Western doctors, Mauro started seeing an alternative practitioner in 2006. Right off the bat she was tested for food allergies—both dairy and wheat came back positive. "Not knowing what I know now, I decided that cutting out both would be too hard," Mauro explains. "So I just cut out the dairy."

But every time she ate, she got terrible stomachaches, "to the point that I didn't want to eat anymore," she says. Her wheat sensitivity, meanwhile, had turned into full-blown gluten intolerance.

She went gluten-free in September 2009, and within the first month, she felt much better. "I thought it was a mental thing," she says today. "But I have a sweet tooth, and I was missing my cupcakes. So I had one, and sure enough, I got really sick." Her chronic joint pain came back for nearly a month and a half after that. "I learned quickly that I could not cheat," Mauro says.

Since then she's been strictly gluten-free and has never felt better. In fact, her rheumatoid arthritis has all but resolved, her platelet and white blood cell counts have returned to normal, and her anemia is going away. Most important, her joint pain and inflammation are gone, her body is healthy, and her Pilates is as thriving as ever—personally and professionally—with her studio named Austin's Best Pilates Studio in *Austin Fit Magazine*'s 2012 "Best of" readers poll.[26]

FAVORITE GLUTEN-FREE FOODS: fruits and veggies; smoothies; cucumber rolls; chips and salsa; fish with kale, broccoli, and potatoes; Pamela's Chocolate Chip Walnut Cookies; Kinnikinnick Donuts

One pronounced difference stood out immediately: Between the two groups, the gluten-free diet of Burkina Faso's rural residents protected those people from inflammation.[27]

As we've said before, such inflammation can inhibit athletic performance and impair or delay recovery. Just ask professional basketball player Kyle Korver.

Korver is a shooting guard (with a mean three-point shot) for the NBA's Chicago Bulls. When he signed with the Bulls from the Utah Jazz in 2010, he gave serious thought to how to maximize his performance. "As I get older, I want to keep on playing basketball as long as I can," he says. Issues such as his energy level, his recovery from games and workouts, and maintaining healthy joints loomed large. "Inflammation in my knees is the biggest thing I fight throughout the year," he explains.

At the advice of a friend, Korver voluntarily made the switch to a gluten-free diet. "I've never had any allergies, food intolerances, anything like that. This was about performance all the way," he says. And did it work? Did he feel the difference in his knees? "Yeah, I have," he says without hesitation. "I do feel healthier."

WEAKENED AND CHALLENGED IMMUNE SYSTEM

Inflammation provides the perfect segue to shift from talking about the gut and the GI system specifically to talking about the body's immune system more generally. They are, after all, quite related—and gluten-induced inflammation and other responses are a common denominator between them.

Just as sports can either help or hinder the GI system, so, too, can they affect the body's immune system. Your body's natural killer (NK) cells, part of the innate immune system, provide a good example. NK cells are part of your body's nonspecific first line of defense against tumor cells and virus-infected cells. In other words, healthy levels of active NK cells protect you from infection and cancer.[28] Suppressed levels of NK cell activity make you susceptible.

This is where exercise and sports come into play. From your resting baseline level of NK cell activity, low to moderate to strenuous exercise stimulates your system, resulting in heightened immune function and inflammation. However, during recovery immediately following activity, NK cell activity plummets to low levels—a period of susceptibility to infection—before returning to the pre-exercise baseline.[29]

Here's the good news: Repeat that cycle enough times, and you can eventually increase your resting baseline of NK cell activity (as studies have shown in well-trained athletes), thus using exercise to boost your immune system.[30]

But in this case, there is such a thing as too much of a good thing. Frequent high-intensity exertion repeatedly places your NK cell activity into the below-baseline recovery rut, putting you into a state of chronic immune suppression.[31] That leaves your body and its immune system less able to cope with the problems caused by gluten: gut and systemic inflammation, leaky gut, cytotoxic effects, and GI distress.

Dr. Allen Lim has seen it happen before. Lim was the physiologist for pro cycling's Team RadioShack and other teams, and today does private sports physiology consulting for cyclists. He's a veteran at working with elite cyclists in the Tour de France and other major Grand Tour races. Such events are a classic example of intense exercise–induced immune system depression, and the impact it can have on gluten intolerance, even in healthy athletes.

Consider the case of Team RadioShack's Levi Leipheimer (now with Team Omega Pharma–Quick-Step), winner of the 2011 Tour de Suisse. In the last few seasons, Leipheimer has adopted a gluten-free diet during training and racing and has responded extremely well to it. Lim has a theory why.

"We see the differences [in performance and response to gluten] when these guys are really stressed out at the difficult training camps and the Grand Tours," such as the Tour de France, Lim explains. "Those events put a lot of pressure and demand on the body, which gets immune suppressed. Riders who normally might not have a problem with gluten in their diet get hypersensitive with an inflammatory response to wheat- and gluten-based products.

"These big races make them like a canary in a coal mine," he continues. "You have a guy who's normally fine on any diet, but in the hard events, the toll it takes on the body is so extreme that going to the gluten-free diet may suppress some of the inflammation associated with eating, and that goes a long way to helping them feel better."

Lim is not the only one to make this observation. Others have seen it before as well. For example, one researcher noted the case of a long-distance runner. Day to day, he did fine with gluten; he had no symptoms, no problems with diet. However, in the heat of competition, when he was pushing his body to the limit, he suddenly wasn't able to tolerate the gluten that otherwise hadn't caused him any obvious problems. During long-distance races, the runner was wracked with abdominal pain and bloody diarrhea. When he removed gluten from his diet, the pain and diarrhea during races disappeared.[32]

Professional triathlete Terra Castro, gluten-free since 2000, has observed this peculiarity, too. "It's crazy. Some athletes go gluten-free just on a performance basis, and it works," she says. "They get more cut, less bloated, don't have potty issues. It's the extreme intensity we put on our digestive system, racing triathlons. You invest so much—it's one day, one race; you get one shot. You don't want anything else in your system challenging it other than the race itself."

Those unwanted and unneeded challenges include gluten.

Xterra professional Jenny Smith feels the difference in her immune system even when she's not competing. "I feel like my immune system is stronger," she says, "and my day-to-day health is better." Since going gluten-free in 2007, she continues, "I rarely get sick, and when I do get hit with a bug, I respond to it and recover pretty quickly. I attribute that to my gluten-free diet."

Just take a step back and consider the sheer prevalence of gluten-free athletes in endurance sports such as distance running, cycling, and half and full Ironman distance triathlons. Irish Olympic marathoner Martin Fagan,[33] Australian Olympic marathoner Kate Smyth,[34] U.S. Olympic marathoner Ryan Hall,[35] and U.S. marathoner Stephanie Rothstein[36] (hopeful of making the 2012 Olympic team as of this writing) are all gluten-free. So are elite triathletes Jesse Thomas,[37] John Forberger,[38] and Desirée Ficker.[39] And you've probably read before about the gluten-free diet of pro cyclist and Team Garmin-Cervélo marquee rider Christian Vande Velde.[40]

They are just the tip of the iceberg; the list goes on and on. Throughout this book you'll read profiles of at least as many *other* elite endurance athletes we're not mentioning by name here, because they'll come up in later chapters. In fact, some 20 percent of the gluten-free athletes we interviewed for this book are elite endurance athletes. Given how many gluten-free athletes are playing and competing in so many different sports, it's a surprisingly high percentage. Is it a coincidence? We think that's unlikely.

This leaves us with an important question: Why? Why do we find so many gluten-free endurance athletes?

There are several possibilities: (a) These are athletes with gluten intolerance who happen to practice an endurance discipline and are proof that you can compete at the highest levels of sport despite gluten intolerance; (b) these are healthy athletes who are cutting-edge and quick to adopt a new diet if it promises the potential of performance improvement, but they were awesome athletes already; (c) they've discovered a genuine performance benefit of the gluten-free diet that helps healthy and gluten-intolerant athletes alike; or (d) the unbelievably high demands they place on their body as elite endurance athletes strains their system, making them more susceptible to gluten—whether

ATHLETE INSIGHT

Jenny Smith

PROFESSIONAL XTERRA OFF-ROAD TRIATHLETE

Born: 1973 • Lives: Colorado • Gluten-Free Since: 2007

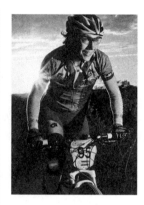

WHEN JENNY SMITH was a child, wheat (and gluten) was something of a Jekyll-and-Hyde food for her and her family back in her native New Zealand. Her father had been diagnosed with Crohn's disease, and her younger sister—two years her junior—was born allergic to gluten and dairy. Smith, meanwhile, "lived on bagels and oats," she says. "I was lucky I got on as well as I did. Gluten was never a good food for me. I didn't feel good when I would eat toast."

It wasn't until the early 2000s, though, that she started to steer her own diet farther from gluten, as her father and sister already had. By then Smith had moved to Colorado for college. She was a runner, but while recovering from an injury, her future husband, Brian, and a friend introduced her to mountain biking. She was a natural, and success came quickly.

Smith became an eight-time member of New Zealand's Mountain Bike World Championship team (2001–2010). She tackled her first Xterra off-road triathlon in 2005 and proved a fierce competitor there, too. Just one year later she took second at the U.S. Xterra National Championship and fourth at the Xterra World Championship, missing the podium by eighteen seconds. She had many other prominent race results throughout the early and mid-2000s.

Along the way, however, various symptoms started to creep in. Her allergies and sinuses began to flare up; she attributed it to environmental factors (pine needles and pollen and such). She became "extraordinarily lactose intolerant." She just didn't feel 100 percent.

In 2007 she cut out gluten for good, having flirted with lower-gluten diets for a few years. Now, her allergies are gone, she tolerates dairy much better, and overall she feels great. And despite the fact that she calls herself "an older athlete" now, her race results have only gotten better; for example, she took first place in 2010 at the grueling Trans Andes Challenge, a multistage mountain bike race in Patagonia; landing on the podium (sometimes, at the very top) in a number of prominent Xterra races; and most recently, in 2011, finishing fourth in the prestigious Leadville Trail 100 mountain bike race, eight minutes under the old course record and seven minutes off the new record.[41]

FAVORITE GLUTEN-FREE FOODS: eggs ("a ridiculous amount"); vegetables, such as squash and sweet potatoes; avocados; bananas; peanut butter and almond butter; dates; rice tortillas (with ham and cheese); limited gluten-free pasta and bread

they're healthy or gluten intolerant—and thus more likely to adopt and benefit from a gluten-free diet.

For any given athlete, several of these are likely to be true, but that last one is worth reiterating, because it also reflects the findings of Lim, and Castro, and Smith. Frequent, intense athletics—through training and competition—suppresses the immune system and other "coping" mechanisms of the body, making athletes more prone to problems with gluten and more likely to feel and perform better by going gluten-free.

An anecdote from pro triathlete Tyler Stewart sums it up well: "I could eat anything and never have any issues. As a kid, through college, even my first couple of years as an amateur triathlete, I never had the bloating or stomach pains. But the more seriously I got into sports, and the more my body turned into a machine, the more important the fuel became. My body became that much more sensitive, and it has gotten more so every single year. Now it's like putting regular gas into a sports car." For Stewart, going gluten-free provides the high-octane fuel her hypersensitive "engine" needs.

SUBTLE EFFECTS

If you're a conventional athlete who currently eats gluten, we can't promise that going gluten-free will make you an overnight Olympian. But you may be surprised how much better you feel and perform on the gluten-free diet. Or the change may be more subtle.

Some athletes who voluntarily go gluten-free looking for a performance edge only see the benefit in hindsight. They may not have noticed any problems when they were eating gluten. Any impact on their performance was too subtle to notice and didn't reach an obvious threshold. Once they've "crossed over" to the gluten-free side, however, they realize that they feel better, perform better, are less bloated, and have improved digestion.

So it was for four-time mountain bike world champion Brian Lopes. "If your whole life you've been doing something one way and been successful, then how do you know it's been impacting you?" he says.

Lopes explains that he was never one to be particularly mindful of his eating habits. "I don't go to McDonald's or anything like that, but I didn't really have a diet," he says. "In the morning I liked having pancakes, waffles, a croissant, some sort of pastry, a cinnamon roll, whatever."

He tried the gluten-free diet, largely on a whim. "I basically started because I was farting . . . every day, all day," he explains. Lopes made the switch during the fall of 2010. Now, he notices a difference in his body retrospectively. "If I do eat a little gluten, I get bloated and gassy for sure. I may have felt that way in the past, but didn't realize it, because that was normal for me."

IS GLUTEN BAD FOR EVERYONE?

By now you might reasonably be asking yourself, *Is gluten bad for everyone? Should everyone go gluten-free?* To which we answer a resounding . . . maybe. Gluten is increasingly being implicated in a host of conditions, not just gluten intolerance—type 1 diabetes, rheumatoid arthritis, irritable bowel syndrome, schizophrenia—and the list is growing.[42] Each week, it seems, researchers find another way that gluten is impacting our health, another disease in which gluten is implicated.

ATHLETE INSIGHT

Brian Lopes

WORLD CHAMPION PROFESSIONAL MOUNTAIN BIKER

Born: 1971 • Lives: California • Gluten-Free Since: 2010

HIGHLIGHTS: BRIAN LOPES'S record as a mountain biker is beyond impressive. He holds more than nineteen major titles, including nine National Championships, six UCI World Cup Championships, and four world championships. He was the ESPY Action Sports Athlete of the Year in 2001, and he won two NEA Awards (World Extreme Sports Award) in 2000 and 2001. Lopes is also featured in Sony PlayStation's Downhill Domination video game.[43]

FAVORITE GLUTEN-FREE FOODS: Pamela's Pancakes, Bob's Red Mill gluten-free oatmeal, Udi's Gluten Free Bread

But as we've said before, and as we revisit in chapter 4, despite important generalizations we can make, a crucial element of individual biology comes into play. Every person, every athlete, is different. Your formula has to match what works best for you.

What we *have* done, so far, is laid out a compelling case that gluten *probably* shouldn't be a part of *your* formula. From demonstrating in chapter 1 how gluten's toxicity has increased over the years and how rates of gluten intolerance are on the rise around the world, to giving in this chapter the specific ways in which gluten can negatively impact your body and your performance—whether you're gluten intolerant or not—we're firm believers that any athlete has the potential to benefit from the gluten-free edge.

That perspective flies in the face of common wisdom that says if you don't have some form of gluten intolerance, then gluten is fine for you; that you have no reason to go gluten-free.[44] We beg to differ. Actually, there are some important reasons to go gluten-free. If you're an athlete looking to get the most out of your body, you ought to be paying extra-close attention to the prospect of going gluten-free. Get off the gluten train and onto the gluten-free edge.

Anita Nall Richesson is certainly on board. She's a U.S. Olympic gold-medalist swimmer and former world record holder (see page 199). She has also worked as the nutritionist for the Jacksonville Jaguars NFL football team. Nall Richesson instituted something of a culture shift in the Jaguars' team cafeteria. She educated players about their nutrition and made sure that gluten-free food options were readily and prominently available. She didn't expect everyone on the team to make the gluten-free switch all at once. But she saw certain players respond very well to the diet, and expects more to follow . . . eventually.

"Do I think everyone would benefit from going gluten-free?" asks Nall Richesson rhetorically. "Absolutely."

DOWN THE RABBIT HOLE

GLUTEN HAS A complicated impact on your immune system. The rabbit hole goes much deeper, and quickly gets more complex and confusing, especially when you start considering not just the main gluten reaction, but also the impact of gluten exorphins (opioids), other gluten/gliadin peptides, and the relationships between them.

For example, in cases of gluten intolerance, and celiac disease especially,[45] different parts of the immune system are simultaneously suppressed and provoked. Certain components of the system go on attack, initiating an autoimmune reaction that in part makes untreated celiac disease so devastating. Meanwhile, NK cell activity drops off, opening the door to infection and cancer, which helps explain why people with celiac disease are at heightened risk for certain cancers and other diseases.

Meanwhile, in healthy athletes, certain gluten compounds—especially the exorphins and other peptides—can have not only a variety of negative effects (including immune suppression and neurotoxin-like effects that impact the cerebellum, motor control, and coordination[46]), but also a stimulatory effect on the immune system.[47] Depending on a wide range of factors, in one instance they may do X, but in another they do Y. Researchers are quick to note this seeming contradiction. The reality is that life just isn't so black-and-white. Although we can accurately describe a large-scale negative response to gluten, when we start looking at the more subtle effects of gluten exorphins and other peptides, it's impossible to say "If A, then B." It's more like, "If A and B, and possibly C, or maybe D, then perhaps E, but also F. Or, neither E or F, but instead G." There's a lot of bad, and potentially some good to gluten, but alas, it's impossible to separate the wheat from the chaff, so to speak.

The human body is incredibly complex, and science is still working to understand how we respond to gluten—in both healthy and gluten-intolerant people. It's a good reminder that, for all of the information in this book, it's important to tie it all back to your individual biology and how *you* respond to the potential gluten-free edge. If you're gluten intolerant, it's a no brainer. But if you're voluntarily gluten-free, it's more food for thought.

NOTHING TO LOSE, EVERYTHING TO GAIN

"There's a bit of Pascal's wager," pro cycling's Dr. Lim says. In Pascal's wager, French philosopher Blaise Pascal argued that the existence of God could not be proven or disproven through reason, but that there was much to be gained by believing in God and living accordingly, and that there was little to be lost by making that gambit. Lim notes that going gluten-free isn't going to hinder an athlete, and that for the right athlete it can be a huge help. Dr. Peter Osborne, who specializes in treating patients with gluten and other food intolerances, agrees. "It's not a detriment to go gluten-free," he says, "but it can certainly, even most likely, benefit someone." From that perspective, embracing the gluten-free edge is a win-win . . . nothing to lose, and everything to gain.

You don't have to be gluten intolerant for the wager to work. Theoretically, gluten can impact any athlete at any time. Take the case of a twenty-nine-year old elite female flatwater kayaker. She started having gastrointestinal symptoms: vomiting, pain, diarrhea, bloating. She started losing weight, and wasn't able to put it back on. She came down with sudden iron deficiency, bad enough to require blood transfusions because oral supplements and injections weren't working. Her symptoms had all the hallmarks of a classic case of celiac disease.

And here's the kicker. She tested negative for celiac disease, negative for gliadin (gluten) antibodies, and negative for villous atrophy in her small intestine biopsy. The only food intolerances doctors documented were soy, coconut, banana, and a few other things, such as MSG. Gluten notably wasn't on that list. Yet a gluten-free diet improved some of her symptoms and completely relieved others.[48] That is Pascal's wager in action. The gluten-free diet won't hurt your performance, and if things go right, it can seriously help.

BEWARE THE TRIGGER

Gluten intolerance is a dark horse. Of the 30 million or more Americans with some form of gluten intolerance, the majority are undiagnosed or misdiagnosed. Many may be asymptomatic. Everything is fine until—surprise!—the gluten intolerance turns on. Unless you've had active gluten intolerance since birth, it's almost always triggered by some mechanism. It could be childbirth (in women), a serious illness, extreme physical exertion, too much stress, or overconsumption of gluten in your diet.

If you're an athlete, sports plus dietary gluten could be the combo that tips the scales. By proactively going gluten-free now, you can hedge your bet and avoid developing gluten intolerance in the first place.

Just consider a series of stories involving elite athletes who had no previous history of gluten problems, and who found themselves in a very different situation after gluten intolerance triggered.

A few short years ago, there was an Olympic track cyclist and world record holder who had a good understanding of diet and nutrition. He was very physically fit and strong. He ate an iron-rich diet and also took iron supplements. Yet he started showing signs of mild anemia. Then he developed problems with malabsorption and, in early 2009, experienced unexplained weight loss and underperformance.[49] Celiac disease that he never knew he had—he never had a reason for suspicion, never had problems with dietary gluten—had turned on.

It was a similar story with an NCAA Division I collegiate female volleyball player. What's so notable about her case is the sudden onset of symptoms, the dramatic change in her health, and the decline in her athletic performance. As intense preseason training got underway, she started losing weight rapidly. She developed diarrhea, vomiting, and lost her appetite. Team coaches and physicians suspected her of having an eating disorder. Soon she was experiencing terrible fatigue, plus bloating and abdominal pain. Things got so bad that she was removed from play and sidelined. Doctors eventually sorted out her problem. Again, it was celiac disease. Hers was a striking example of how an underlying predisposition toward gluten intolerance, coupled with the trigger of gluten plus intense athletics, was all that was needed for her to switch from healthy athlete to struggling and sick.

But her story had a happy ending. Her health experienced a dramatic rebound on the gluten-free diet. She returned to the team for her sophomore year and had a successful volleyball career as a college athlete. Best of all, she didn't just come back to her pre-illness level of play, before the celiac disease switched on. Coaches noted that she exceeded her previous healthy level of performance.[50]

Finally, there was the strikingly similar story of a D-I female collegiate tennis player. Coaches described her as a high-level athlete. Then her health—and performance—fell off the rails, so to speak. Doctors had a long list of potential diagnoses. They eventually discovered it was celiac disease. (Are you seeing the pattern?) They put her on a gluten-free diet and she made a full recovery, returning to elite athletic competition.

ATHLETE INSIGHT

Kristen Taylor

FORMER COLLEGIATE LACROSSE PLAYER, UNIVERSITY OF NORTH CAROLINA

Born: 1988 • Lives: Oregon • Gluten-Free Since: 2007

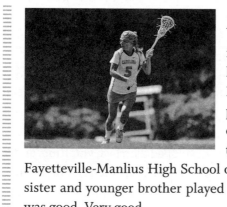

A NATIVE OF upstate New York, Kristen Taylor grew up in a lacrosse family. Both of her parents played for Cornell. Her dad worked for Brine, a prominent lacrosse equipment company. Her mother coached the girl's lacrosse team at Fayetteville-Manlius High School outside of Syracuse. Her older sister and younger brother played lacrosse. So did she. And she was good. Very good.

As a sophomore and junior, Taylor played under her mother, helping lead the team to back-to-back state championships in 2004 and 2005 (and being named tournament MVP both times). As a senior in 2006, Taylor narrowly missed a three-peat, with Fayetteville-Manlius losing the state championship by a single goal. She graduated high school as a three-time All American.

Taylor went to the University of North Carolina, one of the top-ranked collegiate women's lacrosse programs in the country. Her freshman year was nothing short of stellar. She played in twenty-one games, starting in eleven of them. She tallied an impressive forty-three goals, and her dominant play made her one of the top freshman attackers and top freshman overall in not just the Atlantic Coast Conference, but the nation. UNC named her Rookie of the Year and WomensLacrosse.com named her to its nationwide All-Rookie Team.

Her lacrosse star was rising rapidly, and then things changed. During summer 2007 before the start of her sophomore year, Taylor contracted a serious case of meningitis. She recovered, but just three weeks after being cleared for play, she went to the tryouts for the U.S. Women's Developmental National Team. She made the team, but not without paying a price. Her health started a rapid downward spiral.

"My immune system was struggling," she recalls. "At the national tryouts, we went through four days of four sessions per day. It completely wiped my body out." That fall she started getting weaker and sicker. Always a strong runner, she noticed "running was starting to become hard." She fatigued easily. "It was really frustrating," Taylor recalls.

So she started training more, and harder, and that only made things worse. At one point, she was blacking out ten or more times per day. "That's never a good thing on the lacrosse field," she jokes today. Taylor developed extreme headaches and began losing weight. She also developed neurological damage that at one point caused doctors to suspect multiple sclerosis.

Taylor's coach, UNC women's lacrosse head coach Jenny Levy, remembers the change in her talented player. "One of her strengths was her endurance," Levy says. "That fall, her performance had decreased significantly on the field. Talking to her about it, she felt awful."

Iron testing—routine for UNC's student athletes—revealed a major deficiency. Supplementation didn't help. The college's sports medicine team ultimately discovered the culprit: celiac disease, diagnosed through both a blood test and small intestine biopsy. "We understood then, she was malnourished," Levy says. "She wasn't absorbing anything because her celiac disease was such a problem. We shut her down through January, not knowing if she'd even be able to play that spring of 2008 during her sophomore year."

Taylor spent the winter back home in upstate New York. She met with nutritionists, including members of Dr. Peter Green's team at the Celiac Disease Center at Columbia University. Meanwhile, her older sister, Kelly, who also played for the UNC women's team, and her mother and brother were also diagnosed with celiac disease.

Now armed with the knowledge she needed to care for her body with her diet, and with the support of the UNC athletic program, Taylor returned to the field for her sophomore season, ranking second on the team for goals scored and third for assists and points. By her junior year, the team made the Final Four for just the second time in program history, and in her senior year in spring 2010—when she served as a tri-captain for the team—UNC reached the national championship game.

"After being on the gluten-free diet I felt so much better right away," Taylor says. "It's amazing that food you think you're eating to help you is actually hurting you."[51]

FAVORITE GLUTEN-FREE FOODS: lean meats, sweet potatoes, Rice Chex, protein bars, Udi's Gluten Free Bread

As with the volleyball player, the tennis player's symptoms seemingly came out of nowhere. "The immediacy of symptom onset was notable because the athlete had no history of similar complaints," researchers observed.[52]

If you know about gluten and stress as trigger, however, this isn't surprising at all.

In fact, as you read profiles of gluten-free athletes throughout this book, you'll start to notice a common pattern with startling similarities. Many of the people started out as healthy athletes with no obvious signs of gluten intolerance or other digestive or food issues. But then at some point, their athletic career partially or fully derailed. They commonly develop anemia, stress fractures, stomach trouble, or fatigue. In many cases, celiac disease has "turned on." And it has done so for two reasons: (a) the athlete was eating a lot of gluten because of his or her desire for carbs, and (b) the athlete experienced some form of "stress"— either an injury, an illness, or a drastic increase in training load, such as happens when an athlete makes the leap from high school to collegiate athletics, or from amateur to pro levels of competition. The good news is that these parallel stories all have happy endings: the resolution of symptoms and a return to their sport, often with improved performance that exceeds their previous "healthy" days, upon adoption of a gluten-free diet.

Keep this pattern in mind as you read about the athletes, and consider how it might apply to you—now or one day in the future. It is a cautionary tale of the dangers and potency of gluten plus athletics, and an equally promising tale of the powerful effectiveness of a gluten-free diet.

TO THE ATHLETE WITH GLUTEN INTOLERANCE

We've spent most of this chapter talking about the many ways in which gluten can affect *any* athlete, gluten intolerant or not. But if you're an athlete who *does* have gluten intolerance, you likely already know that gluten can affect your body and your performance in more profound ways. Some aspects of gluten exposure are different than they are for conventional athletes (such as the anaphylactic reaction of someone with a serious wheat allergy, or the villous atrophy that frequently occurs in the small intestine during the autoimmune response of celiac disease). Other aspects of gluten exposure are greatly magnified compared to what they'd be for a healthy athlete.

For you, going gluten-free isn't just an edge. It's critical. A recent study published by the American College of Sports Medicine found that athletes with gluten intolerance exposed to gluten experienced a serious decrease in athletic performance.[53] Well, duh. If you have a serious form of gluten intolerance, decreased athletic performance is the least of your health worries if you're chronically ingesting gluten. And if you *are* a gluten-free athlete who's been exposed to gluten, you don't need a formal study to tell you that that's a bad thing.

It's also important to keep in mind that you face some unique concerns related to nutrient absorption and malnutrition, iron absorption and anemia, calcium and vitamin D absorption and risk for osteoporosis, and other concerns. We address those in much greater detail in chapter 5.

Unlike "regular" athletes, you have to sometimes deal with the consequences of getting "glutened." When traveling, you have to think extra about where your food is coming from and what's in it. When your

ATHLETE INSIGHT

Christie Sym

PROFESSIONAL TRIATHLETE

Born: 1983 • Lives: Australia • Gluten-Free Since: 2007

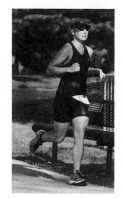

"**WHEN I LOOK** back throughout my life, I see signs," Christie Sym says of her celiac disease. Weak tooth enamel. Nail problems. By sixteen, she developed "really fussy eating habits." "Food made me sick my whole life," she adds. Sym developed intestinal pain and severe stomach cramps. Intense activity, such as track running, caused her "to curl up in a ball on the floor" afterward. She also suffered headaches and flu-like symptoms. "The worst thing was how it affected my training—for three days at a time, I'd feel like I've been sick, wouldn't digest foods properly," she says.

At age twenty-one, Sym found that "sticking away from wheat products and pasta made me feel much better." Then she started seeing great success as an athlete: Australian U18 cross country champion, Australian mountain bike Olympic squad member, three-time Australian national adventure racing champion. Finally, at age twenty-four, she went to an allergy clinic, where she was diagnosed with celiac disease. Sym made the leap to go gluten-free *and* switched to half Ironman triathlons.

Since then she has proven more and more dominant, with many wins and even more podiums. "From my personal perspective, sticking to the gluten-free diet is the key to getting the best out of your body, in your training and your sport," she says. "It's the key to success for me."[54]

FAVORITE GLUTEN-FREE FOODS: gluten-free oats with bananas, raisins, and maple syrup; thin rice cakes with tahini, avocado, and a bit of goat cheese; quinoa; roasted sweet potato with garlic and rosemary or thyme; flourless chocolate cake for a treat

football team is chowing down on a hearty pasta dinner the night before a big game, or your fellow triathletes are munching on toasted bagels as the morning of a race, you may have to fend for yourself and find suitable gluten-free alternatives to eat.

Once you learn how to maximize the gluten-free edge, however, your health—and your athletics—will be full speed ahead.

A CASE STUDY:
GLUTEN-FREE PROFESSIONAL FEMALE IRONMAN TRIATHLETES AND THE 2011 SEASON

As we interviewed athletes for this book, a curious trend started to emerge. We talked to one elite triathlete, and then another, and then another—all of them professional athletes, all women, all accomplished at the half and full Ironman and other endurance distances. They had impressive resumes, with many of their best race results coming in the period of time since they've been gluten-free.

There's Desirée Ficker, who went gluten-free in 2006 after a diagnosis of gluten intolerance—that same year she took second place at the Ironman World Championships in Hawaii. She then won three consecutive Austin Marathons (2008–2010) and has continued on a tour de force of the endurance sporting world.

There's Christie Sym, who went gluten-free in 2007 after a celiac disease diagnosis. She became a prolific Australian Adventure Racing Champion and in 2011 won several half Ironmans and placed ninth at the Ironman 70.3 World Championship.

There's Amanda Lovato, who voluntarily went strictly gluten-free in 2010, and who has since noticed a positive change in how she's feeling. A former World Duathlon Champion, she has proven herself a force to be reckoned with, winning many triathlons at a variety of distances, including one win and three podium finishes in total at three half Ironman races in 2011.

There's Heather Wurtele, who's been gluten-free since late 2009 to deal with long-standing gastrointestinal problems during competition. She burst onto the scene with several notable wins, including one at Ironman Coeur d'Alene, and has since racked up more victories, including back-to-back wins at Ironman St. George (2010–2011) and a victory at Ironman Lake Placid (2011).

There's Tyler Stewart, who went gluten-free in 2007 to feel and perform better. She started out winning Ironman World Championship amateur titles before rocking the professional triathlon world with wins such as Ironman Coeur d'Alene, where she set a new course record in 2009, and an impressive performance at Ironman Texas, where she set a new record for the fastest female Ironman bike split of all time.

And there's Terra Castro, who went gluten-free in 2000 because of some major inflammation problems. She started out as an elite junior on Team USA, and has grown into a consistent Top 5 finisher at the Ironman distance.

Talking with these impressive athletes, each anecdotally seemed to be performing even better since going gluten-free. But was that really the case? We decided to run a statistical analysis on their 2011 Ironman season, examining the competitive field of professional women and the race results for every race that had at least one gluten-free pro female finisher. Were these athletes really performing better than they did before their gluten-free days, and more important, was it giving them an edge on their competition? The results shocked even us.

Over the course of 2011, these six gluten-free triathletes competed in twenty-two half (IM 70.3) and full (IM) Ironman triathlons. Typically one or two of them were in any given race, though their numbers varied from event to event.

At this level of elite Ironman-distance triathlons, among professional female triathletes, the gluten-free set made up 12 percent of the competitors. Some races had a higher percentage, some a little less. This in and of itself was notable.

In the United States, gluten intolerance is believed to affect about 10 percent of the population nationwide (some recent estimates place the number higher, at 12 to 15 percent).[55] But, only 10 percent or so of those with gluten intolerance are correctly diagnosed[56] and therefore on a gluten-free diet.

That means that in theory 1 percent of the U.S. population (10 percent of that 10 percent) is actually gluten-free, and they're gluten-free for medical reasons. Even if we assume higher rates of diagnosis in recent years (thanks to growing awareness and education), even if more athletes are getting sick from gluten, and even if more athletes are simply aware of their body and thus more likely to respond to subtle problems and preemptively switch to a gluten-free diet to enhance their performance, 12 percent of pro female triathletes in any given race being gluten-free is unexpectedly high.

It more closely mirrors recent consumer research suggesting interest in gluten-free foods currently hovers somewhere around 15 percent of the U.S. population, in part because of the perceived health benefits of the gluten-free diet.[57] Many of those consumers are voluntarily gluten-free, though as researchers learn more about nonceliac forms of gluten intolerance, the line between the medically gluten-free and voluntarily gluten-free is growing increasingly blurry.

While an argument could be made that the pro female triathletes represent a similar blend of medically and voluntarily gluten-free, *all* reported symptoms (some reported definitive diagnoses) and *all* reported full resolution or improvement of their symptoms once they removed gluten from their diet. This suggests that their rate of gluten intolerance was at least as high—and possibly higher—than that of the general undiagnosed population. Yet they have all taken the step to go gluten-free, unlike the 90 percent of Americans who are still walking around "glutened."

But for these athletes, was their gluten-free food wager paying off? Or was it an empty promise?

We looked at their rate of Top 5 finishes, podium finishes (first, second, or third place in a race), and race wins. All other factors being equal (all pros, all women, comparable training, etc.), if the gluten-free diet didn't matter, if it didn't affect their performance one way or the other, we'd expect their rate of race results (wins, podiums, etc.) to mirror their representation in the race field: about 12 percent. If their performance fell under that mark, going gluten-free might be a detriment. If it was more than that, it might be evidence of the gluten-free edge we've been talking about.

In the raw data of twenty-two races, our sampling of gluten-free athletes scored seventeen Top 5 finishes in sixteen races. (At IM Lake Placid, the gluten-free women took both first *and* third!) They scored eleven podiums in ten races, and earned six first-place finishes. Put another way, if at least one gluten-free athlete competed in a race, then a gluten-free athlete won the race 27 percent of the time, stood on the podium 45 percent of the time, and finished in the Top Five 73 percent of the time. (Remember, on average the gluten-free athletes comprised just 12 percent of the women's pro race field.)

At first blush, these raw numbers seemed impressive. But they weren't all as straightforward as they seemed. The races had a varying number of pro female competitors, ranging from five to ten in some races, to twenty to twenty-five in other races. A Top 5 finish can have very different meaning in a field of five (a guarantee, short of a DNF) versus a field of twenty-five (a 20 percent shot, all other things being equal). Nevertheless, the percentages seemed high, so we decided to dig deeper.

We ran a statistical analysis. The math on the podium finishes gets quite complicated, but a look at the rate of race wins says everything we want to convey. Basically, in any given race, the chance of a gluten-free athlete's winning the race was in theory a function of the number of gluten-free racers versus the total number of racers (gluten-free plus non-gluten-free). That ratio varied from race to race. We wanted to know, based on that varying ratio, what were the honest chances that the gluten-free athletes would win at least six out of twenty-two races, as they actually did during 2011.

We did a Poisson binomial distribution, which is a way to measure the likelihood of multiple true or false events taking place when the probability of each individual event is different. We treated the races as binary true or false values (the gluten-free women either won the race or they didn't) with varying probabilities of victory (based on the number of gluten-free competitors vs. the total number of entrants in the women's pro category). When we ran the numbers, our jaws hit the floor. Statistically, you would have expected those gluten-free athletes to win six or more races a scant 5 percent of the time. Some 95 percent of the time they *should* have won five or fewer races. Those are 19–1 odds . . . a great payoff if you're into sports betting, but not exactly what you'd call a sure thing, or even a likely thing.

In fact, it was highly *unlikely* that those women would have won as many races as they did. Yet that's exactly what happened. And the only substantive difference between the gluten-free women and their peers was the gluten-free diet. Was it the result of mere chance, or did the gluten-free diet play a starring role in their victories?

Before you say anything, we know: Correlation does not equal causation. You're absolutely right. The fact that the gluten-free women did so well may or may not have been caused by their gluten-free diet, even though the two results were correlated. It could have been a random, if highly unlikely, coincidence. Or the correlation between the two results could have been caused by a third, but unmeasured, variable. We freely admit as much (though we don't think that's the case, and we'll explain why in a moment).

This was only a quasi-scientific study. There were a number of factors we couldn't control for, and more than a few unknown or uncontrolled variables.

For instance, did we accurately measure the number of gluten-free athletes? Were there others in the competitive field we didn't know about, thus skewing the numbers? Possibly. We're convinced there are many more gluten-free triathletes out there than most people realize.[58] *If* there were more gluten-free athletes in the mix, how they performed in those twenty-two races may or may not have skewed the stats, positively or negatively.

Also, were these women elite athletes who would have done well anyway, whether they were gluten-free or not? Maybe. But consider this: We know for a fact that some of these women have "legitimate" forms of gluten intolerance (e.g., celiac disease or gluten sensitivity). They are beating the competition, a lot, *despite* their gluten intolerance. In their cases, the gluten-free diet is not just getting them back to health and competition form; it's getting them into peak condition to smash the competition.

ATHLETE INSIGHT

Heather Wurtele

PROFESSIONAL TRIATHLETE

Born: 1979 • Lives: British Columbia • Gluten-Free Since: 2009

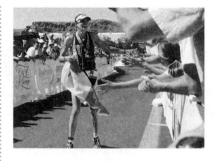

A CONSUMMATE ATHLETE, Heather Wurtele grew up downhill skiing and playing volleyball and basketball. Then she became a varsity rower at University of British Columbia. Wurtele "caught the triathlon bug," she says, following several years of adventure racing with her husband, fellow triathlete Trevor. As her body adjusted to increased training loads with the switch from amateur to pro status in 2007, she gave more thought to training, recovery, *and* nutrition. "I had training and recovery covered. But what about what I was eating? It has a huge impact on performance," she says. "When I cut gluten out of my diet it was amazing. I felt a lot better pretty much right away." Bloating and the need to "look for a Porta-Potty on every run over half an hour, things you assume are normal," went away. And her performance and race finishes have only gotten better since she went gluten-free, including a Top 10 at the Ironman World Championships and numerous impressive wins at other Ironman races, such as her defense of her Ironman St. George title in 2011, where she beat the next-fastest female pro by a whopping thirty-six minutes.

FAVORITE GLUTEN-FREE FOODS: Bob's Red Mill gluten-free pancakes, Udi's Gluten Free Bread, quinoa, brown rice, hemp seeds

We also know that the others who voluntarily went gluten-free did so because they are well attuned to their body, more responsive to subtle and not so subtle signs and symptoms indicating they might not be performing to their full potential. They have gone gluten-free to tap that potential, and have found that they feel better, that their symptoms (bloating, digestive trouble, pain, inflammation) have resolved, and that they are performing better. We can't help but think about something we've said several times in this chapter—that the stress and exertion faced by elite endurance athletes pushes the body to extremes, making them more susceptible to problems with gluten. In this case, not only are these athletes *avoiding* those problems by also avoiding gluten; they seem to be *increasing* their performance with the gluten-free diet.

Are these women disproportionately toppling the competition *because* of their gluten-free diet?

We think so. The trend evidenced in these numbers doesn't lie. It offers compelling evidence of superior performance, in both gluten-intolerant athletes and voluntarily gluten-free athletes. By most other measures, they're on a level playing field with the competition, yet the race results sharply diverge.

We shouldn't expect gluten-free athletes to stand atop the podium as often as they do, but that's exactly what we're seeing. Remember, we should have expected them to win so often with about 5 percent probability.

The seemingly trivial absence of gluten from their diet is resulting in disproportionately more wins. Results like those can't be denied. The proof is in the podium. They are performing better than their peers, distinguished only by their choice of a gluten-free diet. The only difference between them and the competition was gluten . . . or, as the case may be, the lack of it. That, and the medals hanging on their fireplace mantle at home.

In our opinion, this amounts to compelling proof positive that the gluten-free edge exists. It is real.

NEED TO KNOW

- For healthy and gluten-intolerant athletes alike, gluten can cause a range of problems that inhibit performance: impaired digestion, leaky gut, cell toxicity, gastrointestinal problems, inflammation, and neurological effects.
- A chronically challenged and/or suppressed immune system due to frequent, intense athletics or exercise can leave otherwise healthy athletes more susceptible to previously subtle or nonexistent problems with gluten.
- The combination of high dietary intake of gluten plus an increase in athletic exertion (such as that seen transitioning from high school to college sports, or from amateur to pro status) can be a trigger that "turns on" a latent, silently waiting gluten intolerance.
- A proper gluten-free diet greatly reduces and frequently fully resolves such problems.
- In addition, athletes on a gluten-free diet not only regain their health and ability to compete, they are succeeding and winning at the highest levels of elite sports.
- There's growing evidence that gluten-free athletes are even gaining an edge on their competition attributed to the benefits of the diet.

3

Get Your Motor Running:
How the Body Stores
and Uses Energy

THE REST OF this book deals mostly with gluten-free nutrition. After all, food is the fuel that supplies your athletic engine. But before we talk about what to put in that engine, we ought to talk briefly about how the engine works. Like a car that shifts gears, your body has several energy pathways that are called into action at different times, depending on both the duration and intensity of your exertion.[1] Following are the spare nuts and bolts of what you need to know, with some particulars omitted for clarity.

FOOD SOURCES

Pretty much all the food you eat can be classified as containing carbohydrates, protein, and/or fat.

Except under exceptional circumstances, protein—converted into amino acids—doesn't provide significant sources of energy. Your body gets its fuel chiefly from carbohydrates and fat.

Glucose, a simple sugar that accounts for some 99 percent of sugars circulating in the blood, is a major player in the game. Glucose can be stored as glycogen in the muscles and liver, or it can circulate in the blood. Blood glucose comes either from the digestion and absorption of dietary carbohydrates or from the breakdown of glycogen in the liver, which releases glucose into the bloodstream.

Dietary and body fat (adipose tissue), meanwhile, are composed partly of triglycerides, another potential source of energy. Even in lean, elite athletes with a low body fat percentage, both dietary and body fat can be important sources of energy. In addition, excess glycogen beyond that which can be stored in the muscles and liver is converted into fat for additional storage.

ENERGY PATHWAYS

No matter what your diet consists of, or its ratio of carbs to fat to protein, the same energy pathways apply, though which pathway your body recruits when may vary (more on that in chapters 6 and 10).

At the most basic level, all energy that your body uses for athletics comes from adenosine triphosphate (ATP). You probably learned about it in high school biology. When ATP is liberated of one of its phosphate groups, it releases energy and becomes adenosine diphosphate (ADP). Your body uses the energy for activity, and the ADP gets "recycled" by adding back a phosphate group and creating ATP again. It's like a continuously rechargeable battery where the energy "currency" is calories.

ATP AND PCR

Your muscle cells (and all living cells in your body, basically) have a small amount of ATP on hand, ready to go at a moment's notice. The only problem is, those ATP stores are depleted almost immediately.

Then a second source kicks in: phosphocreatine (PCr). Also known as *creatine phosphate*, PCr readily donates a phosphate group to turn ADP into usable ATP. For a short period of time, PCr helps your muscle cells maintain an almost steady supply of ATP. The key word there, though, is *short*. It's a limited mechanism.

Together, initial ATP and PCr can fuel between three and fifteen seconds of intense exercise, such as an all-out sprint or a competitive dead lift. Both of these initial energy pathways happen anaerobically, without the assistance of oxygen. If you're planning to go for more than a few seconds—and except for world-class 50-meter sprinters, who isn't?—then you're going to need to find another gear.

ANAEROBIC GLYCOLYSIS

Anaerobic glycolysis is that next gear. Physical exertion lasting beyond the initial seconds, especially if it's fairly intense exertion, looks to anaerobic glycolysis for its energy. Glycolysis is a metabolic pathway with at least ten discrete steps. It involves the conversion of glucose or glycogen (or both) into ATP and lactic acid. And it does so quickly; it's fast.

Anaerobic glycolysis can provide about one to two minutes of energy at an all-out effort, or at best a few minutes of energy if you're not quite at your max. Track runners in the 400-meter sprint are relying almost exclusively on this system, crossing the finish line with almost nothing left in the tank, having exhausted their anaerobic glycolytic pathway. (This time limitation is also why 10K runners who start their finishing kick too early will run out of gas before they reach the finish line. They'll have turned on their anaerobic glycolysis pathway too soon.)

Aside from the time limitation of anaerobic glycolysis, there's one other major problem with this pathway: the buildup of lactic acid. During anaerobic glycolysis, your body isn't able to get rid of lactic acid in your muscles faster than it accumulates. Too much lactic acid in your muscles increases their acidity, inhibiting further glycogen breakdown and impeding muscle contraction.

Have you ever "felt the burn" during a workout? Have your muscles ever been "pumped"? That's lactic acid at work.

THE OXIDATIVE SYSTEM

Any physical effort lasting more than a few minutes is going to need a more lasting source of energy, one that takes place with the assistance of oxygen: the aerobic oxidative system, which comprises two major components—the oxidation of carbohydrates and the oxidation of fat.

Compared to anaerobic glycolysis, the other source of carb-based energy, carbohydrate oxidation is slower to turn on, but once it does, it's a great source of energy for sustaining long-term output. Like its anaerobic counterpart, it utilizes glycolysis. But unlike its counterpart, it *doesn't* involve lactic acid buildup (intermediate pyruvic acids get

ATHLETE INSIGHT

Christian Vande Velde
PROFESSIONAL CYCLIST

Born: 1976 • Lives: Colorado • Gluten-Free Since: 2008

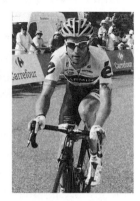

THE YEAR 2008 was a good one for pro cyclist Christian Vande Velde of today's Team Garmin-Cervélo: an impressive showing at the Giro d'Italia, third overall in the Tour de France, third overall in the Tour of California, an overall win at the Tour of Missouri, and champion of the USA Cycling Professional Tour. Certainly, he'd had success before. But by any measure, 2008 was a breakout year. What had changed?

For one thing, his diet. In 2008 Slipstream Sports, the parent organization behind Team Garmin, made a now well-known decision: to have its riders go gluten-free. The premise was simple but revolutionary in the pro cycling world at the time . . . that gluten has an inflammatory effect on the body, hindering digestion, delaying recovery, causing gastrointestinal symptoms, and impairing riders' performance. And Slipstream didn't apply this logic only to its gluten-intolerant riders. In a message posted on the team website, it noted that potentially anyone, Garmin's healthy riders included, could have a "sub-symptomatic inflammatory response" to gluten.

Remove the gluten, Slipstream reasoned, and you could improve performance. Vande Velde was "willing to give it a try," he told *VeloNews*. His chiropractor had suggested the dietary change, too.

Vande Velde's 2008 season seemed to confirm the theory right out of the gate. After the switch, he reported having more energy and feeling fresher mentally and physically. Vande Velde soon became a poster child for the gluten-free diet that was earning a reputation as an anti-inflammatory diet in athlete circles.

Fellow Slipstream rider Tom Danielson responded very well to the diet, too.

Then, in 2010, Slipstream's gluten-free edge became headline news when *Men's Journal* featured the team in its article "Winning Without Wheat." Overnight, going gluten-free had, in a sense, gone mainstream.

Vande Velde has continued his winning ways. At the inaugural and much anticipated USA Pro Cycling Challenge in 2011, which attracted the major Grand Tour teams and some of the best riders from around the world, Vande Velde finished second overall, still sticking with his gluten-free diet, which included pasta and pizza from the Gluten Free Bistro. In fact, three of the top four riders were gluten-free: winner Levi Leipheimer then from Team RadioShack, Vande Velde from Team Garmin-Cervélo, and teammate Tom Danielson in fourth.

The only *non*-gluten-free rider in the top four was Tejay van Garderen from Team HTC-Highroad. Amusingly, in his profile on the website of sponsor Smith Optics, he rants that "I hate all the cyclists who pretend they are allergic to gluten in order to lose weight." As the minority in the Top 4 at the Pro Cycling Challenge, surrounded by three gluten-free riders, you have to wonder if he's thinking of changing his mind.[2]

FAVORITE GLUTEN-FREE FOODS: rice, sweet potatoes, chicken, salad, almond butter, nuts, beans, quinoa, pure maple syrup, raw honey, olive oil

converted before that happens), and *does* involve additional pathways such as the Krebs cycle and the electron transport chain. The result is *much* more energy from the same starting quantity of glycogen, though it doesn't metabolize as rapidly as in anaerobic glycolysis.

Then there's fat oxidation. Triglycerides from fat get converted to glycerol and fatty acids, which provide the body with another excellent source of energy. Per gram, carbohydrates provide 4 calories of energy, while fat provides 9 calories of energy, more than double.* There's no free lunch, however. Fat oxidation requires more oxygen to take place, so it occurs even more slowly than carbohydrate oxidation.

Without replenishment, glycogen stored in muscles and the liver can provide about 1,500 to 2,500 calories of energy via the oxidative system. Fat, even in fit athletes, can provide some 70,000 to 80,000-plus calories of energy.

SHIFTING GEARS

Unlike the gears in your car, these energy pathways don't necessarily shift sequentially, nor do they operate exclusively, one at a time. In practice, multiple energy pathways are contributing to your athletic output at any given time. Depending on the nature of that output, though, one system will tend to predominate.

It comes down to how much energy you need, how quickly, for how long. The ATP-PCr and anaerobic glycolysis (AG) systems offer fast, immediate energy, but they do so at a sacrifice—they don't replenish quickly and they have short time limits on how long they can last. The oxidative system (OS), on the other hand, offers a complementary set of attributes—"slower" sources of energy, but ones that can last for a long time and be replenished throughout exercise.

Thus, duration and intensity are two crucial factors in understanding which systems will come to the fore for you and your sport. Are you going at maximum effort (or near it) for a few seconds or a few minutes? ATP-PCr and AG will dominate. Are you an ultramarathon runner going at 60 percent exertion for ten hours straight? OS will dominate.

Your VO_2 max—the capacity of your blood to carry oxygen to muscles (which is influenced by iron, gluten intolerance, and the gluten-free

---

*A scientific calorie is defined as the amount of heat required to raise the temperature of 1 gram of water by 1 degree Celsius. However, in the context of food and athletics, it is more useful to use the common nutritional calorie, which is 1,000 scientific calories (or 1 kilocalorie, sometimes denoted by the capitalized Calorie). These nutritional calories are the ones you see listed on product packaging at the grocery store. Throughout this book, we use "calorie" to refer to the common nutritional calorie.

diet)—and your lactate threshold—the point at which lactic acid begins to build up in muscles faster than it's broken down, roughly corresponding to the switch from aerobic to anaerobic metabolism—can also influence which energy pathways predominate. (We cover these topics in greater detail in chapters 5 and 10.)

Even within the OS, the relative contributions of carbohydrate and fat oxidation can vary in relation to your level of exertion. For example, one study showed that during training at 75 percent of VO_2 max, 25 percent of an athlete's total energy may come from fat oxidation. But as training intensity decreased to 50 percent of VO_2 max, the contribution of fat oxidation increased to more than 50 percent of the total energy.[3]

Other factors come into play, too, such as diet. In chapters 6, 8, and 10, we talk about how low- and high-glycemic-index carbs and dietary fat can influence your ratio of carbohydrate versus fat oxidation.

Finally, your training (chapter 10) can impact your body's recruitment of energy pathways, by teaching it to burn fat more readily and efficiently,[4] by raising your VO_2 max and lactate threshold, and more.

BONKED: HITTING THE WALL

If you've been around sports at all, then you've almost certainly heard about bonking, about hitting the proverbial wall. It refers to the sudden onset of extreme muscle fatigue. Now that you've read about the body's primary energy pathways, it's easier to understand how and why this happens and, more important, how to avoid it.

Your body only has so much energy at its disposal, either readily available or in storage as glycogen or fat. When those energy supplies are depleted, you're kaput. And depending on which energy pathway is predominating, you may hit that wall sooner than later.

In all instances, muscle glycogen tends to be the limiting factor. When the glycogen runs out, so does your energy and capacity for athletic exertion. Meet the wall.

In short-duration, high-intensity sports, such as sprinting, the ATP-PCr system is primary, with support from anaerobic glycolysis. Because those systems can only last for a short time, you simply can't sustain such maximum effort for long. You *have* to back off the throttle,

ATHLETE INSIGHT

Natalie Jill

FITNESS MODEL AND COACH

Born: 1971 • Lives: California • Gluten-Free Since: 2000

IF YOU WATCH former *The Biggest Loser* trainer Jillian Michaels's *Ripped in 30* video series, Michaels isn't the only ripped body on the screen. She's joined by other fitness professionals who look just as lean and mean. One of those people is fitness model and coach Natalie Jill. She's appeared on magazine covers, in sports and fitness ads, in other fitness video series, and as a model demonstrating exercises in magazine spreads.

Jill has long had an interest in fitness and nutrition, and in helping others eat better and look better, but her own health had a bit of a rocky start. "For as long as I can remember from when I was a kid, I had stomachaches all the time," she says. "I thought that was a normal thing when you ate food." Jill would often become bloated. She'd eat noodles and bread, thinking they would help, but they only made the problem worse.

In her teen years, she started reading fitness magazines and took control of her diet, cutting out processed foods and eating more protein and fruits and vegetables. Curiously, some of her stomach symptoms began to subside. By her early twenties, she was entering fitness competitions. The competitions proved to be a phase—she preferred working *with* people for fitness, rather than competing against them. Having left the fitness competition world, she relaxed her dietary habits, and her stomach started hurting again. At first she thought it was just a difference between her "clean" and less clean eating habits.

After three years of searching, however, she had an answer:

celiac disease. In retrospect, it all made sense: the stomachaches, and how they responded or didn't respond to different foods in her diet. Plus, she realized that autoimmune conditions ran in her family—her sister has type 1 diabetes; another relative has rheumatoid arthritis. Jill was the first celiac diagnosis in the family.

Gluten-free for more than a decade now, she's arguably never looked—or felt—better. And she's helping others achieve similar results, helping clients lose fat and get fit . . . without gluten.[5]

FAVORITE GLUTEN-FREE FOODS: "lots of protein"; nuts and nut butters; fruits and veggies; healthy starches (yams, sweet potatoes, brown rice, quinoa, gluten-free oatmeal); Pamela's Pancakes (sometimes)

sometimes significantly. Your body won't let you do otherwise. This type of bonking is not serious. Although your body forces you to dial back the intensity to reasonable levels, allowing other energy pathways to kick in, you still have plenty of glycogen left to use.

The more serious and classic case of bonking comes in endurance sports where the oxidative system is dominant. As we noted earlier in this chapter, carbohydrate-based glycogen stored in muscles and the liver can only provide up to about 2,500 calories of energy. Even if you successfully shift your body into fat-burning mode (fat oxidation), it will still burn glycogen, too, though at a slower rate. In this way, fat burning takes some of the burden off your glycogen stores, enabling them to last longer before depletion. But it's only a stay of execution. Glycogen is still being burned, and once it's gone, you're going to hit the wall. Hard. Without carbohydrate consumption during the activity—and the glycogen replenishment that goes along with it—the clock is ticking. Eventually, time will run out.

If you've ever watched the Ford Ironman World Championship in Kona, Hawaii, on TV and watched a triathlete collapse across the finish line into the arms of waiting medical staff, you've seen what true glycogen depletion looks like. It isn't pretty.

NEED TO KNOW

- While protein is important for muscles, your energy comes chiefly from carbohydrates and fat.
- Carbohydrates are converted into glucose, which circulates as blood sugar, providing immediate needed energy to muscles and other cells. Excess glucose is stored as glycogen in muscles and the liver.
- Fats, consisting of a glycerol plus fatty acids, can be a rich source of energy, providing 9 calories of energy per gram, compared to 4 calories per gram of carbohydrate.
- The body has four major energy pathways: adenosine triphosphate, phosphocreatine, anaerobic glycolysis, and the oxidative system. The first three take place without the assistance of oxygen.
- The first two pathways provide immediate energy in the initial seconds of activity, but it is rapidly depleted.
- Anaerobic glycolysis kicks in next, providing minutes' worth of energy. Although it is also a rapid system, it is characterized by a buildup of lactic acid, which places limitations on the system.
- The oxidative system comprises two parts—aerobic glycolysis of carbohydrates and fat oxidation. Both take place with the assistance of oxygen. They are slower to turn on, but an excellent source of long-term energy.
- Energy pathways often work in combination, rather than exclusively, although one tends to predominate. The duration and intensity of activity help to determine the balance.
- Bonking, or hitting the wall, involves the sudden onset of extreme muscle fatigue due to high levels of glucose and glycogen depletion.

4

Fueling the Engine:
The Food Foundation

I F YOUR BODY is an athletic engine, then food is the fuel that keeps the motor running. It's the foundation of your performance, whether in sports or an all-around active lifestyle.

For conventional athletes, it might help to think of your body as a flexible-fuel vehicle. You can put in different fuels—meat, fruits, vegetables, gluten grains, gluten-free grains, and so on. No matter what the fuel, your engine will still run. But your performance and your "miles per gallon" will vary.

For athletes with gluten intolerance, the engine isn't nearly so forgiving. Only certain fuels will work. Using a nonconforming fuel—such as one that includes gluten—may not only drastically reduce engine performance; in a worst-case scenario, you may experience total engine failure.

The gluten-free edge is about finding the best-fit fuel match for your genetic predisposition (including potential problems with gluten) and the food you eat. Your genes won't change, but your inherent genetic risk can be turned on and off with the flick of a fork. For example, if you have the genetics for celiac disease but never eat a lick of gluten, your disease won't turn on—end of story. Ditto for the healthy athlete pushing his or her body to the extreme: If you don't stress your system with gluten in the first place, a latent susceptibility to that pesky protein can't bubble to the surface when you're competing at your max and pushing your body to its absolute limit.

ATHLETE INSIGHT

Jenn Suhr

U.S. OLYMPIC MEDALIST AND 10-TIME NATIONAL CHAMPION POLE VAULTER

Born: 1982 • Lives: New York • Gluten-Free Since: 2011

AT THE START of 2012, Jenn Suhr, the queen of American pole vaulting, was riding high as the No. 1 ranked pole vaulter in the world. Six months earlier, though, a very different scenario was playing out.

Suhr had enjoyed phenomenal success as an indoor and outdoor pole vaulter. She is the American record holder in both disciplines. She's a ten-time national champion—the most of any active American track and field athlete—including five consecutive outdoor titles from 2006 to 2010. And she is an Olympic silver medalist from the Beijing Games. In other words, life has been good for Suhr.

By early 2011, she had captured her latest national indoor title (her fifth, for ten total) and was hoping to defend her outdoor title and secure a spot in the World Championships.

But then her health declined. Various news reports noted that she was fatigued, weak, not recovering, dehydrated, experiencing stomach problems, and suffering variously from muscle cramps and muscle twitches. Such symptoms had been surfacing on and off for a few years. She competed when she could, and sat out of events when she couldn't, including early 2011, when she missed four competitions.

During summer 2011, it was different. There was a more fundamental change in her health. Suhr failed to defend her outdoor title and barely qualified for Worlds.

She was diagnosed with celiac disease, one of the latest elite athletes to join the club. Thankfully, on the gluten-free diet, her health and her season pulled a 180 and went on a meteoric rise.

The media and the track and field community were quick to note that Suhr was displaying her best form since 2008. Then she posted the second-best jump of her life—4.91 meters—which ended up being the best height of any female vaulter in the world for all of 2011. By the end of the year, she was in top form, ranked by *Track & Field News* as the top female vaulter on the planet. December 2011 had been her best month of training in three years, she told the *Rochester Democrat & Chronicle*. Looking ahead to the London 2012 Games, her sights are firmly set on one thing: a gold medal.

Finally healthy and gluten-free, she may well find it within reach.[1]

We described in the last chapter how your body recruits energy to keep your engine going. A logical follow-up question for every athlete is, What food should I eat to maximize how I feel and perform?

Running the engine is one thing. Getting the most out of your engine is another. Welcome to bioenergetics, the transformation of food into energy. Answering the question of what to eat starts with understanding the three macronutrients—carbohydrates, protein, and fat—and the relationships between them.

MACRONUTRIENTS

CARBOHYDRATES

Carbohydrates are energy-yielding macronutrients that are classified according to size, from simple sugars (monosaccharides) to slightly less simple sugars (disaccharides) to complex molecules (polysaccharides, such as starches and fiber). You can just call them an athlete's best friend. When you eat carbohydrate-rich foods, which come almost exclusively from plants, your body magically converts those foods into blood glucose for quick energy and into glycogen for stored energy.

If you're active, and especially if you're an athlete, forget anything you've heard about the merits of a low-carb diet. Carbohydrates are *fuel*, and should be the foundation of a well-rounded sports nutrition program. Whereas too many carbs can be a bad thing for people who live a sedentary lifestyle—getting stored as body fat, causing blood sugar spikes, and prompting insulin resistance—in active people, carbohydrates are a cornerstone of peak performance.

SIMPLE CARBOHYDRATES

Simple carbs include both mono- and disaccharides.

Monosaccharides (meaning "one sugar") are the basic carbohydrate unit. They are the building blocks of the carb world, and they come in various "flavors," such as glucose (blood sugar), fructose (fruit sugar, the sugar naturally found in fruits, honey, saps, some vegetables, agave nectar, and corn syrup), and galactose. Glucose is the primary energy source for all the body's activities—every cell in the body needs glucose to function.

Disaccharides ("two sugars") are formed when two monosaccharides come together. Sucrose (also known as *table sugar*) is a disaccharide. Lactose (also known as *milk sugar*) is another.

In terms of athletic performance, glucose is the belle of the ball. Your brain needs it to think clearly, react quickly, and make good decisions. Your muscles need it to keep working. And when you run out of it, things go south pretty fast.

COMPLEX CARBOHYDRATES

Complex carbs are polysaccharides ("many sugars"), and they're just what they sound like—multiple simple carbs (simple sugars) strung together to make complex ones. Three are especially important in gluten-free sports nutrition: glycogen, starches, and fiber.

Two of the three—glycogen and starches—are for energy storage. Humans store carb energy as glycogen; plants store it as starch. When you eat gluten-free grains such as rice, corn, quinoa, or sorghum; gluten-free root vegetables such as parsnips, potatoes, sweet potatoes, taro root, beets, or cassava (aka manioc, yuca, or tapioca); or gluten-free legumes such as beans and lentils, you're consuming starches that get broken down into glucose, which is used immediately for energy now or stored as glycogen for energy later.

That's why athletes love their starches. Which is, ironically, where gluten comes into play. Although gluten is a protein, it's found in starchy grains such as wheat, barley, and rye. And because gluten-based foods such as bread and pasta are full of those starches, many athletes' diets are surprisingly heavy in gluten, too. If you focus solely on gluten-containing foods, it's easy to forget about all the other great sources of complex carbs that are naturally gluten-free.

The other principal complex carbohydrate you get from plants is the structural substance called *fiber*. It's like scaffolding for the plant, and is what allows asparagus to stand at attention and gives you the stringy stuff in celery and the coating on a kernel of corn. Found in all plant-derived foods, fiber can't be broken down by human digestive enzymes, so it ends up sweeping its way through the gastrointestinal tract and performing internal housekeeping duties.

There are different types of fiber: Some slow the digestive process, help balance blood sugar, and keep energy levels stable; some speed up the digestive process and help get rid of toxins. Both types comprise polysaccharides that can't be broken down during digestion. And just as athletes end up eating gluten because they're interested in wheat starch, so do they eat gluten because they desire fiber, found in wheat bran.

Of course, if you're gluten intolerant and/or looking for the gluten-free edge, wheat bran is strictly off-limits. Fortunately, again as with the starches, there are plenty of hearty gluten-free options in the fiber department, such as raspberries, apples, beets, and gluten-free oats.

EMPTY CARBS

Alas, not all carbohydrates are an athlete's best friend. Aside from the obvious problem of gluten-containing carb sources such as wheat, there's also the issue of empty carbs. All carbohydrates provide caloric energy, but empty carbs give you little else. Normally, carbohydrates offer additional benefits, such as vitamins, minerals, and other nutrients. But foods filled with empty carbs are made from refined, highly processed ingredients that have been stripped of additional nutritional value.

NUTRIENT PROFILES OF GLUTEN-FREE GRAINS AND WHEAT

GRAIN 1 CUP RAW	FIBER (G)	CARB (G)	PROTEIN (G)	CALCIUM (MG)	IRON (MG)	MAGNESIUM (MG)	ZINC (MG)	SELENIUM (MCG)	THIAMIN (MG)	RIBOFLAVIN (MG)	NIACIN (MG)	FOLATE (MCG)
Amaranth	18	129	28	298	15	519	6.2	36.1	0.16	0.41	2.5	96
Buckwheat	17	122	23	31	3.7	393	4.08	14.1	0.17	0.72	11.9	51
Corn	9	94	10	7	4.2	155	2.2	18.9	0.47	0.24	4.4	30
Millet	17	146	22	16	6	228	3.36	5.4	0.84	0.58	9.4	170
Oats (GF)	17	103	26	84	7.4	276	6.19	n/a	1.19	0.21	1.5	87
Quinoa	12	109	24	80	7.7	335	5.27	14.4	0.61	0.54	2.6	313
Rice (Brown)	7	143	15	43	2.7	265	3.74	43.3	0.74	0.17	9.4	37
Rice (White)	2	148	13	52	1.5	46	2.02	27.9	0.13	0.09	2.9	15
Rice (Wild)	10	120	24	34	3.1	283	9.54	4.5	0.18	0.41	10.8	152
Sorghum	12	143	22	54	8.4	365	3	n/a	0.45	0.27	5.6	38
Teff	15	141	26	347	14.7	355	7	8.5	0.75	0.52	6.5	135
Wheat	n/a	137	26	65	7	276	8	172	0.8	0.23	13	83

All information, unless otherwise noted, was obtained from the USDA Agricultural Research Service Nutrient Data Laboratory. Data for the nutrient composition of magnesium, zinc, and folate in sorghum grain, and folate levels in teff, were obtained from *Gluten-Free Diet: A Comprehensive Resource Guide*, by Shelley Case, RD. The selenium value for amaranth is from *SELF* magazine's Nutrition Data database.

n/a – not available

Classic examples are such ingredients as white sugar and cornstarch. To some degree, they have a limited place in an athletic diet because they provide easily digestible carbs that can be quickly converted into energy. But they also typically have a higher glycemic index, causing bigger swings in blood glucose and insulin levels, and they lack many of the micronutrients that play important supporting roles in your athletic performance.

FIBER-RICH GLUTEN-FREE FOODS

Rasberries	Brown rice
Apples	Celery
Citrus fruits	Asparagus
Beets	Artichokes
Cauliflower	Avocado
Gluten-free oats	Buckwheat
Broccoli	Greens
Brussels sprouts	Nuts
Legumes (such as beans and peas)	Quinoa

PROTEIN

The word *protein* comes from the Greek, meaning "of prime importance." When it comes to physical strength and structure, protein certainly lives up to its name. Some 60 to 75 percent of all protein in an average adult is found in skeletal muscle.[2] It's responsible for keeping you strong and upright. Structurally more complicated than carbohydrates or fats, protein plays a variety of roles in the body.

The human body has about fifty thousand different protein-containing compounds.[3] The function of each protein depends on the length and sequence of its individual amino acid combinations. There are twenty different known amino acids—some the body can make (called *nonessential*), and some that must be provided by the food you eat (called *essential*). When the body's need for a nonessential amino acid becomes greater than its ability to produce it, the amino acid becomes *conditionally* essential. (This occurs during periods of growth in young people, for example.)

Both animal- and plant-based proteins contain essential amino acids. Strictly speaking, there's no biological advantage to eating one over the other. Animal proteins, because they contain all nine essential amino acids, are known as *complete proteins*. With the exception of a few plant sources, most plant-based proteins are deficient in at least one essential amino acid. For example, many grains don't contain sufficient levels of the essential amino acid lysine. (Two exceptions are naturally gluten-free quinoa and soy, both of which *do* contain complete proteins, which is why you will commonly find soy protein isolate in commercial protein bars, and why quinoa has been called the "supergrain of the Andes." Buckwheat and amaranth are also gluten-free plant sources with near-complete proteins, and they're rich in the amino acid lysine, often missing from other plant sources, including wheat.) However, by combining different plant sources in a well-rounded diet of nourishing whole foods, even gluten-free vegetarian and vegan athletes can get all the protein—and essential amino acids—they need.

PLANT-BASED SOURCES OF PROTEIN
(1 CUP RAW)

FOOD	PROTEIN (G)
Hemp seeds	53
Lentils	50
Kidney beans	43
Black beans	42
Pinto beans	41
Pumpkin seeds	39
Chickpeas (garbanzo beans)	39
Lima beans	38
Tempeh	31
Flaxseeds	31
Almonds	33
Chia seeds	30
Amaranth	26
Teff	26
Sesame seeds	26
Oats	25
Quinoa	24
Wild rice	24

Millet	22
Sorghum	22
Tofu	20
Buckwheat groats	19
Brown rice (long-grain)	15
White rice (long-grain)	13
Corn (yellow kernels)	5

ANIMAL-BASED SOURCES OF PROTEIN

FOOD	PROTEIN (G)
Tuna, 4 oz	28
Ostrich, 4 oz	25
Venison, ground 4 oz	25
Salmon, wild 4 oz	25
Greek yogurt, 8 oz	23
Pork, ham 4 oz	22
Bison, ground 4 oz	21
Beef, ground 4 oz	21
Pork, ground 4 oz	20
Chicken, ground 4 oz	20
Turkey, ground 4 oz	19
Lamb, ground 4 oz	19
Shrimp, 4 oz	15
Cheddar cheese, 2 oz	14
Eggs, 2 large	13
Goat cheese, 2 oz	12
Yogurt, low-fat plain, 8 oz	12
Yogurt, whole milk plain, 8 oz	8
Whole milk, 8 oz	8

FAT

Let's get this out of the way immediately: Fat is *not* a four-letter word. In fact, contrary to what many American athletes learned growing up—the mantra that "fat equals bad"—your body needs it. The brain uses fat for proper neuron firing, and your body uses fat as an excellent energy source during athletic exertion, especially in aerobic endurance sports.

A study that looked at varying levels of dietary fat intake in runners found that both men and women on a low-fat diet suffered from compromised athletic performance, compromised health, insufficient calorie consumption, and inadequate intake of calcium, zinc, and essential fatty acids. Athletes on moderate- and high-fat diets (30 to 45 percent of their daily calories), fared better across all measures.[4] In other words, the fat was good for them.

As with the issue of simple versus complex versus empty carbohydrates, for the athlete, the issue of fat comes down to what type of fats you're eating.

All fats consist of triglycerides, which are a glycerol plus three fatty acids. Fatty acids, in turn, contain chains of carbon and hydrogen. When the chain of carbon is fully packed with all the hydrogen bonds it can possibly hold, you have a saturated fat (such as that found in cream, cheese, butter, coconut oil, and cottonseed oil). Saturated fats are typically solid at room temperature.

When the carbon chain contains fewer than the maximum number of hydrogen bonds, the carbon atoms form one or more double bonds, forming either mono- or polyunsaturated fats, respectively (such as those found in olive oil, avocados, and nuts). Unsaturated fats are typically liquid at room temperature and are the healthiest of the group.

Meats may contain either saturated or unsaturated fat or both.

Sometimes, artificial processes are used to make unsaturated fats behave more like saturated fats. During hydrogenation, hydrogen atoms are added to unsaturated fats to make them more solid and shelf-stable at room temperature. This process is used to create margarine, for example. Such fats can either be fully hydrogenated, or they can be only partially hydrogenated, the latter of which also results in the creation of trans fats, the least healthy of the lot.

High-quality, healthy fats are essential to good health and are often underestimated as a beneficial nutrient for athletes. They provide twice as much calorie energy per gram as either carbs or protein, can easily be stored in the body (even in lean athletes with low overall body fat percentages), and play a crucial role in the absorption of fat-soluble vitamins A, D, E, and K.[5] Without fat as a carrier, these vitamin levels become deficient. Fat is also an important component in cell membranes, protects body structures and organs, provides the body with essential fatty acids, and is an essential building block for hormones.

FAT FACTS

Lipids: a family of compounds that includes fats (triglycerides), cholesterol, and waxes

Fats: a subset of lipids found in the body and food as triglycerides

Oils: fats that are liquid at room temperature

HEALTHY FATS

Avocados

Coconut (oil, milk, and meat)

Ghee (clarified butter)

Nuts

Olives and olive oil

Pastured, organic butter

Seeds and their oil (including chia, flax, hemp, and sesame)

MICRONUTRIENTS

Macronutrients—the carbs and proteins and fats—are the big guns of sports nutrition. They do, after all, provide the energy that sustains your efforts. But there's an equally important supporting cast of characters called *micronutrients*: vitamins, minerals, phytochemicals (plant chemicals), and antioxidants. Although they don't directly provide caloric energy in the same way that macronutrients do, they help release that energy and keep you strong and healthy. Needed in small amounts, they're critical to energy production and help support growth, maintenance, and repair of body tissues. They also work as cofactors in the production of enzymes, hormones, and other regulating agents, and help fight inflammation and disease. You can't function without a steady supply of micronutrients, which, for the most part, must be obtained from the food you eat.

VITAMINS

Derived from the Latin word *vita*, meaning "life," vitamins are organic (carbon-containing) substances necessary for normal biological functions. There are thirteen vitamins, classified as either fat-soluble (they must be in the presence of fat to be absorbed) or water-soluble (the B complex of vitamins and vitamin C).

MINERALS

Minerals are inorganic substances necessary to nearly every system in your body. While there are almost two dozen dietary minerals, the focus in overall health and sports nutrition is usually on the major minerals: calcium, phosphorus, magnesium, potassium, sodium, chloride, and zinc. Minerals come from the Earth and can't be made by living organisms. Plants get minerals from the soil—then you eat the plants to get the minerals you need. You also get minerals from the water you drink and, indirectly, from animal sources.

CHLOROPHYLL

CHLOROPHYLL IS THE pigment that gives plants and algae their intense green colors. It's rich in magnesium, which is an energy-production mineral. Muscles contain about 25 to 30 percent of all magnesium in the body; bones contain about 60 percent. Green is good, especially for athletes.

PHYTOCHEMICALS

Phytochemicals (also known as *phytonutrients*) are the health-promoting nutrients found in plants. They're the plant's natural protection against disease and provide health benefits to you when you consume the plant. They're the plant's immune system. By eating a wide variety of colorful fruits and vegetables, you transfer that immune-boosting power from the plant to your body. An example is resveratrol, a compound found in grapes, red wine, peanuts, blueberries, and cranberries, and which is thought to have anti-inflammatory and cardioprotective properties.

ANTIOXIDANTS

Oxygen may be essential for human life, and it may play a crucial role in aerobic energy pathways during exercise, but it can also be a troublemaker in the form of oxidative stress. Electrons normally like to hang around in pairs, like Hansel and Gretel. But when oxygen interacts with certain molecules, it "steals" an electron, leaving the target molecule with an unstable, unpaired electron. The result is a free radical. That free radical molecule goes off looking to in turn steal an electron for itself, restoring its own balance but leaving the next molecule down the line with an electron imbalance. This chain reaction passes the electron imbalance down the line, so to speak, leaving damage in its wake. Such free radical oxidative stress has been implicated in muscle injury and aging, to name two processes of great relevance to athletes.

Here's a way to visualize basic free radical oxidative stress: When you slice an apple and leave it exposed to the oxygen in the air, it turns brown. That is the process at work before your very eyes.

Fortunately, there's something of an antidote to the free radical problem: antioxidants. As their name implies, they fight (anti) the oxidative stress (oxidant). They neutralize the free radical chain reaction, like pouring cold water onto a hot fire. Vitamin C is a potent antioxidant, for instance. And you know how, if you squeeze lemon juice over that sliced apple, the lemon juice will prevent it from turning brown? Well, guess what? Lemon juice is rich in vitamin C. Sure, it's brightening up the flavor of that apple pie you might be baking. But it's also protecting those apples from oxidative stress and free radical damage.

Antioxidants can have a similar effect in your own body. This is good news, because some free radical damage is a simple fact of life. Your cellular mitochrondria, for example, are constantly busy using oxygen to synthesize ATP, the basis for your energy and athletic output. An unavoidable by-product of that process is oxidative stress. Furthermore, research suggests that as you increase your metabolism through exercise, the rate of free radical damage accelerates, too. Your body gradually responds in kind and adapts to the oxidative stress, but a nourishing diet high in natural antioxidants can give your body the boost it needs to bolster the immune system, slow down the effects of aging, fight off disease, and perform at your athletic best.

ANTIOXIDANTS

THE MAIN ANTIOXIDANTS are vitamins A, C, and E, and the minerals selenium and zinc. Flavonoids and carotenoids, chemicals found in abundance in plants, also function as powerful antioxidants. Eat vegetables and fruits daily to keep your antioxidant levels topped off.

WHAT *SHOULDN'T* YOU EAT?

Now that macro- and micronutrients are out of the way, let's start talking details. If you're going to take advantage of the gluten-free edge, your first step is to get the gluten out of your diet.

Avoid the following grains:

Wheat	Spelt
Barley	Durum
Rye	Semolina
Einkorn	Triticale
Emmer	Oats (if not certified gluten-free)

You'll also want to avoid foods traditionally made from the flours of those grains:

Bread	Cookies
Pasta (including couscous)	Beer
Pizza	Noodles
Bagels	Breakfast cereals
Cakes	Pancakes

Waffles	Bulgur
Pies	Farina

Gluten can also hide in products under ingredients label terms such as:

Modified food starch	Barley malt
Wheat gluten	Malt
Hydrolized wheat gluten	Malt flavoring

In addition to the usual suspects, you may also find gluten in products such as:

Processed meats	Canned soups
Imitation crabmeat	Sauces and marinades
Soy sauce	Seitan

Please note that these lists are not exhaustive. Gluten can potentially be found in almost any food with an ingredients label. If it has a label, read the label!

A QUICK GUIDE TO SHOPPING FOR GLUTEN-FREE FOODS

AFTER MISSING ITS original deadline, the U.S. Food and Drug Administration is at last moving forward on a gluten-free labeling standard likely based on the widely recognized international standard of 20 parts per million (ppm) gluten maximum for a product to be labeled gluten-free. Until that new labeling law gets passed, however, here's what you need to know: Thanks to the Food Allergen Labeling and Consumer Protection Act, companies must declare if a product contains one of the eight major allergens, which include wheat (e.g., "Contains wheat"). However, keep in mind that wheat-free does not necessarily mean gluten-free if a product contains barley, rye, or oats. Some companies also employ voluntary advisory labeling, warning consumers about the potential for cross-contamination (e.g., "May contain wheat" or "Processed in a facility or on machinery that also processes wheat"). If you're especially sensitive to gluten, you may choose to buy only foods made in dedicated gluten-free facilities, or which have been reliably tested to confirm their gluten-free status. As a final measure, there are several third-party gluten-free certification programs, including that of the Gluten-Free Certification Organization, part of the Gluten Intolerance Group, as well as a new program from the National Foundation for Celiac Awareness and Quality Assurance International.

WHAT *SHOULD* YOU EAT?

Now that you know what *not* to eat, let's focus on what you *should* eat. As you'll quickly begin to notice, the following list should look surprisingly familiar—it contains many commonsense sports nutrition recommendations, except for one big omission: gluten.

Do eat the following foods:

Gluten-free grains, such as rice, corn, sorghum, millet, quinoa, buckwheat, amaranth, and teff (preferably whole grains, such as brown rice vs. white)
Nuts and seeds
Whole meats
Whole fish
Dairy (including cheese and yogurt)
Eggs
Fresh fruits
Fresh vegetables
Legumes (beans, lentils, and peas)
Root vegetables (cassava, potatoes, sweet potatoes, taro, beets, etc.)

In subsequent chapters we'll go into greater detail on many of these food categories, talking about excellent gluten-free food sources of carbs, protein, healthy fats, iron, calcium, dietary fiber, and more. For now, we're building a foundation of knowledge.

If you reread that list of what you *should* eat, you'll notice that shopping for those foods and ingredients will take you to either the periphery of your supermarket, to your local farmers' market, or to your local farm or ranch. You won't spend much time shopping the central aisles of your grocery store, where many gluten-containing, processed products are found.

While it's true that you can increasingly find gluten-free versions of traditionally gluten-containing foods—pasta, bread, pizza, bagels, and so on—the degree to which those foods ought to be a part of your athletic performance diet will vary. Some can be an excellent source of easily digestible carbohydrates and micronutrients. Others aren't worth the box they're sold in (despite the pumped-up price). More on that soon.

DIETARY FLEXIBILITY

WHILE WE DESCRIBE our particular version of a whole-foods, nutrient-dense, gluten-free diet for athletes and an active lifestyle in this book, you can apply the principles of the *Gluten-Free Edge* to a wide variety of gluten-free diets: Paleo, grain-free, high-carb, low-carb, dairy-free, and vegan or vegetarian. The gluten-free edge can be tailored to your dietary needs and preferences.

SEPARATE, BUT NOT EQUAL

For better or worse, all gluten-free diets are not created equal, especially when it comes to fueling your body for sports or an active lifestyle. Sure, it would be simpler to just say, "Eat gluten-free," but the reality is more complicated. These days, *gluten-free* is a big umbrella term that captures a wide range of dietary habits. And unfortunately, some of those habits aren't quite up to par.

For example, some studies have shown that—compared to the U.S. Recommended Daily Allowances—certain gluten-free diets are deficient in a range of micronutrients, such as nonstarch polysaccharides, vitamin D, calcium, iron, fiber, riboflavin, B_6, B_{12}, folate, and more. Such studies are a bit misleading, as it turns out that much of the average, gluten-eating U.S. population isn't getting enough of those micronutrients, either. The situation isn't unique to the gluten-free diet. In fact, the gluten-free diet is sometimes more, and sometimes less, deficient than the average American diet (which isn't saying much).[6]

How would this give you an edge? Answer: It won't. Not any old gluten-free diet will do—only the right gluten-free diet. As an athlete, you're not eating for the average, and you're not eating the diet of the masses. You're eating for performance. You want to meet your body's nutritional needs and give it the best fuel you can, gluten-free or otherwise.

The gluten-free diet can be—and should be—incredibly healthy and nutrient dense. But to succeed in following such a gluten-free diet, you have to avoid some common pitfalls.

POTENTIAL PITFALLS

Once upon a time, making the switch to a gluten-free diet meant that you more or less abandoned all processed foods, ate a diet heavily dependent on fresh fruits and vegetables and meats and fish, and made most food from scratch for yourself at home. Times have changed.

By mid-2011, gluten-free products comprised a $3 billion per year industry in the United States alone, with tens of thousands of products available. Chances are, if you ate gluten-containing foods before—pasta, cakes, cookies, doughnuts, pizza, beer, cereal, you name it—you can buy gluten-free versions of them now, made with different ingredients.

On the one hand, such choice is great. But it's a rose with thorns. Many gluten-free products are more highly processed, with refined gluten-free starches and added sugars and fats, to improve taste and texture. These days, if you want to trade the Standard American Diet for a gluten-free junk food diet, you can do that. Don't expect to gain any gluten-free edge, however.

NUTRITIONAL COMPARISON OF COMMERCIAL ALL-PURPOSE GLUTEN-FREE FLOUR BLENDS AND BAKING MIXES

PRODUCT	CALORIES	FAT	CARBS	FIBER	SUGARS	PROTEIN
Simply Gluten-Free	428	0	100	0	0	4
Tom Sawyer	440	0	104	8	0	4
Better Batter	396	0	92	4	4	4
Gluten-Free Pantry	480	0	139	5	0	5
Bisquick	420	1.5	93	3	9	6
Namaste Foods	450	1.5	102	6	0	6
Arrowhead Mills	560	2	128	4	0	8
King Arthur	587	0	128	0	0	11
Pamela's	480	10.5	81	4.5	9	12
Bob's Red Mill	400	4	88	12	4	12
Gluten Free Bistro	400	4	88	12	0	12
Wheat Flour (white, bleached, enriched, all-purpose)	455	1	95	3	0	13
Wheat Flour (whole-grain)	407	2	87	15	0	16

All values are based on the manufacturer's nutrition labeling on the product and were accurate as of May 2011. They have been scaled to 1 cup of dry mix to standardize the values. All values (except calories) are in grams and have been rounded to the nearest half gram. The flour blends are in order of protein content. Two versions of wheat flour (*not* gluten-free) are included as well for reference. Wheat values are based on those of the USDA Agricultural Research Service Nutrient Data Laboratory.

ATHLETE INSIGHT

Diana Rolniak

COLLEGIATE BASKETBALL PLAYER, UNIVERSITY OF UTAH

Born: 1990 • Lives: Utah • Gluten-Free Since: 2008

HIGHLIGHTS: DIANA ROLNIAK started out as a figure skater, "but I got to be too tall," she says. "So they kicked me out." She began playing basketball around age eight, following in footsteps of her grandfather and great-aunt, who both played collegiate ball. She went to Regis Jesuit High School in Colorado, where she was ranked No. 83 nationally on ESPN's HoopGurlz 100. Rolniak helped lead the team to a 2009 state championship and set a state record for career blocked shots and most blocks in a game. At Utah, she quickly established herself as one of the team's lead blockers, and as a sophomore (2010–2011) played in all thirty-five games with twenty-four starts.[7]

FAVORITE GLUTEN-FREE FOODS: chicken; mashed potatoes; sweet potato fries; lasagna with gluten-free rice noodles; steak; chicken fried rice; nutrition shakes; eggs, gluten-free toast, and fruit for breakfast; KIND bars and apples for snacks. Pregame dinner is always grilled chicken, mashed potatoes, and vegetables (three plates' worth of food).

Just ask professional Xterra off-road triathlete Jenny Smith. "You have to be careful with processed gluten-free food," she says. "Much of it is not high quality. They don't have a place in an athletic diet. You could end up pretty nutritionally depleted if you do that." Smith notes that, the gluten status aside, a gluten-free bagel typically has less nutritional quality than a whole wheat bagel.

Fitness model Natalie Jill, gluten-free since 2000 due to celiac disease, agrees. "A gluten-free muffin or doughnut can be worse for you than a real muffin if you're not gluten intolerant," she explains, noting that refined gluten-free starches can give the product a higher glycemic index, causing an insulin spike in you, the athlete.

Powerlifter Ginger Vieira is of one mind with Smith and Jill. "I don't need or want junky carbs," she says. "Gluten-free products can be so carb dense." The carbohydrate density in and of itself isn't necessarily bad, especially if you need those carbs to fuel endurance performance, compared to powerlifting. But a problem slowly starts to creep into your diet when those gluten-free carbs come with little else in the way of nutrition.

Nevertheless, such specialty gluten-free foods can be tempting. "I remember, the day I was diagnosed, I went to the grocery store and bought all the things that were labeled gluten-free," says collegiate lacrosse player Kristen Taylor. Recreational runner Kendra Nielsen was in a similar boat following her own diagnosis. "It was quite easy to eat gluten-free junk food. It was a problem for me when I was first diagnosed," she says. "Anything with 'gluten-free' on it I wanted to try, even if I normally wouldn't eat it, such as cookies."

U.S. Olympian and national champion distance runner Amy Yoder Begley adds, "You have to be careful now, with so many gluten-free alternatives. You almost feel like you want to try them all."

They're gluten-free. You're curious. You feel enabled and empowered. They're an option. They're convenient. They're . . . there. You may want to buy them and eat them just because you can. That's not necessarily a formula for athletic success, however.

Professional gluten-free triathlete Christie Sym—who has celiac disease—has been mindful of that slippery slope. "I'm not really a fan of gluten-free products off the shelf. I hardly eat junk food," she says. "But when I was first diagnosed, my mum—because she found all these gluten-free products—would buy them. I'd say, 'Mum, I wouldn't eat those normally!' And I felt bad, because she was making an effort. It's great that products like those are coming out, but they're not going to make up the bulk of your diet, and they're expensive. You might eat them as a treat, but not in your day-to-day training diet."

Fellow triathlete Heather Wurtele concurs. "Just because something is gluten-free doesn't mean it's healthy," she says. "There's gluten-free crap; really badly processed things. I would never eat plain white bread. Why would I do that even if it's gluten-free?"

It's good cautionary advice to keep in mind.

WILL GOING GLUTEN-FREE HELP YOU LOSE WEIGHT?

Ah, the million-dollar question. We don't mean to be noncommittal, but it depends. Despite common misconceptions that the gluten-free diet is a new form of weight-loss diet, research and real-world anecdotes don't back up such a perspective. Will *some* people lose weight switching to a gluten-free diet? Undoubtedly. But the reality for athletes, especially, is highly individualized, influenced by a wide range of factors, including increased digestion and absorption, reduced inflammation, daily calorie intake adjustments, and changes to the quality and content of your diet.

If you've been eating a junk-food, gluten-containing diet and switch to a whole-foods, gluten-free diet, you'll likely lose weight, thanks to purging your diet of processed, refined foods filled with empty calories—food calories from simple sugars and unhealthy fats that come without the benefit of nutrients, vitamins, minerals, and so on.

If you eat a healthy gluten-containing diet, on the other hand, and switch to eating a healthy gluten-free diet, you may see little change in your body weight. Aside from issues related to gluten-induced inflammation, you're basically making a one-for-one dietary swap in the weight department.

And if you fall into the trap of swapping your current diet for the gluten-free equivalent of a junk food diet, you're probably going to gain weight. Not only will you be eating refined, processed junk food with empty calories and higher glycemic index values, but many such gluten-free versions have added sugars and fats to improve taste and texture.

GLUTEN MYTH-BUSTING

Gluten gets a bad rap, and for good reason, but when it comes to weight gain versus weight loss and gluten's influence on obesity, gluten sometimes unnecessarily gets thrown under the bus. So let's bust a few interrelated myths before we go any further.

MYTH #1: GLUTEN STIMULATES APPETITE

There exists a complex relationship between the brain, peptides, and the gut in regulating hunger and appetite.[8] That much is true, but when it comes to gluten, appetite stimulation doesn't seem to come into play. This gluten-related myth arises from research related to how endogenous opiates (endorphins made by your own body) influence appetite, and how appetite responds to naloxone, a drug that blocks the opiate effect. Studies have shown that administering naloxone to healthy adults leads to reduced daily calorie and food intake,[9] demonstrating the role of endogenous opiates in the regulation of appetite and eating. As the logic goes, ingesting gluten creates gluten exorphins (true), which are exogenous opioids (opiates that come from outside your body, also true), and since endogenous opiates stimulate appetite, so should gluten-based exorphins. Right? Wrong. Although gluten may create opiate-like exorphins, they don't always behave exactly like endorphins.

Consider one study with naloxone that found that opiates play a role in dietary intake of high-sugar and high-fat foods, but not in salty or savory foods.[10] Gluten did not correlate consistently with appetite. In the study, the intake of some gluten-containing foods increased, others decreased, and others remained relatively unchanged under the influence of naloxone. If gluten caused increased appetite and naloxone blocked that effect, you wouldn't expect the study participants to eat even more glutenous foods under the influence of naloxone. But that's exactly what happened. For example, participants consumed 40 percent more gluten-containing bread sticks.

Another study definitively put this myth to rest. Researchers examined gluten and its exorphins and their effect on appetite both with and without naloxone. Their conclusion? "Although a number of studies have suggested a role for endogenous opiates in appetite regulation, we could not demonstrate any effect of 'exorphins' on the amount of calories ingested nor on the perception of satiety."[11]

MYTH #2: GLUTEN FAILS TO SATISFY HUNGER

This myth follows from Myth #1. And as you might guess, it's also false. The premise is that if gluten causes you to stay hungry, you'll eat more and gain weight. We've already seen that gluten doesn't stimulate appetite, nor does it have an effect on calories ingested or satiety. But here's more evidence: One study looking at satiety in response to both gluten-containing and gluten-free grains found no major differences.[12] Both kinds of grains more or less satisfied the appetite equally well. (There were three exceptions—gluten-free oats, buckwheat, and quinoa all did a better job of satisfying hunger.)

In addition, whole grains satisfied hunger better than refined grains. And since whole wheat will have more gluten than refined wheat starch, according to the myth, whole wheat shouldn't satisfy hunger. But it does.

In fact, some studies have shown the same or even *reduced* food intake as a result of gluten intake (and other proteins, such as whey, soy protein, egg albumin, casein, and pea protein), because protein combined with carbs, rather than carbs alone, stabilizes or increases satiety (satisfies hunger). This was true even when comparing wheat with gluten and gluten-free isolated wheat starch.[13] Satisfying hunger comes down to eating protein with your carbs, rather than carbs alone, as well as eating whole grains instead of refined grain starches.

MYTH #3: GLUTEN CAUSES YOU TO EAT MORE CALORIES PER DAY

This one is only partly true. We'll explain. Consider one study that compared a control population of healthy adults with no gluten problems to a population of healthy people with celiac disease who had been on a strict gluten-free diet. Because the latter population (those with celiac disease) were on a strict gluten-free diet and deemed healthy by researchers, their disease was essentially turned off. In essence, then, researchers were comparing two populations of healthy individuals—one eating gluten, the other on a gluten-free diet. Compared to their so-called normal counterparts, the gluten-free set—men and women alike—had a lower body mass index (BMI) and had a lower daily calorie intake (to the tune of 14 percent fewer calories).[14] (They also got more of their calories from fat and less from carbs.) This does seem to support the myth. However, we have a hypothesis to explain the results: The "normal" population was suffering from both impaired digestion (requiring them to eat more calories to get the same nutrients) and inflammation (causing the higher BMI) due to gluten. It's a combination seen frequently in obese and overweight celiac disease patients, and at first it seems counterintuitive—a person who can simultaneously be malnourished (or thereabouts) *and* overweight.

Another study offers an insightful window into this mechanism. Researchers looked at two populations of people with celiac disease: One was on a strict gluten-free diet, the other "cheated" and ate some gluten. The strict gluten-free diet group consumed 400 fewer calories per day, yet they had slightly *higher* body weight and *more* muscle. That's because the gluten-free diet was promoting healthy digestion and absorption; they were getting the nutrients they needed from less food. The "cheating" group, on the other hand, was effectively poisoning themselves. They needed to eat more to try to get nutrients, and *still* weighed less and had less muscle.

So can gluten cause you to eat more calories? Possibly. But will you gain weight from those calories? Only if you're absorbing them.

Gluten does a lot of things to the human body, many of them negative, but automatically causing weight gain isn't necessarily one of them. If we're going to point fingers at wheat and the other gluten grains for negatively impacting body weight and contributing to obesity, then we should look not at the gluten, but instead at the starches and their impact on blood glucose and insulin (in combination with a host of other lifestyle factors). (For more on that topic, check out our discussion in chapter 6.)

CELIAC DISEASE EXAMPLES

When we look at more examples from within the celiac disease community, we begin to quickly see the varied ways in which body weight responds to gluten and the gluten-free diet. There is *not* a one-size-fits-all pattern for weight management.

Some studies show a "migration to the middle" when switching from a gluten-containing to a gluten-free diet—people with normal BMIs tended to stay that way, people who were underweight tended to gain weight, and people who were overweight tended to lose weight. For example, one study of 215 celiac disease patients—including people who were underweight, normal weight, overweight, and obese—looked at the switch to a gluten-free diet. Among men, 31 percent gained weight, while 41 percent lost weight. Among women, 35 percent gained weight, while 36 percent lost weight. Weight *gain* among ninety-one individuals averaged 16.5 pounds. Weight *loss* among twenty-five individuals averaged 27.5 pounds.[15]

Likewise, a study of 369 celiac disease patients also supported the "migration to the middle" trend. In this population, 61 percent had a normal BMI, 17 percent were underweight, 15 percent were overweight, and 7 percent were obese. Of those that started underweight, 66 percent gained weight. Of those that started overweight or obese, 54 percent and 47 percent lost weight, respectively.[16]

A third study of celiac patients—this time children—included 75 percent with a normal BMI, 13 percent who were overweight, and 6 percent who were obese. After three years on a gluten-free diet, the overweight children had lost weight (including 44 percent who normalized their BMI), while many of the normal-weight children increased their BMI (including 13 percent who became overweight).[17]

Other studies show strong trends toward weight gain on the gluten-free diet. For example, one prominent study examined 371 celiac disease patients, with a distribution of 4 percent underweight, 57 percent normal weight, and 39 percent overweight. After two years on a gluten-free diet, 81 percent of patients had gained weight, including 82 percent of initially overweight individuals.[18] Another study, of more than 140 children with celiac disease (11 percent of whom were initially overweight, and another 3 percent of whom classified as obese), looked at their weight at diagnosis and again after at least twelve months of being on a gluten-free diet. The number of children who were overweight doubled.

What do we make of these studies? What's going on?

It's clear that in an overwhelming majority of cases, the switch to a gluten-free diet is repairing the GI system and increasing digestion and absorption of nutrients, enabling sick people with low BMIs to finally get nutrients from their food and put on healthy weight. In cases of weight loss, we're seeing drastic reductions in inflammation and other negative physiological responses to gluten, plus—in some cases—a switch from a diet of heavily processed, refined gluten-containing foods to healthier, whole gluten-free foods.

But there are other factors to consider, especially in the cases of weight gain among normal BMI and overweight individuals, such as the impact of lifestyle (active vs. sedentary), the nature of the gluten-free diet to which a person switched (healthy whole foods vs. gluten-free junk food), and the need to decrease caloric intake to account for increased nutritional absorption.

REAL-WORLD ATHLETE EXAMPLES

In terms of the weight-loss/weight-gain balance, there are additional factors to consider as well, especially for athletes with gluten intolerance. Athletes, by their very nature, tend to eat healthier and are more active than your average study participant. Once you sort out issues of digestion and nutrient absorption, inflammation, and portion sizing, a gluten-free diet can be part of a formula for a lean, mean athletic machine. Let's look at some real world examples.

In some instances, the reduced inflammation and bloating caused by removing gluten from the diet can result in weight loss. That was the experience of professional triathlete Terra Castro, who experienced extreme inflammation and bloating when she was eating gluten regularly. "I looked very swollen," she recalls. "I was gaining a lot of weight. My immune system was freaking out." No matter how hard she trained, she wasn't seeing performance gains . . . and wasn't seeing the added weight melt away. But after four weeks of eating gluten-free, she had lost 20 pounds, and the weight has stayed off. "Since then I've been a very healthy weight," she says.

Conversely, some gluten-intolerant athletes that switch to the gluten-free diet may see significant weight gain. If they were seriously malnourished because of gluten's negative impact on their system, they may finally be putting healthy weight back onto an undernourished body. Consider the case of Diana Rolniak, who plays Division I basketball for the University of Utah. She's been gluten-free since July 2008, when she was diagnosed with celiac disease. "Weight was always an issue for me," she says. "I was very active, but not able to keep on weight."

At one point during her senior year in high school, the 6-foot, 4-inch forward weighed just 100 pounds. "I was very, very sick," she recalls. "Getting my celiac disease under control was a major health issue." And she did, thanks to the gluten-free diet.

During the summer of 2009 alone, prior to starting her freshman year at Utah, Rolniak put on 30 desperately needed pounds.

Collegiate distance runner and outdoors enthusiast Alex Borsuk experienced similar weight problems. In the span of a single summer, just before her diagnosis with celiac disease, she lost 12 pounds, "without even trying." That's not good "for someone who wants to stay healthy and be active and do the kinds of things that I do," she says.

But even for athletes not emaciated by nutrient deficiency from celiac disease, there can be unexpected weight gains on the gluten-free diet. Traditionally, the weight-gain/weight-loss equation at its most basic comes down to the number of calories consumed versus the number of calories burned. If you burn more than you eat, you lose weight. If you eat more than you burn, you gain weight.

However, for athletes with gluten intolerance, there's an added component to the equation: calories consumed versus calories *digested and absorbed* versus calories burned. When your GI system heals on the gluten-free diet, you may suddenly find yourself getting more calories and nutrients from the food you've been eating, thanks to improved digestion and absorption. The result can be surprising and unexpected weight gain.

Just ask Michael Danke, a recreational runner diagnosed with celiac disease in 2003. "In college I was running 6 to 8 miles a day. And I was eating easily 6,000 calories per day, but I wasn't gaining any weight," he recalls. "As it turns out, I was only absorbing about 1,500 calories per day. Now, I may eat 4,000 calories per day and absorb 3,500 with my healed intestine." Suddenly, his portion sizes were all wrong. He was eating the same amount as he was before, but now that amount was too much.

For Danke, the solution was to buy a kitchen scale and weigh his portions of food until he retrained his mind and his stomach to new portion sizes that matched his recovered body and increased nutrient absorption.

Professional triathlete Christie Sym had a similar experience. She stands 5 feet, 9 inches tall, but at her sickest due to celiac disease was down to about 110 pounds. "I was skin and bones, down to nothing," she says. Once diagnosed and on a gluten-free diet, she started putting on more weight . . . rapidly.

Her body weight shot up to near 155 pounds. "That was so hard to deal with," she says, "from being underweight and told to put weight on, to the opposite and wanting to lose some of it."

And it wasn't just an issue of weight. There was also her appetite to contend with. Initially, "I still had the same hunger," she says, because her body hadn't adapted to the amount of food she was eating and how much of it she was absorbing. When she was sick, "my coach told me to eat more and more, but I would still be losing weight, not absorbing it. When I started absorbing more, my hunger was still the same, but I didn't need to eat that much."

Today, she eats half as much as she did then and is at a healthy weight, right where she wants to be: somewhere in the range of 138 to 147 pounds.

The same thing happened to Amy Yoder Begley. "The strangest thing for me was—and this is still a problem from time to time—when I had active celiac disease and was not absorbing, I would eat and eat all the time, and not absorb nutrients," she says. "After taking out the gluten, I want to eat all I was eating before, but now I'm absorbing everything. It's the hardest thing ever."

ATHLETE INSIGHT

Terra Castro

PROFESSIONAL TRIATHLETE, TEAM LUNA CHIX

Born: 1980 • Lives: Texas • Gluten-Free Since: 2000

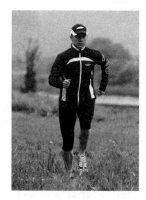

TERRA CASTRO ran cross country in high school. "I had plenty of 'number two' problems," she recalls. "I thought it was nerves or stress or eating too close to a run." She experienced inflammation and bloating, rashes, cramping in her muscles, and anemia. When Castro switched to a gluten-free diet, her symptoms cleared up; in particular, her iron levels increased greatly. She was inspired to get into triathlons watching her grandfather race. "I was getting up at four a.m. to watch him and thought, 'This is silly. I should just do it,'" she says today. Castro experienced almost immediate success and became a member of Team USA's junior elite squad. She turned pro in 2003 and signed with Team Luna Chix in 2005, the same year she found her niche at the Ironman distance. Today she's a consistent Top 5 finisher.

FAVORITE GLUTEN-FREE FOODS: gluten-free Luna protein bars (mint chocolate chip and cookie dough flavors), Clif Shot Bloks, Udi's Blueberry Muffins (with a cup of coffee), toasted whole-grain gluten-free bread with almond butter, quinoa pasta, white rice ("Brown rice pasta is difficult for my stomach to digest"), sweet potatoes

EATING RIGHT

For now, don't worry about the body-weight issue. Focus on eating the right types of gluten-free foods: whole, fresh, nutrient-dense foods. And skip refined, overly processed gluten-free snack foods. The rest will come as your body recalibrates and you adjust your food intake to match your improved digestion and absorption, decreased inflammation, and overall better health and performance.

Such mindful gluten-free eating is a natural fit for athletes and anyone living an active lifestyle. It's not just about ensuring that what you're eating is gluten-free, but also about being aware of what you're putting into your body.

Terra Castro certainly thinks so. As a triathlete, she's been around her fair share of night-before, prerace, gluten-heavy communal pasta dinners. "I can't eat the pasta dinner. I never have, and I'm never going to have that," she says. "But honestly, whether you're gluten-free or not, why put your nutrition, your race, in other people's hands? A lot of age group competitors will spend $700 to enter an Ironman. Yet they won't spend five minutes to go to the grocery store and fill up a bag of food to take with them to the race. You get excited, you get caught up in the event, want to participate, but forget details like your nutrition."

Xterra pro Jenny Smith is of the same mind. "You can't be lazy with your gluten-free diet," she explains. "Regardless of whether you're a conventional athlete wanting to improve your diet, or a gluten-free athlete who's been diagnosed with a condition, the preparation and thought you give your diet is key . . . whole foods, whether they contain gluten or not; staying away from processed gluten-free food."

It often comes down to making intelligent choices about the food you're using to fuel your body's athletic engine.

MAKING THE SWITCH

If you're feeling intimidated by the gluten-free diet, don't be. Like any diet, it has a learning curve, sure. But you can do it, and once you do, being gluten-free will feel like second nature.

That's not to say you won't potentially have hiccups along the way, missteps here and there where you accidentally eat something with gluten in it. That's okay. Cut yourself some slack. You're making an adjustment.

Depending on your current diet, making that adjustment can be a big change. Depression is a possible side effect of gluten exposure, but it

ATHLETE INSIGHT

Michael Danke

RECREATIONAL RUNNER AND TRIATHLETE

Born: 1968 • Lives: Texas • Gluten-Free Since: 2003

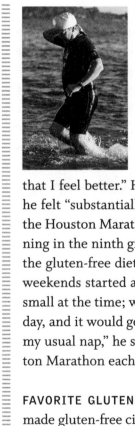

"I HAD BEEN borderline anemic my whole life. I was getting sick about once a month," Michael Danke says. "I didn't think it was any big deal at the time. I didn't even realize that was out of the norm." He wasn't diagnosed with celiac disease until his midthirties, after an especially bad bout of illness that sent him to the hospital. On the gluten-free diet, he says, "within weeks, I realized this is different— that I feel better." His symptoms began to resolve. By six weeks, he felt "substantially" better; by six months, he was training for the Houston Marathon, which he runs every year. "I started running in the ninth grade and it stuck with me," Danke recalls. On the gluten-free diet he also had more energy, and lots of it. "My weekends started at five a.m. with a 15-mile run. My kids were small at the time; we'd go from adventure to adventure on Saturday, and it would get to ten p.m. and I'd realize that I didn't have my usual nap," he says. Now, he looks forward to the next Houston Marathon each year.

FAVORITE GLUTEN-FREE FOODS: pizza, baked potatoes, homemade gluten-free cinnamon chocolate cake

can also surface when you're first going gluten-free, especially if you're focused on all the gluten-based foods you're no longer going to eat and think you're going to miss.

"It was huge," says track and field distance runner and outdoors enthusiast Alex Borsuk, diagnosed with celiac disease in September 2010.

"I was eating whole wheat pasta, whole grains, wheat toast, crackers, pretzels."

"It can be difficult for some people; it's a dramatic change," adds Xterra's Jenny Smith. "If you're used to eating a lot of wheat products, and a lot of processed foods in your diet . . . cereal for breakfast, sandwiches . . . you can wonder, 'What am I going to eat?'"

As it turns out, you can eat plenty. But it's easy to leave the gluten blinders on.

That's how it was for recreational runner Michael Danke. "Was it a big adjustment? Yeah. It was brutal," he says. "For the first few weeks I was gluten-free, I knew that wheat, barley, and rye were killing me, literally. I had to get off gluten. But the issue I had, and I think a lot of celiacs have, is you say to yourself, 'I can't have this and can't have that.' I went through my typical breakfast, lunch, and dinner and thought I couldn't have any of it. I took two sacks of groceries to the curb for a food drive—food I couldn't eat anymore. I really struggled for three or four weeks. It's funny in retrospect . . . that I thought I was going to starve to death."

For professional arena football kicker Craig Pinto, it was difficult initially, too . . . despite how good he felt on the diet. He switched to gluten-free in 2000 after a celiac disease diagnosis. Previously, doctors couldn't figure out what was ailing him. Pinto thought something was seriously wrong. He had resigned himself to a label of "sickly." Despite his background as a successful athlete in high school and early college, he thought he was doomed to have health problems, even as young man. "I remember after a few weeks being gluten-free . . . I was feeling better when waking up. I was less sluggish, more lively in my body. No more headaches," he says. But the gluten had "damaged me more psychologically than physically," he explains. "It took a little while for me to think that I wasn't this really sick young adult."

For others, the dietary switch can be entirely natural, hardly worthy of batting an eyelash. It was that way for powerlifter Ginger Vieira. "Athletes eat a clean diet," she says. "We want to take good care of our health. We eat so that it supports our sport, rather than eating for pleasure or eating for the hell of it." For her, a gluten-free diet was part of a formula of eating for performance in her chosen sport.

ATHLETE INSIGHT

Craig Pinto

FORMER PROFESSIONAL KICKER, NEW JERSEY REVOLUTION INDOOR/ ARENA FOOTBALL

Born: 1977 • Lives: New York • Gluten-Free Since: 2000

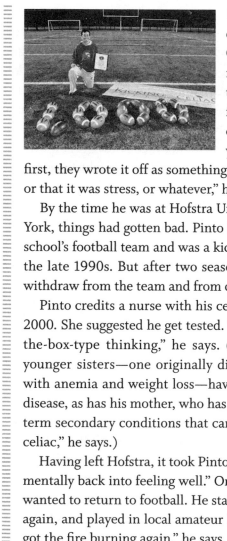

DIAGNOSED WITH CROHN'S disease at the age of twelve, Craig Pinto always had trouble managing his symptoms. "I thought they were recurring flare-ups," he says. Doctors couldn't figure out their cause, yet Pinto kept feeling sick. "At first, they wrote it off as something they thought was in my head, or that it was stress, or whatever," he explains.

By the time he was at Hofstra University on Long Island, New York, things had gotten bad. Pinto had been a kicker for his high school's football team and was a kicker for Hofstra's team, too, in the late 1990s. But after two seasons, his health forced him to withdraw from the team and from college.

Pinto credits a nurse with his celiac disease diagnosis in early 2000. She suggested he get tested. "Back then, it was outside-of-the-box-type thinking," he says. (Since then, both of Pinto's younger sisters—one originally diagnosed with IBS, the other with anemia and weight loss—have been diagnosed with celiac disease, as has his mother, who has osteoporosis and other "long-term secondary conditions that can go wrong with undiagnosed celiac," he says.)

Having left Hofstra, it took Pinto a while "to get physically and mentally back into feeling well." Once he did, he decided that he wanted to return to football. He started training and working out again, and played in local amateur leagues in 2007 and 2008. "It got the fire burning again," he says.

The next year, the New Jersey Revolution, an indoor/arena football team, was holding tryouts. "I went to the open tryout, worked my butt off, and got signed in 2009 right out of the tryout," Pinto says. "It was huge for me. Especially with how down and out I had felt, to be an athlete like that again." By the start of that first season, he had been named team captain. "Only the quarterback was older than I was," he jokes, noting that most players were either fresh out of college or in their midtwenties. He played in 2010 as well, before the team dissolved.

Since then he's been busy with his new nonprofit, the Kicking 4 Celiac Foundation. The group's first project was a solo fundraising effort in 2010. Pinto took to a local football field and set a new twelve-hour field goal Guinness World Record: 717. In 2011 he was at it again, this time to set a new twenty-four-hour record: 1,000. He was successful then, too. "It's funny. I missed almost 500 kicks that day, so in total, I took 1,500 kicks," he says. "I don't think I will ever kick that many footballs again throughout the rest of my life span, let alone in one day."

These days, the former middle and high school football coach is busy full-time with the foundation, setting up new fund-raisers to help channel money to celiac research, and—new for 2012—launching a scholarship program for graduating high school seniors with celiac disease, to help offset the cost of being gluten-free in college.[19]

FAVORITE GLUTEN-FREE FOODS: quinoa pasta ("definitely a favorite"), gluten-free pizza, Udi's Bagels ("I have my shelves stocked"), grilled cheese on gluten-free bread

For triathlete Christie Sym, the switch was similarly inconsequential, though for different reasons. "The doctor was so somber, so sorry for me," she says of her diagnosis and switch to the gluten-free diet. "But I was so happy. I finally had an answer. I had a diagnosis." Her biggest change was always reading labels—being conscious of "every single food that went into my mouth."

College athletes may miss the beer and pizza parties thrown by friends. Other athletes may miss the social aspect of sharing the same food, not wanting to be "different." Athletes in team sports may fear losing a sense of bonding and "oneness" with teammates. Others may worry, *How will I eat at home? How will I eat on the road?* These are questions we'll answer in subsequent chapters.

If your experience with the gluten-free diet is anything like ours and that of the dozens of prominent gluten-free athletes we've interviewed, once you start to feel healthy and perform better in your sport and in life, it'll be full speed ahead. The concerns will fade to the background, and the gluten-free edge will come to the fore.

You can do this. And you don't have to take our word for it. Listen to Allen Lim, who's served as sports physiologist for pro cycling's Team RadioShack: "Some people think it's logistically hard to pull off being on a gluten-free diet. If we can pull it off in the midst of the Tour de France, anyone can."

NEED TO KNOW

- Macronutrients include carbohydrates, fat, and protein.
- Simple and complex carbs, plus fat, provide athletic fuel.
- Empty carbs are made of processed, refined starches that have calories but little in the way of additional nutrition. In limited quantities, they can have a role in athletic nutrition, but for the most part, avoid them.
- There are tons of options for great gluten-free foods rich in fiber, complex and simple carbs, healthy fats, and animal- and plant-based sources of protein.
- Meats, as well as quinoa and soy, have complete sets of essential amino acids. Most plants are typically deficient in at least one, so combine sources to make complete sets.
- *Don't* eat wheat, barley, rye, their ancestors, their hybrids, and foods made from them.

- *Do* eat fruits, vegetables, whole meats and fish, dairy, nuts and seeds, legumes, root vegetables, and gluten-free grains.
- Beware of the gluten-free equivalent of junk food, typically made with refined starches and other processed ingredients, plus added fat and sugar, minus many nutrients.
- Switching to a gluten-free diet may or may not result in weight loss, depending on a number of factors related to diet, inflammation, digestion and absorption, and other issues.
- Making the switch to a gluten-free diet can initially create a blend of positive and negative emotions. Don't be intimidated, and focus on the positive. It gets better and better, especially as your health and performance improve and you start living the gluten-free edge.

5

Special Considerations

BOTH THE GLUTEN-FREE diet and gluten intolerance in athletes warrant special consideration of several dietary factors: nutrient absorption, iron, and calcium.

NUTRIENT ABSORPTION

Gluten causes digestive problems for all people, but if you're an athlete with one of the more serious forms of gluten intolerance, such as celiac disease, the situation is more dire. In that case, exposure to gluten causes an autoimmune reaction that damages the villi of the small intestine. The effects are twofold: the loss of certain digestive enzymes that your body makes on those villi, resulting in decreased digestion, and diminished ability to absorb what nutrients you are able to digest.

The immediate risk, then, is nutrient malabsorption. Nutrient malabsorption can result in nutrient deficiencies, which can result in malnourishment, which can seriously inhibit athletic performance, or even basic quality of life. It's a nasty sequence of events. It doesn't take a degree in exercise physiology to realize that being malnourished is no way to live an active, healthy lifestyle, or to compete as an athlete.

For athletes with gluten intolerance, several potential nutrient issues loom largest:[1]

- Fat malabsorption, decreased uptake of fat-soluble vitamins (A, D, E, and K), and steatorrhea (excess fat in stools)
- Iron absorption problems, iron deficiency, and anemia
- Calcium and vitamin D absorption problems, subsequent deficiency, and concerns regarding bone density, osteopenia, and osteoporosis

These are separate issues entirely from the sufficiency or deficiency of the gluten-free diet. As we noted in the last chapter, all gluten-free diets are not created equal. Poor forms of the diet can be deficient in nutrients critical to athletes. Other forms of the diet can offer ideal fuel for elite athletic performance.

What we're talking about here are unique problems that gluten causes for gluten-intolerant athletes. Take iron, for example. All athletes should know about and care about iron, for reasons we're about to describe. But if you're an athlete with gluten intolerance, and gluten has been impacting your ability to absorb iron, and your gluten-free diet isn't rich in natural sources of iron, you're going to be doubly behind the eight ball, or worse.

On the other hand, if you've been on the gluten-free diet long enough to permit your intestines and your body to heal, and if you're eating a whole-foods, nutrient-dense, healthy form of the diet, these special nutrient concerns will dissolve and your body—and your athletic performance—will respond in unbelievably positive ways.

Meanwhile, if you're a conventional athlete embracing the gluten-free diet for its performance-enhancing benefits, such as the diet's anti-inflammatory properties, it pays to know how the gluten-free diet can help—or hinder, if you make the wrong food choices—such factors as iron levels, which play a crucial role in athletic performance.

IRON

Iron is many things: a metal, the fourth-most common element by mass in the Earth's crust, the stuff of your grandmother's well-seasoned skillet. But it's also crucial to your body's functioning and to peak athletic performance. Iron is a critical component of hemoglobin, the part of your red blood cells responsible for transporting oxygen throughout the body. It's also a critical component of myoglobin, the hemoglobin equivalent in your muscles.

Hemoglobin and myoglobin both contribute heavily to your body's ability to transport and utilize oxygen. In athleticspeak, this ability is known as your VO_2 *max*. We talk more about it in chapter 10. But at this juncture it's important to keep in mind that VO_2 max is one of several important predictors of your peak performance.

As we noted in chapter 3, oxygen is a central component of your body's energy pathways, especially the aerobic pathways that fuel endurance activity. And because your VO_2 max is dependent on oxygen transport and utilization, which in turn are dependent in part on iron, it logically follows that iron is of prime importance to athletes, gluten-free or not.

Inadequate iron intake, poor iron absorption, and/or iron loss can lead to iron deficiency, reduced hemoglobin levels, or even anemia (low red blood cell counts). On a functional level, the result can be decreased energy, decreased aerobic capacity, increased heart rate, delayed recovery, shortness of breath, inability to exercise, poor immune function, dizziness, headaches, and reduced maximum performance.

DID YOU KNOW?

RED BLOOD CELLS, which carry the much-needed oxygen for optimal performance in sports, only last about 120 days before they need to be replaced. They have a tough job, squeezing in and out of tiny capillaries delivering oxygen to working muscles. To maintain sufficient numbers, new red blood cells must be produced at the rate of about two million *per second*. And each red blood cell is home to about 280 hemoglobin molecules.[2] We need iron to crank out those red blood cells at the same rate we're losing them.

IRON AND ALL ATHLETES

Any athlete, gluten-free or not, is at risk of iron deficiency or even anemia. The greater the demands of your sport, the more likely it is that your current iron stores will become insufficient. Some iron may be lost through sweat and urine, especially in men.[3] In impact sports, iron can be lost through acute injury. In sports such as running, gastrointestinal bleeding and other mechanisms of subtle injury can also deplete iron.[4] In general, athletes require more iron than your average American does.

Yet, despite this well-known risk, many conventional athletes do find themselves iron deficient, even anemic. Exercise-induced iron deficiency is more prevalent than it ought to be. According to some studies, at least 10 to 20 percent of all athletes are iron deficient. One study of high-level athletes found that a whopping 70 percent had functional iron deficiency by the end of their competitive season.[5] And you don't have to be an elite athlete to have iron-related problems, either. Collegiate athletes[6] and recreational athletes[7] alike face performance problems related to iron deficiency and/or anemia.

What's more, you don't have to be full-on anemic to experience decreased athletic performance. Basic iron deficiency is enough to make a difference. For example, in one study of collegiate rowers, iron-depleted athletes had slower times compared to teammates with sufficient iron levels.[8]

IRON AND THE GLUTEN-INTOLERANT ATHLETE

In gluten-intolerant athletes, these iron-related concerns are compounded. If you have gluten intolerance *and* compete in a sport, you face a sort of double jeopardy when it comes to iron. In your case, exposure to gluten damages the part of the small intestine responsible for absorbing iron. In other words, you're not able to absorb the iron you're eating. As a result, iron deficiency and anemia are commonly found among people with untreated celiac disease and other similar forms of gluten intolerance.[9]

It's a story all too familiar to athletes such as high-altitude mountaineer Dave Hahn and U.S. national champion distance runner Amy Yoder

ATHLETE INSIGHT

Dave Hahn

HIGH-ALTITUDE MOUNTAINEER, CLIMBING GUIDE, PROFESSIONAL SKI
PATROLLER

Born: 1961 • Lives: New Mexico • Gluten-Free Since: 1999

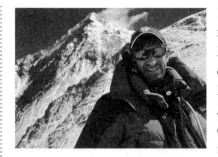

IN 1999, WHILE leading a difficult climbing expedition up
Mount Everest to find and recover the bodies of George
Mallory and climbing partner
Andrew Irvine, who mysteri-
ously disappeared on the
mountain in 1924, Dave Hahn
found himself in dire straits. Although the team discovered the
body of Mallory at 27,000 feet and Hahn made his second successful summit of Everest's 29,035-foot peak two weeks later, he was
unaccountably weak, physically stressed, and extremely short of
breath. Everyone is short of breath at 29,000 feet—up in the so-
called death zone—but Hahn had been there before and knew this
time around that something was wrong.

"I had a great deal of difficulty going to the summit on May 17
with Conrad Anker," he says, "and afterward I felt I had been ir-
responsible in putting my climbing partners at risk. I needed to
know what was going on."

One month later he was diagnosed with celiac disease, the cause
of his ongoing gastrointestinal problems and pronounced anemia.
His body wasn't adequately producing the oxygen-carrying red
blood cells he so desperately needed as a high-altitude mountain
guide. The air up there is thin enough as it is.

"In retrospect," he says, "it was a problem that had been getting
progressively worse for about two years. I thought I was getting old
and began to believe that my career of taking climbers to remote,

cold, and high environments was almost at an end. Instead, my best days in the mountains began after my diagnosis."

Hahn felt dramatically better after switching to a gluten-free diet, but it took almost two years to regain the strength he needed to add another eleven summits of Everest to his growing list of accomplishments. Now fifty years old, he's stronger, feels younger, and is in his prime as one of the most well-respected and sought-after guides in mountaineering history. To date he's summited Mount Everest a record 13 times, Mount McKinley 20 times, Mount Rainier 270-plus times, and Mount Vinson (in Antarctica) 27 times. Humble and quick to admit he wasn't the best athlete growing up, his achievements not only include a staggering number of high-altitude summits, but a stellar list of daring mountain rescues as well.

Had he not found out what was sabotaging his health and zapping his strength, his life would have been very different. "I could not have continued climbing had I not been diagnosed," he says. What he once called fuel (pasta, cereal, bread), he now calls poison. "Luckily, I only get noticeably poisoned about two times a year," he says, "but the results aren't pretty. In about three hours, I begin to sweat profusely, faint, and vomit."

The downside of long expeditions and maintaining a gluten-free diet is that the freeze-dried meal choices can get somewhat monotonous. But, as he says, "luckily I don't go climb big mountains for the food." He's also lucky his job of guiding clients up Mount Everest lands him in the rice bowl of the world. "Sometimes I get to feeling like I'm having beans with rice and then rice with beans and after that beans with rice," he jokes.

But he's not complaining. "I have never felt like the diagnosis was the finding of an illness," he says, "more like a key to being strong and healthy."

FAVORITE GLUTEN-FREE FOODS: Larabars, cashews, Pamela's Peanut Butter Cookies

Begley, both of whom have celiac disease. As a matter of fact, it's a story familiar to many of the gluten-intolerant athletes we interviewed for this book—an overwhelming majority of them faced iron deficiency and anemia issues prior to their switch to the gluten-free diet. (And without exception, *all* of them are performing *much* better with recovered iron levels since going gluten-free.)

For athletes like these, the gluten-free diet restores the ability to absorb dietary iron, thus replenishing hemoglobin and red blood cells.

IRON AND THE GLUTEN-FREE DIET

The gluten-free diet can be something of a mixed bag when it comes to iron. It all depends on what sort of gluten-free diet you're eating. If it's a poor gluten-free diet, you're setting yourself up for iron-related problems. If it's a good gluten-free diet, you're setting the stage for a full recovery from any iron-related issues you've been facing. Allow us to explain.

On the one hand, a poor gluten-free diet can place you at greater risk for iron deficiency, beyond that to which you're already predisposed as an athlete. Here's at least one reason why:

Regular, unbleached whole wheat flour contains about 3.6 milligrams (mg) of iron per 100-gram serving.[10] Much of the wheat flour consumed in the United States, however, is in the form of bleached, enriched, refined white wheat flour. To make refined, white wheat flour, whole wheat flour is processed, which strips it of many micronutrients. But thanks to mandates from the federal government, such nutritionally depleted flours are fortified, enriched by adding back a handful of the lost nutrients, including iron. (It's backward logic—you remove one to two dozen nutrients, only to add back a handful under the guise of making the flour "more nutritious"—but that's another topic for another day.) As a result, enriched, bleached, all-purpose, white wheat flour typically contains 4.64 mg of iron per 100-gram serving.

Gluten-free flours, on the other hand, typically aren't enriched. And if you're eating gluten-free processed foods made from refined gluten-free starches (as opposed to more nutritious whole-grain gluten-free flours), they've similarly been stripped of their iron content, without having the iron added back in through fortification.

Consider one prominent gluten-free, all-purpose flour blend (which shall remain nameless) made from white rice flour, potato starch, and tapioca starch. It contains a scant 1.3 mg of iron per 100-gram serving,[11] roughly 36 percent of that found in whole-grain wheat flour, and 28 percent of the iron in fortified, refined wheat flour. Given that per capita wheat flour consumption in the United States was 136 pounds in 2008, if you assumed a similar consumption of refined gluten-free starches in the gluten-free community, you'd have to pop twenty to thirty 65 mg iron supplement pills, or fifty to seventy-plus 28 mg iron supplement pills, just to make up the difference.[12] All of those pills just get you back to square one for iron in the diet of the standard sedentary American. They don't even begin to address the added iron needs of athletes, let alone of gluten-free and gluten-intolerant athletes.

But it doesn't have to be that way. Whole-grain gluten-free flours can be just as iron rich as their whole wheat and fortified, refined wheat counterparts. For example, another prominent gluten-free all-purpose flour blend (which shall also remain anonymous) made from whole gluten-free grain flours, bean flours, and a bit of starch, contains 3.6 mg of iron per 100-gram serving, identical to the iron content of standard whole wheat flour.[13]

Even better, an athletic gluten-free diet can—and should—be filled with many iron-rich, naturally gluten-free foods that have nothing to do with flours and baked goods. (Check out the text box on page 124 for more details.) Researchers have been working on iron-fortified gluten-free breads,[14] but to date, many fortified, processed gluten-free foods remain insufficient in their levels of many micronutrients.[15] More nutritious gluten-free products are coming down the pipeline, but frankly, you don't need them. There are plenty of other, better, naturally gluten-free sources of iron and other micronutrients out there.

The net effect of choosing such iron-rich, gluten-free foods and gluten-free and whole-grain bean flours over refined gluten-free starches is that most cases of gluten intolerance–related iron deficiency and anemia resolve completely on their own, without the need for iron supplementation.[16] (Men have an easier time than women getting the iron that they need, however.[17])

These nuances underscore the importance of choosing the proper gluten-free diet. Again we come back to what is becoming a familiar mantra: All gluten-free diets are not created equal. You've got to choose the right foods if you're going to benefit from the gluten-free edge.

And finally, iron supplements are not out of the question. Proper iron supplementation has been shown to significantly improve VO$_2$ max and performance in iron-deficient and anemic athletes.[18] However, supplementation should be done under the guidance of a medical professional, since too much iron is not a good thing.[19] Plus, if you suspect that you may have celiac disease or another form of gluten intolerance, premature iron supplementation can mask celiac-induced iron deficiency or anemia.[20] It's best to get a definitive diagnosis first, then embark on an iron plan that will work for you.

IRON-RICH FOODS

IRON COMES FROM two primary dietary sources. Heme iron comes from the meat of animals and is readily absorbed. Nonheme iron comes from plants and is somewhat less bioavailable. Both plant and animal sources can be great ways to get the iron you need to support your athletic performance and active lifestyle.

Animal Sources of Iron

Organ meats (liver, giblets)	Pork
	Eggs
Clams	Lamb
Bison	Poultry
Beef	Fish

Plant Sources of Iron

Kelp	Parsley
Blackstrap molasses	Almonds
Pumpkin and squash seeds	Dried prunes
	Cashews
Sunflower seeds	Beet greens
Millet	Swiss chard

Kale

Walnuts

Dates

Beans

Sesame seeds

Lentils

Peanuts

Green peas

Brown rice

Olives

CALCIUM

The body contains more calcium than any other mineral. Around 97 to 99 percent of the calcium in the body combines with phosphorus to form your bones and teeth. What's left over plays an important role in nervous system function, muscle contractions, and blood clotting.[21]

While we tend to equate calcium with bone strength,[22] there's more to the story. The small percentage of calcium that's not tied up in bones and teeth is critical to several metabolic functions, including muscle contractions, where this mineral is required to help trigger ATP for energy. It helps turn the muscles on, so to speak.[23]

Because calcium is vital to so many bodily functions, proper balance is a high priority. If blood calcium levels drift too high or too low—in concert with vitamin D and a system of hormones—it impacts more than bones. Muscle contractions can be compromised, too.[24] And when the levels of calcium in your blood aren't appropriately sustained by your diet, the calcium in your bones provides a bank account for withdrawal and deposit.

So what happens when you add gluten to the mix? If gluten-induced damage has occurred in the upper area of the small intestine where calcium is absorbed, low-level deficiencies start to take place. You can't access and assimilate the mineral if the absorptive lining of the small intestine is inflamed and damaged. If this goes on, your body withdraws more and more calcium from your bones to deposit it in your blood. Skeletal material is stripped away to get to the needed calcium. If you can't absorb calcium, or you're not getting enough of it in your diet, the bank account eventually runs dry and the bones become porous, brittle, and prone to breaking. Osteoporosis is the eventual end result, which you see quite frequently in cases of undiagnosed, untreated celiac disease.

ATHLETE INSIGHT

Amy Yoder Begley

U.S. OLYMPIAN AND NATIONAL CHAMPION DISTANCE RUNNER

Born: 1978 • Lives: Oregon • Gluten-Free Since: 2006

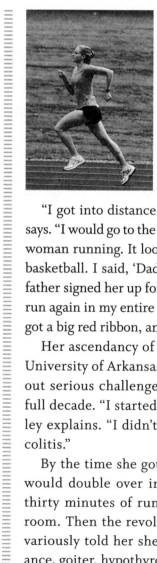

MOST PEOPLE KNOW Amy Yoder Begley as one of the modern-day stars of the U.S. running community—U.S. Olympian from the 2008 Beijing Games, six-time national champion distance runner, NCAA national champion distance runner, fifteen-time NCAA All American, and USATF Junior 5K and 10K national champion in high school.[25] Her impressive resume is long, but her running has humble roots.

"I got into distance running when I was eight years old," she says. "I would go to the park to walk my dog, and I'd always see this woman running. It looked like fun! But I was doing softball and basketball. I said, 'Dad! I want to run!'" When she was ten, her father signed her up for a 5-miler. "He thought if I ran it I'd never run again in my entire life," she says. "He was wrong. I ran 45:44, got a big red ribbon, and that was all it took."

Her ascendancy of the running ranks in high school, at the University of Arkansas, and as a professional hasn't been without serious challenges. In fact, those challenges lasted for a full decade. "I started having symptoms around sixteen," Begley explains. "I didn't say anything at first—my dad had IBS, colitis."

By the time she got to college, things were pretty bad. She would double over in pain. She couldn't handle more than thirty minutes of running without needing to use the bathroom. Then the revolving door of diagnoses started. Doctors variously told her she had IBS, ovarian cysts, lactose intolerance, goiter, hypothyroidism, anemia, osteopenia, and more. "I was sick," Begley recalls. "I couldn't run like that, let alone live like that."

She was running 50 miles per week and getting stress fractures in her tibia. "At twenty-six years old, having the bone density of someone in their forties or fifties was really concerning," she remembers. Her iron levels, meanwhile, were anemic, despite the fact that she was eating red meat three to four times per week *and* taking supplements.

And yet, "doctors didn't take me seriously . . . endurance athletes do have some of those problems sometimes."

In a way, her running may have both accelerated her problems *and* her search for answers. "If I hadn't been a runner, I might not have noticed symptoms for many more years. I think it did speed the process, for sure. I really thought there was something very wrong. Every year, it was something new."

Finally, in 2006 at age twenty-eight, she got a definitive answer: celiac disease.

Within two or three weeks of starting the gluten-free diet, she felt significantly better. Bloating and swelling decreased. ("When you drop two jeans sizes, that's pretty cool.") Her iron levels "skyrocketed," she says. The osteopenia began to turn around. She regained the ability to tolerate dairy.

Then, two and a half years later, she made the U.S. Olympic team. "For the first time I felt like my body was healing and really healthy," Begley says.

"When I was eight or ten, I drew out this whole thing—two goals: to make the Olympic team or open an animal sanctuary." That first goal had been realized, thanks in part to the restorative power of removing gluten from the equation.

FAVORITE GLUTEN-FREE FOODS: Generation Ucan sports drink; Bob's Red Mill gluten-free oats; Nature's Path Mesa Sunrise Flakes; bison steak, fajitas, and burgers (for iron); spaghetti squash, sweet potatoes, tomatoes, and other veggies; lentils and hummus; edamame; quinoa; brown rice; corn tortillas; bananas and other fruit; peanut butter; soy milk; yogurt; and the list goes on . . .

BONE DENSITY

Osteoporosis: literally meaning "porous bones," a
  condition in which the bones lose tissue and become
  brittle, fragile, and at greater risk for fracture

Osteopenia: a reduction of bone mass of a lesser severity
  than osteoporosis

Osteomalacia: a condition in which the bones are soft and
  decalcified

In this context, maintaining strong, healthy bones and muscles comes down to a three-part equation: sufficient dietary intake of calcium and vitamin D (which will vary by sex, age, and sport), proper absorption, and appropriate physical activity.

Even among "standard" athletes, however, calcium and vitamin D intake is often deficient. This is especially true during winter, as reduced exposure to natural sunlight causes your body to produce less of its own vitamin D.[26]

Now here's some good news, both for athletes in general and for those with gluten intolerance: Moderate exercise has a positive impact on intestinal calcium absorption.[27] Not only that, but leisure activity—not to mention regular moderate athletics—also has a positive impact on bone density.[28]

There are, as you might guess, differences between men and women, and between young and old. (In both instances, the latter group tends to have more issues with calcium and bone-related problems.)

There are also differences across sports. High-impact sports such as gymnastics, running, and many team sports tend to yield improved bone density, whereas low-impact sports such as cycling and swimming show little positive effect on bone density.[29] In fact, frequent intense exercise through nonimpact sports such as cycling can result in bone problems. (If you practice a low-impact sport, it's a good idea to include weight training and/or high-impact cross-training to help out your body's bones.)

Those who engage in high-impact sports aren't immune to bone issues, either. Bone fatigue and stress fractures can come into play if you're not careful. Such was the case with a fifty-one-year-old runner with a four-year history of celiac disease. He'd been on a gluten-free diet, but not long enough for his bones to recover before running a half marathon. He ended up with stress fractures in his tibia.[30]

That example and others like it notwithstanding, as with recovery from iron deficiency and anemia on a gluten-free diet, so, too, can going gluten-free have a tremendously positive impact on recovering bone density in athletes with gluten intolerance.[31] Again, of the many gluten-intolerant athletes we spoke to, quite a few faced bone density problems, and in almost every case, those bone density issues resolved once the athlete went gluten-free. Bone loss due to celiac disease may be reversible; with a gluten-free, nutrient-dense, calcium-rich, whole-foods diet, bone mass can be increased.

Finally, just as with iron deficiency, supplementation—this time with calcium—is an option. But before going that route, we first advocate incorporating calcium-rich foods into your diet. And if you're one of the many people who are both gluten intolerant and dairy intolerant, not to worry. There are plenty of dairy-free, high-calcium food sources out there for you, too!

CALCIUM-RICH FOODS

Dairy Sources of Calcium

Swiss cheese	Buttermilk
Cheddar cheese	Yogurt
Goat's milk	Whole milk

Nondairy Sources of Calcium

Kelp	Tofu
Carob flour	Sunflower seeds
Collard greens	Beet greens
Turnip greens	Buckwheat
Molasses	Sesame seeds
Almonds	Broccoli
Parsley	English walnuts
Dandelion greens	Spinach
Brazil nuts	Raisins and dried apricots, currants, dates, and figs
Watercress	

VITAMIN D

Calcium and vitamin D work together in the bone density equation. Vitamin D is a fat-soluble vitamin, which means it needs dietary fat to shuttle its way into circulation. It's important to note that vitamin D is often deficient in people with gluten intolerance, because of poor fat absorption. If you can't absorb fats, the vitamin D in the food you eat can't hitch a ride to work.

Interestingly, vitamin D isn't even strictly a vitamin; it's a hormone—one that we can synthesize on our own. How do we make vitamin D? We do it with the help of sunlight. The same ultraviolet light that we're warned of because of skin cancer also helps us to make vitamin D. (That's why many pediatricians say to give babies at least some unprotected exposure to the sun, to help with the generation of vitamin D. Some research even suggests that chronic sunscreen use blocks the sunlight spectrum responsible for the synthesis of vitamin D.[32])

VITAMIN D-RICH FOODS

Cod liver oil

Salmon

Steelhead trout

Halibut

Sardines

Mackerel

Soy milk with added calcium and vitamin D

Sunflower seeds

Liver

Eggs

Mushrooms

ATHLETE INSIGHT

Erin Elberson Lyon

FIGURE COMPETITOR AND PHYSICAL THERAPIST/PATIENT ADVOCATE

Born: 1974 • Lives: Florida • Gluten-Free Since: 2004

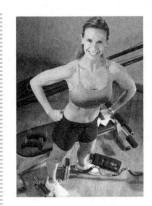

OF THE 700-PLUS riders in 2011's Livelong for Livestrong charity bike ride, not many made more of an effort to be there than Erin Elberson Lyon. Just eleven weeks after her tenth knee surgery, she was back on her bike participating in the 100-kilometer ride to benefit the Lance Armstrong Foundation. Not one to be deterred, Erin considers her repeated postsurgery comebacks as some of her most significant accomplishments. "I like to say that every day upright and breathing is a good day, and recognizing that and being grateful to your body for cooperating with you on a daily basis is quite an achievement," she says.

Erin's achievements are impressive, especially under the circumstances. Another comeback was a four-day, 500-mile bike ride for charity. Riding that many miles with chronic knee problems is no easy task. A cartilage disorder that causes potholelike lesions in her knees makes her active lifestyle difficult. The end result has been pain, limited movement, experimental surgeries, and even time in a wheelchair. But that's just one part of her story.

The second part started with her first figure competition. "I occasionally like to step onstage in a sparkly bikini and high heels," says Erin with a laugh, adding that she also "loves lifting heavy stuff." She prepared for her first competition by spending long hours in the gym and by following a whole-foods, clean diet. No sweets, no processed food, no junk—and by default, largely gluten-free. "I noticed the GI issues I'd had all my life got better," she says. "Prior to that, I thought all the gas and bloating was normal and that having an upset stomach was something every-one experienced."

Once the competition was over and she returned to her regular diet, the symptoms returned. She felt much better on her competition diet, but she wasn't exactly sure why. Doctor after doctor diagnosed her with IBS—irritable bowel syndrome. She knew she had an irritable bowel; she wanted to know *why* it was irritated. Finally, in 2004, a curious doctor tested her for celiac disease and she found her answer. "Prediagnosis, I always felt tired, had less energy, slept worse, had unpleasant GI symptoms, but still managed to perform decently," she says, "although not at my best."

Along with her celiac disease diagnosis came a diagnosis of osteopenia, less severe than osteoporosis, but with reduced bone mass nonetheless. At age thirty, that didn't make sense . . . until she learned that unmanaged celiac disease had robbed her of the necessary nutrients to maintain strong bones.

With a master's degree in physical therapy, a committed yoga practice, and a serious interest in nutrition, Erin got herself back on track. "Now my diet comprises mostly veggies, fruits, meats, poultry, eggs, seeds, some dairy, and some nongluten grain products like certified gluten-free oatmeal and rice," she says. "And if a food won't spoil, it worries me."

Although she still has occasional problems with her knees, she has renewed energy, her bone density scan is now normal, and her recovery time is much shorter. "Without being gluten-free, I doubt I would have been able to heal and recover from my multiple surgeries the way I have."

FAVORITE GLUTEN-FREE FOODS: apples, beef, eggs

NEED TO KNOW

- Fat malabsorption, iron deficiency, and calcium and vitamin D deficiencies (and associated bone issues) can cause problems for all athletes, but especially for athletes with gluten intolerance.
- Iron plays a crucial role in hemoglobin, red blood cells, and VO_2 max, an important predictor of peak athletic performance.
- Calcium and vitamin D are important for bone density and bone strength, as well as muscle function.
- A whole-foods, nutrient-dense, gluten-free diet is important, not only for healing the intestine and promoting proper fat, iron, calcium, and vitamin D absorption, but also for avoiding basic dietary deficiencies in these important macro- and micronutrients.
- In some cases, iron, calcium, and vitamin D supplementation may be warranted, but should be undertaken in cooperation with a medical practitioner.

6

High Octane:
Gluten-Free for
Maximum Performance

HAVING COVERED WHY gluten causes problems for both conventional and gluten-intolerant athletes, the body's energy pathways, and the basic ins and outs of the gluten-free diet and thinking about food as fuel for athletic performance, it's time to dig one level deeper—to talk not about gluten-free carbs and protein and fat on a superficial level, but get more specific about how the gluten-free diet can be further tweaked to bring out your maximum possible performance.

ATHLETES, THE GLUTEN-FREE DIET, AND THE GLYCEMIC INDEX

The glycemic index (or GI) is a general measure of how rapidly and how substantially your body's blood sugar responds to a certain food. Foods with a high glycemic index value (or GI value), such as white bread and table sugar, result in a blood sugar "spike" you've probably heard or read about (or even experienced). Such foods also cause the infamous "crash" that often goes along with high-GI foods. In response to the rapid, dramatic increase in blood sugar, your body releases a major burst of insulin, which serves to just as quickly shuttle all that sugar into your cells, muscles, and liver, causing a dramatic drop in blood sugar. Such up-and-down swings usually aren't desirable (although there are exceptions for athletes, as we'll come to in a bit). On the flip side, low-GI foods cause less of a blood sugar response, one that is more of a slow release. Think of these foods as moderating, stabilizing forces on your blood sugar that help you keep an even keel.

It's not an exact science. For example, different brands of gluten-free oatmeal may have different GIs. In addition, a particular food's glycemic index is also dependent not just on its own properties, but on the method by which it has been cooked and the other foods with which it has been eaten. Take the common potato. It can have a drastically different glycemic index depending on whether it's been baked, boiled and mashed, or fried, not to mention whether it's eaten alone or with a hearty piece of steak or a side of green, leafy vegetables.

Foods with a high glycemic index tend to get a bad rap. With the prevalence of type 1 diabetes and the nation's epidemic of type 2 diabetes stemming from poor diet and obesity, such a view is understandable. But within athletic circles, the issue is not nearly so cut-and-dried. Although there are times when low-glycemic-index foods are the way to go, there are also times when you *want* the high-glycemic-index foods. For instance, when you need to metabolize food quickly—get it digested, absorbed into the bloodstream, and into your muscles for immediate energy—high-glycemic-index foods can be the way to go.

Also, as an athlete, your body has unique, brief periods of time following exercise and competition when it craves and needs high-glycemic-index foods. More on that shortly.

PERFORMANCE AND LOW- VERSUS HIGH-GLYCEMIC-INDEX FOODS

The glycemic index refers principally to carbohydate-based foods, which—as we noted in chapters 3 and 4—are a main source of fuel and energy for athletes. So which should you choose—high or low—if you want to maximize your performance? The answer is . . . both.

Whether you emphasize low- or high-glycemic-index carbs will depend in part on personal preference, your sport, and whether you're eating those carbs before, during, or immediately after your activity.

As a general rule, basing your gluten-free athletic diet on low- versus high-glycemic-index foods will have little impact on your performance.[1]

You'll perform more or less equally well on a diet dependent on one, the other, or somewhere in between.

The exception is endurance athletes. Compared to high-GI carbs, an athletic diet rich in low-GI foods has been repeatedly shown to maintain higher rates of fat oxidation. And because fat oxidation is a better source of long-term aerobic energy, it's often a preferred energy pathway among endurance athletes who have been shown to perform better in certain studies. (A second reason to recommend low-GI carbs is that such meals have been shown to help inflammatory cytokines return to normal faster after exercise or competition, during the recovery phase.[2] In other words, you might think of high-GI carbs as mildly inflammatory, and low-GI carbs as mildly anti-inflammatory.)

At the end of the day, don't stress too much about the glycemic index of your diet. And don't spend too much time—or lose too much sleep—calculating GI values for the foods you're eating. Unless you have diabetes, insulin resistance, or another condition that warrants watching the numbers more closely, keep the glycemic index in the back of your mind as a general framework for approaching the carbohydrate part of your gluten-free diet. For the athlete, both low- and high-GI foods have positive roles to play.

Also, studies show that eating good carbs, regardless of their GI values, is more important for your athletic performance than whether or not they're high or low on the chart.[3] Experiment with different gluten-free carbohydrates in your diet, and go with what works for *you*.

THE GLYCEMIC INDEX AND GLYCEMIC LOAD OF COMMON FOODS

ALTHOUGH THE GLYCEMIC index is a well-known and commonly used measure, a more useful indicator of a food's impact on blood glucose and insulin levels is the glycemic load. It takes the index and basically prorates it against a typical serving size for the food and the portion of that serving size that's actually made up of available carbs. As a result, some foods with a high glycemic index can have a low glycemic load—and thus, lower impact on blood sugar and insulin. A classic example is watermelon. At 76, its GI value is relatively high, but thanks to low amounts of carbs (it is, after all, mostly water), the glycemic load calculates to a low 8.

In the following table we note the respective GI values and glycemic loads for a range of common foods, including a handful of gluten-containing foods (in italics) for reference. Values (based on a "glucose = 100" baseline) are taken from the oft-cited "International Table of Glycemic Index and Glycemic Load Values," published in a 2002 issue of the *American Journal of Clinical Nutrition*. In reality, many foods have an average value with a plus or minus range. We've omitted the range for clarity. What the values mean:

Glycemic Index (GI)

55 and under = low
55 to 70 = medium
70 and over = high

Glycemic Load (GL)

10 and under = low
10 to 20 = medium
20 and over = high

FOOD	GI	GL
White jasmine rice	109	46
Gluten-free buckwheat pancakes, from a mix	102	22
Glucose (blood sugar)	100	10
Parsnips	97	12
Baguette	95	15
Rice Chex	89	23
Baked potato	85	26
Corn Chex	83	21
Gluten-free multigrain bread	79	10
Gluten-free corn pasta	78	32
Gatorade	78	12
English muffin	77	11
French fries	75	22
Cheerios	74	15

FOOD (continued)	GI	GL
Instant Cream of Wheat	74	22
White-wheat-flour bread, hard, toasted Italian	73	11
Bagel, white	72	25
Millet, boiled	71	25
Whole-wheat-flour bread	71	9
Skittles	70	32
White-wheat-flour bread	70	10
Ocean Spray cranberry juice cocktail	68	24
Sucrose (table sugar)	68	10
Chocolate ice cream*	68	8
Beets	64	5
Healthy Choice Hearty 100% Whole Grain Bread	62	9
Boiled spaghetti, durum wheat	61	27
Sweet potato	61	17
Sweet corn	60	20
Basmati rice, white	58	22
Honey	55	10
Kiwi fruit	53	6
Orange juice	52	12
Banana	51	13
Brown rice, steamed	50	16
Bulgur	48	12
Green peas, frozen, boiled	48	3
Carrots	47	3
Lactose (milk sugar)	46	5
Black beans	42	13
Orange	42	5
PowerBar, Ironman, chocolate	39	10
Apple	38	6
Quinoa, cooked*	35	18
Lentils	29	5
Chickpeas (garbanzo beans)	28	8
Milk, full-fat	27	3
Fructose (fruit sugar)	19	2
Peanuts	14	1
Agave nectar, organic, light, 97% fructose	10	1

*Value derived from SELF magazine's NutritionData database

ATHLETES, GLUCOSE TOLERANCE, INSULIN SENSITIVITY, AND THE GLUTEN EFFECT

As an athlete—and for your health in general—you want to have good glucose tolerance and high insulin sensitivity. The two go hand in hand. When your insulin sensitivity is high, it means that your body's insulin is effective at moving glucose from your blood into your muscles' cells. If you have all the glucose in the world circulating in your blood but your muscles can't access it, they'll run out of energy. Fast. Glucose tolerance and insulin sensitivity are crucial for maximum performance.

As insulin sensitivity declines, you develop what is known as *insulin resistance*. Your body stops using insulin as efficiently or properly. Your pancreas ends up needing to produce even more insulin just to try to handle the same amount of blood glucose. Eventually, the pancreas can't keep up with insulin demand, and your blood sugar will rise. Meanwhile, your muscle cells aren't getting the glucose energy they need. This can give rise not only to decreased athletic performance, but also to formal insulin resistance and prediabetes, and it can set the stage for the onset of type 2 diabetes.[4]

All grains (and both gluten-based and gluten-free diets) can affect blood glucose and insulin in several ways: through their starches, through their protein, and in the case of gluten-containing grains, through the "gluten effect." For the purposes of this discussion, starch is an important thing to consider and, as we'll also see, so is gluten.

Grains store their starches in primarily two forms: amylose, which is more slowly digested and causes a smaller blood sugar rise;[5] and amylopectin, which is more easily and rapidly digested, causing a greater blood sugar spike. Wheat, on the average, contains about 25 percent amylose and 75 percent amylopectin. It turns out that many gluten-free starches, including rice, corn, and potatoes, fall in that range as well, though there is some variability from variety to variety. Most starches— whether they contain gluten or not—contain 15 to 30 percent amylose and 70 to 85 percent amylopectin. However, some, such as certain durum wheat pastas, glutinous sticky rice, and waxy potatoes, may consist of nearly 100 percent amylopectin.[6]

These high-amylopectin, high-glycemic-index starchy foods, when chronically consumed—especially by sedentary and/or overweight nonathletes—could result in consistently elevated blood sugar, a situation that can strain the pancreas, lead to insulin resistance, and eventually result in diabetes. Amylopectin is not the whole story, however.

Many factors influence the glycemic response to grain-based foods,[7] including their method of preparation, cooking temperature (which serves to gelatinize the starches, partially breaking them down due to elevated heat in combination with water), the presence of protein[8] (whether grain based or other), and more. As a result, you'll find a wide range of glycemic indices for both glutenous and gluten-free breads. The index for whole-grain breads, cakes, bagels, baguettes, and other baked goods can range from the 50s (moderate) to the 90s or even close to 100 (high).[9] If we compare apples with apples, so to speak, we find that gluten-free and "regular" pasta tend to have a similar glycemic index, but that gluten-free breads made from refined gluten-free starches tend to have a higher glycemic index and cause larger blood glucose and insulin responses than do breads made from refined wheat flour. No surprise there.

But here's where the body's response to gluten-containing and gluten-free grains begins to diverge sharply.

As we noted in chapter 2, gluten impairs digestion, including inhibiting the digestion and absorption of wheat starch. Consequently, gluten-free breads regularly exhibit greater digestibility and greater starch absorption.[10] Predictably, breads made from refined gluten-free starches caused a greater blood sugar rise in studies than did comparable gluten-containing breads.

Now is when it gets *really* interesting. Despite the fact that glutenous and gluten-free breads, grains, and starches have parallel amounts and ratios of amylopectin and amylose, and despite the fact that many gluten-free breads made with refined starches cause greater glycemic responses than wheat breads do, research studies consistently show that the gluten-free diet has a *protective* effect against diabetes. We call this the "gluten effect." Gluten is an X factor that increases your risk for insulin resistance and diabetes. (Not only that, but gluten exorphins, the opiate-like compounds that "invade" the body and cross the blood-brain barrier, also stimulate heightened insulin release from the pancreas.[11] Gluten provokes hyperinsulinemia, which can eventually can lead to insulin resistance, prediabetes, and type 2 diabetes.)

Although researchers are still working to understand exactly *why* gluten is causing such a problem, the *what* of the benefits of a gluten-free diet are clear: A gluten-free diet has been shown to improve insulin sensitivity (including in muscle cells, athletes!), to improve insulin response and secretion, to maintain glucose tolerance, and to overall improve glycemic management.[12]

Not only that, but the gluten-free diet is associated with a dramatically reduced risk of developing type 1 diabetes, as well as improved management of existing type 1 diabetes. In several prominent studies with mice with a genetic predisposition toward diabetes, a gluten-based diet resulted in a 47 to 64 percent chance of developing diabetes. Contrastingly, in mice on a gluten-free diet, that risk dropped to 5 to 15 percent.[13]

These findings are significant. Gluten impairs glycemic management. The gluten-free diet benefits it. And there are implications, not just for the population at risk for type 1 diabetes (where the pancreas doesn't secrete needed insulin), but also for those at risk for type 2 diabetes (where the body's cells lose their sensitivity and responsiveness to the insulin the pancreas is secreting).

When we factor exercise into the equation, the story gets even better. Regular exercise helps to maintain glucose tolerance and keeps insulin sensitivity high. And such benefits don't just accrue during the exercise itself. There's a window of elevated insulin sensitivity during the recovery period following a workout, and that increased sensitivity can last well into your resting period between workouts.[14]

If you're gluten intolerant and showing signs of insulin resistance, or at risk for diabetes because of family history or celiac disease, this is important information. The combination of an active lifestyle (via regular exercise) and a gluten-free diet can be an important way to manage your health and mitigate glycemic risk.

On the other hand, if you're an athlete looking to boost your performance, there's also reason to pay attention. The gluten-free diet's beneficial impact on glucose tolerance and insulin sensitivity can help your body more efficiently shuttle energy into muscles where it's needed to support maximum output.

ATHLETE INSIGHT

Ginger Vieira

POWERLIFTER

Born: 1985 • Lives: Vermont • Gluten-Free Since: 2000

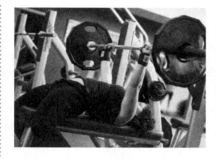

GINGER VIEIRA is both a testament to the common link between gluten intolerance and other autoimmune diseases, and a cautionary tale of an athlete with active yet asymptomatic celiac disease. She switched to a gluten-free diet in 2000, after routine testing related to a 1999 diagnosis with type 1 diabetes revealed celiac disease as well.

"Doctors caught it before it started doing severe damage to my body," she says. Even so, Vieira has not been in the clear. Although "I can cheat . . . if there are crumbs . . . I don't get sick," she says, both her blood tests and her intestinal biopsy have consistently come back positive. "My symptoms are so silent," she explains. This can be a blessing and a curse. She doesn't go through the pain and discomfort and other negatives of a more traditional celiac experience, but her body also doesn't give her visceral feedback that lets her know when she's ingested gluten that could cause her harm.

As it is for many people with asymptomatic celiac disease, it was tough for Vieira to stick with a strict gluten-free diet, especially in college. "During my junior year I was eating a lot of gluten, not taking care of my body," she admits. It was the one time when she really noticed some gluten-related symptoms: some "fogginess," she says, and mild fatigue.

By that fall of 2007, she was ready to reclaim her health. She started working out in the gym, hired a personal trainer, and started taking yoga classes. Within a few months, she became serious about fitness, enrolling in a bodybuilding training program and yoga instructor training program. She eventually became a certified personal trainer and certified yoga instructor.

Meanwhile, in the span of a year and half, her strength had doubled, maybe even tripled. "Someone suggested I try competing at powerlifting," Vieira explains. She had no idea what a reasonable strength was for competition. She entered her first competition—an American Powerlifting Association event in May 2009—and promptly set seven new records across two age divisions (women's open and women's junior, as she was still under age twenty-five at the time), for bench press, dead lift, squats, and combined total score.[15]

Vieira eventually set a total of fifteen women's powerlifting records, though she hasn't bothered to keep track of how many are still standing.

Since she has taken to powerlifting, the gluten-free diet has come much more easily. "I do it not because I'm being told to by a doctor, but because it's a form of 'clean eating' that will help my powerlifting," she says. "My diabetes and my celiac disease have never held me back athletically. I've learned how to work with them."

FAVORITE GLUTEN-FREE FOODS: chicken, lean ground turkey, lean beef, peanut butter, any kind of nuts, apples, low-fat cheese, gluten-free oats, eggs, turkey bacon, chocolate

A BENEFIT, BUT NOT A SILVER BULLET

All of this said, the gluten-free diet is not a silver bullet, and diabetes is nothing to screw around with. We've said this before about other topics, and it's true again here: Multiple factors come into play with diabetes, and the gluten-free diet is only part of a bigger picture. Lifestyle (active vs. sedentary) looms large as a risk factor. So does body weight (healthy vs. overweight). Timing and magnitude of first exposure to gluten in early life also appears to play a role, though researchers are far from understanding the exact specifics.[16]

Then there's the issue of dietary choices. As we've noted several times throughout this book, not all gluten-free diets are created equal, and poor gluten-free diet choices can leave you at risk for type 2 diabetes. Case in point: white rice. In places such as Japan, where the diet was historically based on naturally gluten-free rice, rates of type 1 diabetes are very low. Rates of type 2 diabetes, on the other hand, are higher, and diabetes of both types are on the rise.[17] Researchers point to a number of factors, including a more sedentary lifestyle, an increasingly Western diet with rising rates of gluten consumption, and heavy consumption of white rice. Recent studies have shown that switching from white rice to brown rice and other whole grains can reduce the risk of developing type 2 diabetes by 16 to 36 percent.[18] (Wheat bread and gluten, on the other hand, are a different story. Surprisingly, studies show that whole wheat bread can cause just as great a blood sugar and insulin spike as does white bread.[19])

Reaping the diabetes-protective effect of the gluten-free diet is about not only avoiding gluten, but also about making wise choices about living an active lifestyle and consuming appropriate starches and gluten-free grains.

GLUTEN INTOLERANCE
AND DIABETES

IF YOU'RE AN athlete with gluten intolerance, take note. Certain forms of gluten intolerance, celiac disease especially, are associated with heightened risk for type I diabetes.[20] Even in people with celiac disease without diabetes, researchers are finding higher blood glucose levels and signs of potential insulin resistance, compared to a sampling of people from a healthy population.[21] When comparing blood sugar and insulin response to eating gluten-free breads made from refined starches, those with celiac disease had greater response curves than healthy controls. (This is one possible reason—among many theories—why counterintuitively and unexpectedly we find people with celiac disease who are simultaneously overweight and malnourished. Because insulin isn't shuttling glucose into their muscles properly, the body perceives their sustained high blood glucose levels as an oversupply, and stores the glucose as fat rather than as glycogen.)

KEY METABOLIC WINDOWS: WHAT TO EAT BEFORE, DURING, AND AFTER ACTIVITY

Now that you're versed in the unique behavior of the glycemic index in the context of a gluten-free diet, it's time to tackle key metabolic windows for athletes—namely, how to eat before, during, and immediately after exercise and competition. As a general rule, the longer and more intense your exercise or sport, the more important your nutrition and these metabolic windows become.

BEFORE ACTIVITY

As we've previously noted, the differences between low- and high-glycemic-index, gluten-free carbs don't so much come down to performance as they do to which energy pathways your body chooses to use.[22] Both types of carbs (and those anywhere in between) will fuel great athletic performance. High-glycemic-index foods favor carbohydrate oxidation, which is good for short to moderate distance and duration events and sports with moderate to high intensity. Low-glycemic-index foods favor the addition of fat oxidation to the energy pathway equation, which can be a benefit for endurance athletes in long-duration, moderate-intensity sports. Whether you opt for low- or high-glycemic-index carbs, or some combination of the two, when we talk about "before activity," we're talking specifically about the night before, the morning of, and/or a few hours before your event. (For more information on what to eat in the twenty-four hours or more preceding an athletic event, check out the section on whether or not you should carb-load on page 151.)

DURING ACTIVITY

What you eat during your chosen sport—whether it's a game, a race, or some other competition, or any given training day—will depend on a number of factors specific to you and your sport. We recommend planning your gluten-free nutrition using the theory of "twigs, sticks, and logs." It's a way to think about not only low- and high-glycemic-index, gluten-free carbs, but also fats. The philosophy is akin to burning wood in a fireplace or campfire.

Twigs are your high-glycemic-index index simple carbohydrates. They flare up. They ignite easily, burn quickly, and are quick to burn out, too.

Sticks are somewhat "beefier" than twigs. They're your low-glycemic-index complex carbohydrates. Rather than being a flash in the pan, they provide more lasting but still easy-to-activate energy.

Finally, *logs* are your fats. They're big. They're more difficult to ignite. But they're filled with lots of fuel, and once you get them going, they'll burn slowly for a long time, providing sustained energy.

If your chosen sport is short duration, with high intensity (such as sprinting), focus your nutrition on the twigs end of the spectrum. You need a lot of energy, and you need it now.

If your chosen sport is moderate duration, with low to high intensity (most team sports), build more sticks into your nutrition plan. The twigs aren't going to help you last, so you need more substantial sources of energy. But you still want that energy to be relatively easy to digest and access.

Finally, if your chosen sport is long duration (endurance events, backpacking), make sticks your foundation and consider adding logs to your dietary mix. Regular consumption of sticks (low-glycemic-index complex carbs, plus some simple carbs) will help replenish muscle glycogen stores, while logs (fats) will provide a source of energy for ultraendurance events and help keep your body in fat-burning (fat-oxidation) mode.

Keep in mind that these are just guidelines. Eat what you think you need, and eat what your body and mind want (within reason, of course . . . overall, stay with whole, nutrient-dense foods as the foundation). Your body—and your performance—will follow.[23]

And also remember that during-activity nutrition is contingent on participating in a sport whose duration is long enough to warrant eating during the event, such as a marathon, where you'll need to replenish glycogen. If your sport is short enough in duration, you're not going to need or want to eat during the event. When's the last time you saw a 100-meter sprinter munch on an energy gel as he or she was hurtling down the track? Never—because the event is over too soon for active food consumption to come into play. If you don't have the stored energy that you're going to need in your system already when you toe the starting line, it's too late. For such short-duration sports, consider this during-activity nutrition to be a guideline for what to eat in the thirty minutes to two hours immediately *preceding* your event.

AFTER ACTIVITY

Here's where everything we've told you up until now more or less goes out the window. In the postexercise or postcompetition period, your body switches gears from action mode to recovery mode. Recovery is all about two things: rebuilding your muscles and replenishing depleted muscle glycogen. (Okay, we admit it: Recovery is about *more* than that—managing inflammation, restoring immune system strength, and a long list of other subtle issues. But if you adequately address your muscle recovery, much of the rest will naturally follow.)

Your body has a magic metabolic window immediately following activity. Miss that window (thirty to forty-five minutes or so, and up to ninety minutes in some cases), and you'll lose an opportunity to boost your overall performance.

During that magic window, your body has unusually high levels of insulin circulating in the blood. Not only that, but during the window—some effects of which can last for twelve hours or more[24]—you have increased insulin sensitivity.[25] In essence, your body is *asking* you to give it tons of blood sugar, so that it can convert all that sugar into glycogen and replenish depleted stores in your muscles.[26]

Where does that immediate blood sugar come from? High-glycemic-index carbohydrates.[27] Not only does a high-glycemic-index carb meal consumed immediately following exercise improve glycogen replenishment;

it also improves overall recovery *and* subsequent performance, even compared to a low-glycemic-index meal.[28] This is one of the only times in life when you'll have full sanction to eat such an exclusively high-glycemic-index meal, and it's all because you're an athlete in recovery mode during a key metabolic window. (When you do have that carb-rich recovery shake or meal, note that a single big carbohydrate meal can restore muscle glycogen while maintaining your body's fat-burning mode, whereas having multiple smaller high-carb recovery meals will shift your body into carb oxidation mode, and your fat oxidation will turn off until your diet and training adjust to turn it back on.[29])

It's not all about sugar and glycogen replenishment, though. Rebuilding broken-down muscle fibers—by consuming protein and its component amino acids—is also important. The increased insulin sensitivity and insulin release that follow exercise play a role here as well, aiding amino acid uptake for muscle rebuilding and recovery.

Certain amino acids rate more highly in the recovery process than others. One of them is leucine, a branched-chain amino acid that's gotten a lot of press lately for its important role in muscle rebuilding after exercise.[30] Whey, a by-product of cheese making, is high in leucine, which is why whey protein powder is popular in bodybuilding circles, and why you'll often find whey protein in over-the-counter sports recovery drinks (which also typically include high- and low-glycemic-index carbohydrates for glycogen replenishment).

Another important amino acid is glutamine, which plays a role in gut health and immune system strength. Like leucine, it is popular in bodybuilding and other athletic circles for its potential roles in muscle regeneration and glycogen synthesis. Those roles haven't been strongly supported by the peer-reviewed literature.[31] Consumed postexercise for recovery, however, it *has* been shown to reduce delayed onset muscle soreness;[32] to increase plasma glutamine and branched-chain amino acids, such as leucine (supporting the idea of a role in muscle recovery);[33] and to enhance immune strength and prevent infection in athletes.[34]

A word of caution especially to gluten-intolerant athletes: If you take glutamine supplements, beware the difference between glutamine peptide and pure glutamine. Glutamine peptide is typically derived from wheat gluten, a major red flag. Pure glutamine, on the other hand, should be safe for athletes on a gluten-free diet. Keep in mind, though, that compared to glutamine peptide, pure free-form glutamine breaks down quickly in solution. If you're adding glutamine to a recovery drink, drink it soon for maximum benefit.

Ultimately, recovery meals or shakes containing all of these factors—high-glycemic-index carbs, leucine, and glutamine—have been shown to be very effective for recovery in athletes, better than any individual piece of the recovery puzzle taken alone.[35] This is why chocolate milk, naturally high in all three factors, is a very effective recovery drink alongside more "scientific," formulated recovery beverages.

The balance of low- and high-glycemic-index carbs and amino-acid-rich protein in your recovery beverage or meal of choice will also influence whether your recovery period favors muscle rebuilding or glycogen replenishment, and how long your period of increased insulin sensitivity lasts.

The take-home lesson is thus: If your workout involved anaerobic activity, short-duration aerobic activity, or strength training—basically, anything that would tax your muscles without depleting glycogen in any major way—your recovery nutrition should emphasize protein (amino acids), low-glycemic-index carbs, and lower amounts of carbs in general. This will help sustain heightened insulin sensitivity and fat oxidation for longer.[36] On the other hand, if your workout involved aerobic activity—especially prolonged, sustained activity that depleted muscle glycogen—your recovery nutrition should favor high-glycemic-index carbs for glycogen replenishment. And make it a single recovery meal consumed within the magic window, then switch back to a more regular, balanced diet, to help maintain fat oxidation and other beneficial metabolic changes.

DIETARY SOURCES OF LEUCINE

Whey protein	Salmon
Soybeans	Shrimp
Lentils	Chicken
Beef	Almonds
Peanuts	Eggs

DIETARY SOURCES OF GLUTAMINE

Beef	Yogurt
Pork	Cheese
Chicken	Raw spinach
Milk	Cabbage

A DAY-TO-DAY DIET FOR TRAINING AND FITNESS

What to eat before, during, and after exercise is one thing, but what about how to eat on a day-to-day basis, whether to support your training efforts or just to maintain overall physical fitness? What should be your ratio of carbohydrates to protein to fat? How much of each do you need at a minimum? How much of each should you ideally eat?

Advice and recommendations in this regard are much like parenting. The prevailing wisdom of previous generations has been overturned numerous times, and today there is no prevailing wisdom, replaced instead by multiple complementary (and sometimes divergent) points of view.[37]

Consider the seemingly straightforward issue of carbohydrates, in all their athletic glory (and confusing disparity). Not all that long ago, conventional wisdom held that a "good" athletic diet consisted of 60 percent carbohydrates (plus 20 percent each proteins and fats). One study found that the actual macronutrient consumption of athletes ranged between 33 and 57 percent carbs, 12 and 26 percent protein, and 29 and 49 percent fat.[38]

Today, more athletes seem to be leaning toward a 40 percent carbohydrate diet (plus 30 percent each proteins and healthy fats). Some researchers advocate a diet comprising 40 percent carbs, 30 percent fats, and 15 percent protein, with the remaining 15 percent up to athletes to allocate as they see fit to match sport and dietary needs.[39] Yet, the Tarahumara Indians of Mexico and the Kalenjin tribe of Kenya, both known for their prowess as ultraendurance runners, eat a diet consisting of 70 to 80 percent carbohydrates, exceptionally high by modern standards and current recommendations.[40]

You'll find similar variability if you look at recommended and real-world rates of consumption for proteins and fats in athletes.

What all this variety means is that each athlete needs to find his or her dietary sweet spot. There's no one-size-fits-all magic formula. You are an individual, and the diet that gives you the best gluten-free edge is going to have match *you*.

SHOULD YOU CARB-LOAD?

Within some athletic circles, carb-loading has gained a loyal following. The idea is to maximize muscle glycogen stores in advance of a major competition in order to boost performance. Between one day and one week before the event, you shift your dietary balance (carbs to protein to fat) so that carbohydrates comprise 50 to 60 percent or more of your daily caloric intake. Meanwhile, you taper your training schedule, gradually reducing your exercise workload leading up to the event, and completely rest the day before.

Together in combination, this increase in carbohydrate consumption coupled with a reduction in training load allows your muscles to "top off" their glycogen stores, so that you start your event fresh and with a full tank of gas, so to speak.

But does it work as advertised? And if so, should you do it? As usual, our mantra applies: It depends. Although some studies question the efficacy of carb-loading for improved athletic performance,[41] many demonstrate greater peak power, longer times to exhaustion (delayed onset of muscle fatigue), and overall improved performance following a carb-loading diet regimen.[42] (Plus, as we've previously noted, both low- and high-glycemic-index, carbohydrate-based meals eaten prior to exercise and competition yield improved performance.)

That said, there's more to consider. Although as little as one day of carb-loading has been shown to greatly increase muscle glycogen stores,[43] additional carb-loading may provide little added benefit in the muscle glycogen department. Additionally, it can, in fact, shift your body into carbohydrate-oxidation mode and away from fat-oxidation mode, which may be undesirable in ultraendurance athletes, bodybuilders, and other athletes who depend on active fat-burning energy pathways.

HOW OFTEN SHOULD YOU EAT?

What foods to eat is one thing. But *how often* to eat is another. In this department, the research is clear. Eating smaller, more frequent meals throughout the day offers numerous benefits: greater satiety (that content feeling you have when your hunger is satisfied, giving you decreased hunger and improved appetite control), greater fat oxidation, more stable blood glucose and insulin levels, decreased obesity, beneficial changes to cholesterol, decreased gastrointestinal discomfort associated with large meals, greater compatibility with the timing of training sessions, and the list goes on.[44]

Rather than eat "three square meals a day"—a limited number of larger meals spaced apart by many hours in what amounts to a binge-and-fast cycle—aim to eat at least five times per day: a moderate breakfast, a healthy snack, a moderate lunch, a healthy snack, and a moderate dinner, for example. If you're an elite athlete or a particularly active athlete of any type, don't be shy to eat even more frequently than that. Taylor Mokate, a member of the U.S. men's rugby national team who's voluntarily gluten-free for the performance benefit, eats on average *nine times* per day. And he's not alone. Many athletes, intentionally or not, adopt a "nibbling" pattern of eating and drinking, taking in calories eight to ten times per day.

IS GOING GLUTEN-FREE ENOUGH?

Normally, only wheat, barley, and rye have been considered the offending gluten-containing grains. The gluten-free grains—a much longer list—are considered safe whether you have gluten intolerance or not,[45] assuming you are careful to avoid cross-contamination. But in a small number of cases, going traditionally gluten-free may not be enough. Sometimes a person may have the same or a similar reaction as to gluten, but initiated by a gluten-free grain. Or they may have a separate food intolerance to a gluten-free grain in addition to the primary gluten issue. Researchers have demonstrated this effect with corn,[46] rice,[47] and oats,[48] for example.

ATHLETE INSIGHT

Dana Vollmer

U.S. OLYMPIC MEDALIST AND WORLD CHAMPION SWIMMER

Born: 1987 • Lives: California • Gluten-Free Since: 2011

DANA VOLLMER'S pretty much been a household name in the American swimming community for more than a decade, ever since she showed up as the youngest swimmer (age twelve) at the U.S. Olympic trials preceding the Sydney Games in 2000. Since then, her record has been impressive. In Athens in 2004, she won gold as part of the 4x200m freestyle relay, breaking a seventeen-year-old world record in process. She missed the Beijing Games in 2008, but rebounded in a big way one year later, when she was named NCAA Swimmer of the Year and received an ESPY Award nomination.

Her journey had been plagued, though, by chronic lower abdominal pain. "I always thought it was nerves or stress or 'my stomach,'" she told *Sports Illustrated*. Extreme fatigue became a part of the equation, too. Then the symptoms started to affect her training, often reaching levels of unbearable pain. The problems landed her in the hospital three times.

Her coach recommended she connect with Anita Nall Richesson, former swimmer, Olympic gold medalist, and nutritionist for the Jacksonville Jaguars NFL football team (in addition to her PhenomeNall Nutrition private practice). Nall wondered if Vollmer's fatigue and health issues might be related to her diet. Nall had Vollmer tested for food sensitivities. Gluten was near the top of a list that includes several food intolerances, though Vollmer didn't have celiac disease.

Nevertheless, "I have been able to link the stomach cramping and extreme fatigue to gluten," she told *Gluten-Free Living*. Richesson gave Vollmer a shopping lesson at Whole Foods Market and introduced her to the wide array of gluten-free grains.

On the gluten-free diet, Vollmer's physical and mental energy got better, and she found a greater ability to push harder in training, and to recover faster and better from it.[49]

The widely publicized results speak for themselves. At the 2011 FINA World Championships she won gold in the 100-meter butterfly, setting a new American record in the process. It was the elusive individual gold she'd been chasing for years. (She also won team gold and silver at the event.)

Now, along with many other elite gluten-free athletes, she's focused on London 2012.

FAVORITE GLUTEN-FREE FOODS: rice crackers; rice cakes with peanut butter and agave nectar; Venice Bakery pizza crusts; gluten-free flatbread; for recovery, a fruit and vegetable smoothie with protein; for traveling, almonds, banana chips, and gluten-free NoGii bars

For these athletes, it may be prudent to take their gluten-free diet one step further and go completely grain-free.

Dr. Peter Osborne advocates such an approach. Osborne specializes in treating patients with gluten and other food intolerances. A few years ago, he started noting a curious trend among some patients in his practice. "When I had patients go traditionally gluten-free, a lot of times they would improve and get better, but some of them would hit a plateau, or they would later have some of their symptoms recur," he says. "They were having a gluten-free whiplash, a back-treading."

But when he had those patients go completely grain-free, their improvement was greater and their recovery more lasting. They felt better and stayed better. In response, Osborne today draws a distinction between the regular gluten-free diet and what he calls the "true gluten-free diet," which is a grain-free diet.

"It's hard to make generalizations about individuals," he concedes. That's why Osborne does genetic and food allergy testing on his patients. "It comes down to their individuality, what's unique to them, what they should and shouldn't eat. I build from there with sound principles of nutrition."

IS THERE HIDDEN GLUTEN IN YOUR DIET?

As if you didn't have enough to worry about with getting all the obvious and less obvious sources of gluten out of your diet, there's more to think about.

For instance, Osborne's perspective on his "true gluten-free diet" extends beyond the straightforward consumption of grains. He's worried that gluten can also pop up in some very unexpected places, including ones that are generally considered naturally gluten-free, such as cow's milk. How? Most dairy cows in the United States, he notes, are fed a grain-intensive diet that may, but doesn't always, include wheat—and thus, gluten. Meanwhile, studies have shown that intact gluten comes across in the breast milk of human mothers who eat gluten.[50] Osborne is worried the same thing is happening in our dairy milk supply, too. And he's not alone. Dr. Rodney Ford, well known in gluten intolerance and food allergy circles, mirrors Osborne's concern.[51]

However, although relatively few studies have explored the possibility of gluten in milk, those that examined gluten in human breast milk found average concentrations at levels of parts per billion, with the highest levels coming in at single-digit parts per million, well below the 20 ppm international standard for gluten-free status. In addition, one of the only studies to look at the potential for gluten in cow's milk found no reason for concern.[52] Milk, it seems, remains just fine from a gluten-free standpoint.

But there's another cautionary tale to be told, too; one where the evidence is more damning. Researchers are finding gluten in gluten-free grains and products, including some that are explicitly labeled as gluten-free.[53] There are many reasons why this may be the case. Some gluten-free grains are crop rotated with gluten grains in the field, so that a small amount of "rogue" gluten grain grows amidst the gluten-free grains. Gluten-free and gluten grains may be shipped in trucks and containers that haven't been appropriately cleaned between shipments, or may be processed at the same grain mills. Food companies may make gluten-containing and gluten-free products in the same facility, or even on the same production line. Despite adherence to the FDA's Current Good Manufacturing Practices, gluten is getting into naturally gluten-free foods, especially ones that haven't been tested and/or certified to ensure their gluten-free status.

ATHLETE INSIGHT

Pip Hunt

PROFESSIONAL FREESKIER

Born: 1987 • Lives: Utah • Gluten-Free Since: 2007

FROM THE TIME when she first learned to walk, Pip Hunt's youth was defined by two things: big-mountain skiing and stomach troubles. Her parents were big skiers and had tiny Hunt on "the hill"—as she affectionately refers to Crested Butte in Colorado—at just one and a half years old. Her mom in particular was influential, starting a ski program that encouraged kids to learn to navigate and ski the whole mountain . . . groomers, the steeps, glades.

Hunt remembers "stomach sensitivities" being part of the experience from an early age. "But with my family's English heritage, you don't complain about it. You suck it up. That's the environment I was raised in," she says. "As a small child I would say, 'Mommy, my tummy hurts.' And she would say, 'You're fine.' We ignored it."

For a while that strategy worked. She attended a ski academy during high school, skiing four to five hours per day, up to seven days per week. "That led me to be seventeen years old and totally burned out," Hunt says. She returned to her roots—big-mountain skiing, including hucking off cliffs that would spell doomsday for most other skiers. In 2005 she took first place in the junior division at the U.S. National Extremes held at Crested Butte, at the time the only junior-level extreme skiing competition in the country. "I loved it," Hunt says. She turned pro that same year.

Meanwhile, though, she'd been battling new dietary demons, or at least old ones that had come back with a vengeance. In 2004 she ruptured her spleen, and something fundamentally changed.

"I went from being a normal teenager to someone who all of a sudden, without a conscious explanation, started to not feel awesome," she remembers. By 2006, her slow decline had hit bottom. "I was exhausted all the time; I had no energy," Hunt says. During that summer's mountain bike racing season she went from winning races to tenth-place finishes.

Finally in 2007—after three years of seeing different doctors— "it took a homeopath to say, in our first ten minutes together, 'Have you tried taking gluten out of your diet?'" Hunt recalls. "No one had ever suggested food to me." She went cold turkey, and short of unintentional cross-contamination from time to time, hasn't gone back since.

Her health—and her skiing—rebounded. In 2009 Hunt grabbed second place at the U.S. Extreme Freeskiing Championships. Her current gastroenterologist thinks celiac disease was the culprit but doesn't think it's worth it for her to go back on gluten to get a positive test result. "I don't need that official diagnosis," Hunt says. Her energy levels are up, and she feels "less bloated and swollen."

Because of the hard toll big-mountain freeskiing takes on the body, in the most recent seasons Hunt has dialed back her competition schedule to focus on more filming and photo shoots. She's appeared in *Skiing, Powder, Ski Journal, Ski Press,* and a number of other publications. She films in Utah's Wasatch Mountains in and around her adopted "home" resort, Snowbird, where she's one of the mountain's pro athletes. And she's enjoying shopping at her local farmers' market and cooking delicious gluten-free fare in her kitchen, often with friend and fellow gluten-free pro freeskier Angeli VanLaanen (see page 186).[54]

FAVORITE GLUTEN-FREE FOODS: butternut squash with garlic and ginger, potatoes, tomatoes, almonds, chicken-fennel-apple sausages, cinnamon, buckwheat waffles

Consider the alarming results of a recent study from 2009. Researchers looked at twenty-two inherently gluten-free grains, seeds, and flours that weren't specifically labeled as gluten-free. Shockingly, *one third* of those supposedly gluten-free foods had gluten levels *over* the international standard of 20 ppm.[55]

Depending on your reason for being gluten-free (for instance, voluntarily for performance, or medically due to celiac disease) and how sensitive you are to gluten (not very vs. extremely), this news is either water under the bridge or a major red flag.

LIVE A LITTLE

We don't mean to get potentially "doom and gloom" on you. These are just the facts of gluten-free life, and if you have to be gluten-free for serious medical reasons, it pays to be in the know.

But we're not all serious. There's also some lighthearted news to share. When it comes to the gluten-free edge and your athletic diet, you can live a little.

If you're voluntarily gluten-free for the performance benefit, don't lose sleep if you accidentally eat a little gluten here or there. You might even intentionally "cheat" from time to time. Whether you do or not is up to you. It's a personal choice. Your body may notice it right away, or it may take repeated, regular consumption of gluten to make a difference for your performance.

Professional triathlete Amanda Lovato provides a great example and perspective. She's voluntarily gluten-free. Lovato started exploring the gluten-free diet in 2007, and really committed to it in 2010. She noticed that previous gas and bloating disappeared, her acid reflux resolved, she started racing better, she got faster, and she now has more energy. But she doesn't have celiac disease or another form of gluten intolerance. And so she strays from time to time.

"If I have a little gluten, I'm okay. That's why I say I'm 95 percent gluten-free," she explains. "I try day in and day out to be gluten-free, but if I have a cookie, I might get a little bloated or a little constipated, but I can deal with that. The more gluten I eat, the more it affects me. I feel it around my intestines. If it doesn't make you feel good, then why do it? But around the holidays, I definitely splurge—a piece of apple pie or pumpkin pie. I might not feel great the next day, but I don't beat myself up over it. It won't kill me. It just makes me feel uncomfortable. I can deal with that—not every day, but a couple of days out of the year."

Kyle Korver from the Chicago Bulls and Jay Beagle from the Washington Capitals—both voluntarily gluten-free for the performance benefit—share Lovato's perspective. "I'm pretty strict with my gluten-free diet, but I don't sweat a meal with gluten here or there," says Korver. Beagle adds, "When I have control over what I'm eating, I definitely eat gluten-free, and I plan to stick with it. I feel better and digest food better. It's beneficial to my body. But I'm not going to go crazy with it. Sometimes when I'm on the road, I'll eat what I can get."

Climber, mountaineer, and snowboarder Michelle Smith has a similar point of view. "I stay gluten-free most of the time, but I do have the occasional piece of pizza, pasta dish, or sandwich. As long as I don't overdo it with the gluten, I can have some in my diet without bad results," she says. "It would probably take a few weeks of eating gluten before I would start to get in really bad shape again . . . bloated, loose stools, very lethargic."

Says pro triathlete Heather Wurtele, "Occasionally after a big race I'll say, 'Okay, I'll have a treat.' And I'll have maybe a gooey cinnamon bun," she explains. "But then it makes me feel miserable. And it's not really a treat then, is it? You have to think of your overall health and how you feel. That becomes the priority."

In other words, if you're voluntarily gluten-free, you don't have to get neurotic about the diet. Although you should maybe think about how it will make you feel, especially if it's going to impact your performance.

If you *do* have to be gluten-free because of serious gluten intolerance, we're afraid there's no cheating on the diet for you. But you can (and should) live a little, too, though in a different way. Follow in the footsteps of professional freeskier Pip Hunt and abide by the "80/20 rule." It refers to the balance of superhealthy, whole, nutrient-dense gluten-free foods to gluten-free "treats" and other indulgences.

"If 80 percent of what I eat is really good, I'm okay with the other 20 percent and I'm not going to get frustrated with myself," she says. "If I'm in the midst of competition, I'll aim for more like 90/10, but to have a nice piece of chocolate or a glass of wine once a week is better than to get to the end of a season and binge."

ATHLETE INSIGHT

Amanda Lovato

PROFESSIONAL TRIATHLETE

Born: 1972 • Lives: Colorado • Gluten-Free Since: 2010

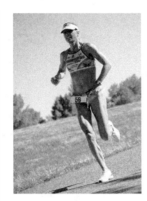

AMANDA LOVATO grew up on a horse farm in Maryland. Her father was a steeple-chase jockey; her mother, an equestrian rider who'd made it to the Olympic trials. "When I was born there was a pony waiting for me," she says. She competed in her first horse event at age three. When her parents divorced when she was twelve, "the horses dissolved." A teacher took her under his wing after seeing her on the playground and perceiving talent. He suggested she try out for the cross country team. "I happened to be really good at it, and when you're good, you want to keep doing it. So I embraced it. And the more I ran, the faster I got," she recalls.

Lovato went to college on scholarship, but toward the end got burned out. Postcollege, though, she realized she missed athletics, but didn't want to return directly to running. A friend encouraged her to do triathlon. Lovato entered her first tri in 1997.

By 1999, she won her age group at Duathlon World Championships. In 2000, she was named a USAT All-American Triathlete; in 2001, she placed sixth in her age group at the Ironman World Championships in Hawaii; and in 2002, she won the overall women's title at the Duathlon World Championships and was named *Triathlete Magazine*'s Duathlete of the Year.

Numerous victories in triathlons of varying distances followed, including a hard-fought win at Ironman Pucón 70.3 in 2010. "I've had a long career, with lots of proud moments," she says. "I love racing." Fueled by her gluten-free diet, Lovato shows little sign of slowing down anytime soon.

FAVORITE GLUTEN-FREE FOODS: organic rice cereal with blueberries, raisins, or blackberries, or some agave nectar ("that's my pre-workout fuel . . . I just love it"); First Endurance Ultragen for recovery, Liquid Shot during racing; cappuccino with sugar-free, dairy-free coconut milk; for lunch, chicken, rice, and an "açai superfood salad with blueberries and kale"; lots of fresh fruits and vegetables, organic as much as possible; for dinner, more rice (or rice pasta) with a protein and sides ("A typical diet for me is rice-based more than anything . . . that's how I feel I've been the healthiest and happiest.")

Plus, indulgences such as dark chocolate and red wine come with their own health benefits, not to mention that they can serve as a nice psychological relief from the rigor of a strict athletic diet. You could even make them a motivational reward for a job well done in your training and diet the rest of that day or week.

NEED TO KNOW

- The glycemic Index and glycemic load are ways of measuring blood sugar and insulin response to eating a particular food. Foods with high values are associated with blood sugar and insulin spikes and crashes, while chronically elevated blood sugar—as a result of regular consumption of high-GI foods—can contribute to the development of type 2 diabetes.
- Both low- and high-GI foods have a place in the diet of successful athletes and active individuals.
- Exercise and the gluten-free diet both increase insulin sensitivity and glucose tolerance, and decrease risk of diabetes.
- Your body has several metabolic windows that favor the consumption of certain ratios of macronutrients and high- versus low-GI carbs.

- Before activity, low- and high-GI carbohydrate consumption are both associated with improved performance, though their effects on the balance of carbohydrate versus fat oxidation vary.
- During activity, tailor the principle of "twigs, sticks, and logs" to you and your sport.
- After activity is a unique window of opportunity to feed your body high-glycemic-index carbs plus protein rich in the amino acids leucine and glutamine, which aid glycogen replenishment and muscle recovery.
- Day to day, eat a balanced diet of gluten-free carbs, protein, and healthy fats roughly in the ratio of 40:30:30, tweaking the ratio to suit your body and needs.
- Carb-loading—increased carbohydrate intake coupled with decreased exertion in the days or week leading up to a major event—is a strategy for maximizing muscle glycogen stores.
- Eating frequent, smaller meals rather than fewer, larger meals each day offers a variety of metabolic benefits.
- Depending on your individual biology and dietary choices, you may opt to go beyond the traditional gluten-free diet, eliminating other grains such as corn or rice, whether due to cross-contamination or cross-reactivity.
- Cut yourself some slack and live a little. If you're gluten-free voluntarily for performance reasons, don't sweat a little gluten in your diet here or there. If you're gluten-free for medical reasons, eat a healthy gluten-free diet 80 percent of the time, but allow yourself 20 percent gluten-free indulgences, such as a piece of dark chocolate or a glass of wine.

7

Channel Your Inner Camel: The Importance of Proper Hydration

W E'VE SPENT A lot of time talking about gluten-free nutrition, about the gluten-free foods we eat to fuel our body for sport and an active lifestyle. We don't know about you, but all this talk about food and sports has made us thirsty. It's time to quench that thirst and get down and dirty with the important topic of hydration. It's another critical component in the athletic equation.

WATER, WATER, EVERYWHERE?

There's fluid in your body, and lots of it. Did you know that, depending on your age and sex and a few other factors, water accounts for some 40 to 70 percent of your body weight?

The reason for the fairly wide range is body fat. It has a pretty low water content, with 10 to 25 percent of its mass accounted for by water weight. By comparison, muscle mass contains 65 to 75 percent water by weight. The more muscle you have, the more water weight you carry as a percentage of your total body weight. (This is one reason why burning body fat doesn't necessarily correspond with weight loss. You may look and feel great and have less body fat and a trimmer physique, but if you've traded low-density fat for high-density muscle, your fitness improvement won't necessarily be reflected on the scale.)

All that fluid in your body can be divided into two parts: intracellular fluid (ICF) and extracellular fluid (ECF). ICF, the fluid inside your body's cells, accounts for about two thirds of your body's total water content. ECF—primarily plasma and interstitial fluid, the fluid between your body's cells—accounts for the remaining third of total body water.

THE WAYS OF WATER AND ELECTROLYTES

Proper hydration is crucial for your body's functions and overall athletic performance. Water serves as a transport medium, a vehicle for waste, a lubricant for joints and organs, a tool for adjusting to temperature changes, and more.[1]

It's not just about the water, though. It's also about what's *in* the water, namely electrolytes. Electrolytes are substances containing free ions, which make them electrically conductive. Table salt (NaCl) is a good example. When dissolved in water, table salt's sodium and chloride ions disassociate, forming positive and negative ions.

In the human body, five electrolytes are worthy of mention here: sodium, chloride, potassium, calcium, and magnesium. All are important in athletics, but the first three are especially notable. They play central roles in mechanisms that move nutrients (such as glucose), oxygen, other electrolytes, and more across cell membranes. They pump fluid, help transmit nerve impulses, and help stimulate muscle contractions.[2]

Too great a shift in the balance of water between ECF and ICF, or too great a shift in the balance of electrolytes across cell membranes, can disrupt cell function in dramatic ways, causing disastrous consequences for athletic performance and overall health.

FOOD SOURCES OF POTASSIUM

Kelp	Dates and figs
Sunflower seeds	Avocados
Almonds	Pecans
Raisins	Yams
Parsley	Swiss chard
Peanuts	Soybeans

Garlic

Spinach

Millet

Beans, cooked

Mushrooms

Potatoes with skin

Broccoli

Bananas

FOOD SOURCES OF SODIUM

Kelp

Green and black
olives

Dill pickles

Soy sauce (gluten-
free)

Sauerkraut

Cheddar cheese

Scallops

Lobster

Swiss chard

Beet greens

Celery

Eggs

Cod

Spinach

Lamb

Pork

Chicken

Beef

Beets

Sesame seeds

Watercress

DEHYDRATION

On a fundamental level, being in a state of dehydration means that your body doesn't have as much water and other fluids as it should. Dehydration can happen in such a way that electrolyte concentrations stay relatively constant, despite an overall loss of body fluid, or can occur in concert with shifting concentrations of key electrolytes.

In athletes, two major mechanisms contribute to the loss of water and eventual dehydration: fluid loss via sweat and via water vapor exhaled while breathing heavily. Of the two, sweat loss is by far the greater concern.

Dehydration can impact an athlete in myriad ways: sweat cessation, decreased ability to regulate body temperature, increased body temperature (hyperthermia), higher perceived effort, elevated heart rate, elevated breathing rate, low blood pressure, insatiable thirst, headache, constipation, kidney failure, brain dysfunction, and, in extreme cases, even death.

It doesn't take much water loss for dehydration to start rearing its ugly head. Fluid losses of just 1 to 2 percent of your body weight are enough to result in decreased athletic performance; losses of 3 to 5 percent body weight result in a progression of worsening symptoms; and beyond that, you'd better be close to your favorite EMT or hospital ER.[3] (The plot thickens, however. Some recent studies have shown no decrease in performance in endurance sports despite fluid losses of 3 to 4 percent.[4] Even so, dehydration is nothing to flirt with, as any endurance athlete who's gone into kidney failure as a result will tell you.)

SPOTLIGHT ON SODIUM

SODIUM GETS A bad rap these days, and for good reason. Americans on the whole eat *way* too much of it. That's why we're seeing recommendations left and right to watch and reduce our sodium intake. But athletes need sodium. It's crucial for good athletic performance. In fact, some athletes are experimenting with consuming slightly elevated levels of sodium. Their rationale is thus: Water retention caused by mildly elevated sodium concentrations may fend off dehydration. Does the strategy work, and is it healthy? The jury's still out . . .

SHADES OF DEHYDRATION

Dehydration can take many forms. The most relevant to athletes and the most common in sports is known as *hyperosmotic dehydration*. When sweating, you're obviously losing water. Sweat also contains sodium chloride, and a bit of potassium, magnesium, and calcium, too. But you lose the water faster via sweat than you do the electrolytes. The result is hyperosmotic dehydration.

At first, because you're losing water faster than the electrolytes, your extracellular fluids have decreased volume and develop elevated concentrations of electrolytes. This yields an imbalance in electrolyte concentrations between your intra- and extracellular fluids. Next, to attempt to balance this discrepancy, fluid flows out of your cells (from your ICF into your ECF). Your cells then have reduced fluid volume (basically, intracellular dehydration). Meanwhile, without properly rehydrating, you're still losing ECF via sweat, further dehydrating your extracellular fluids. The net effect is an overall decrease in both ECF and ICF fluids.[5]

GLUTEN AND DEHYDRATION: ADDED CONCERNS

Gluten impacts hydration and electrolyte balance in several ways.

First, the upper small intestine is the site where electrolytes are readily absorbed.[6] If gluten is causing problems there—whether in healthy athletes or in athletes with forms of gluten intolerance, such as celiac disease—it will negatively impact electrolyte uptake.

Second, in people with untreated celiac disease, researchers have found alterations to a cell structure known as the *sodium-potassium pump,* resulting in excess salt losses into the bowel.[7] With sodium's obvious importance as a critical electrolyte for athletes, it's good to be aware of this potential source of sodium loss (in addition to sodium loss via sweat). Consider it another line item to add to the already long list of reasons for gluten-intolerant athletes to be strictly gluten-free.

And third, in gluten-intolerant athletes (and in healthy athletes, if gluten causes similar gastrointestinal effects), gluten-induced diarrhea can cause a second form of dehydration known as *isosmotic dehydration.* Unlike water lost via sweat, which eventually results in electrolyte imbalances, water lost via diarrhea causes an overall reduction in extracellular fluids without a change in the concentration of electrolytes. Since the electrolyte concentrations don't change, there's no osmosis (water movement) across cell membranes from ICF to ECF. Intracellular fluids maintain their volume and electrolyte concentrations, while extracellular fluids lose volume. Like hyperosmotic dehydration, unchecked isosmotic dehydration can cause a cascade of problems for the athlete.

Fortunately, a gluten-free diet addresses and resolves all three of these potential gluten-related dehydration and electrolyte balance concerns.

ATHLETE INSIGHT

Andie Cozzarelli

COLLEGIATE CROSS COUNTRY RUNNER, NORTH CAROLINA STATE UNIVERSITY

Born: 1990 • Lives: North Carolina • Gluten-Free Since: 2009

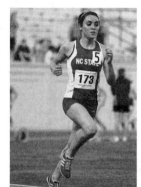

LIKE MANY KIDS in America, Andie Cozzarelli started out playing youth soccer. Apart from the mile run in physical education class, running was something she did simply as part of being a soccer player. But when her older sister started middle school track, Cozzarelli caught the bug, going so far as to wager that she'd beat her sister the following year.

She remained committed to soccer, however, and almost didn't run cross country in high school. The coach convinced her, and thank goodness. That same season, she placed second in the cross country state championship. (Cozzarelli went on to become a four-time runner-up for the state championship.) She also won four state championships in indoor and outdoor track and field (3,200-meter and 1,600-meter events).

During her senior year in high school, things started to change. Cozzarelli came down with mono, and after that she noticed daily stomachaches and constipation. By her freshman year at NC State, the situation had gotten worse. She was gaining weight, despite poor digestion. Her iron levels dropped until she was anemic, even with supplements. She started developing stress fractures. And she was tired all the time.

Sports nutrition consultant Michelle Rockwell, who'd worked with NC State's Athletics Department, suggested Cozzarelli go gluten-free. It was fall 2009, during the beginning of her sophomore year. "With the dietary change, everything felt better right away. It was an amazing change," Cozzarelli says. "I never went back from there." In fact, she went forward . . . in a big way. During the next season, in 2010, Cozzarelli "shattered her previous collegiate-best times" in the mile and 3,000-meter run, notes NC State's Athletics Department.

She lost the weight she'd gained, returning to a healthy racing weight. Her iron levels recovered. Her bones, while still weak, were getting better. And "I felt so much better, a whole lot stronger," she says.

The improvements in her performance have only continued since going gluten-free. In 2011 she set a new collegiate-best in the 3,000 meter and placed fifth in the 5,000 meter at the ACC Outdoor Championships, fourth at that distance at the ACC Indoor Championships, and thirteenth at the NCAA Championships, earning All-America honors.[8]

FAVORITE GLUTEN-FREE FOODS: Udi's Gluten Free Blueberry Muffins, a handful of nuts, and coffee (before races and hard workouts); Udi's Gluten Free Bread for sandwiches; carrots; apples; quinoa pasta

REHYDRATION: MULTIPLE ROLES FOR FLUID INTAKE

Rehydration—or perhaps more accurately, maintaining hydration (since *rehydration* implies that you became dehydrated and needed to rehydrate)—should play several important roles.

First, it should avoid the effects of dehydration by maintaining your body's fluid levels. Second, proper rehydration should also help replenish depleted blood glucose and muscle glycogen levels through the inclusion of carbohydrates in your sports beverage of choice. And third, it should help to maintain or restore electrolyte concentrations, which are influenced by both dehydration *and* how you choose to rehydrate. Allow us to explain.

THE DANGERS OF HYPONATREMIA

When it comes to maintaining hydration or rehydrating, water might seem like an obvious choice. And it is, within limits. After all, water has been called the elixir of life—that is, unless it causes a dangerous condition known as *hyponatremia*, in which case it becomes a matter of "H_2 Uh-Oh . . ."

Also known as *water intoxication* or *water poisoning*, hyponatremia refers to a potentially life-threatening condition in which there is not enough sodium in the extracellular fluids surrounding your body's cells. As a result, those cells dangerously swell with water.[9] In athletes, it is typically the result of two interrelated processes. First, sodium and other electrolytes are gradually lost through sweat. Without replenishment, electrolyte levels slowly fall. Second, rehydrating with too much water as the beverage of choice then boosts plasma and other extracellular fluid levels without replenishing the lost electrolytes, diluting the sodium and other electrolytes further. In combination, these two processes can cause electrolyte concentrations to drop to dangerously low levels.

Most sporting events don't last long enough for this type of concern to come into play. You're not losing enough sodium, and not rehydrating for long enough with only water, for it to matter. Your body has enough electrolytes to get you through the race, the game, whatever. There are two important exceptions, however: elite athletes competing in ultraendurance events, such as 50- and 100-mile ultramarathons, and amateur athletes competing in "normal" endurance events, such as marathons. In both cases, you have the potential for athletes to be out there for five or six (or many more) hours, sweating the whole time, and, if they're making the wrong hydration choices, sipping exclusively water along the way.[10] Even certain sports drinks may not do enough to stop the decline of blood sodium for competitors in ultraendurance events. With such beverages, sodium concentrations decrease more slowly, but they decrease nonetheless.[11] For athletes depending on these beverages, the clock is ticking, and they probably don't even know it.

ATHLETE INSIGHT

Jeff Spear
SABRE FENCER, TEAM USA FENCING

Born: 1988 • Lives: New York • Gluten-Free Since: 2004

AS A GROWING teenager (today he's 6 foot 1) and passionate sabre fencer, Jeff Spear got concerned when he suddenly started losing weight. His concerns fell on largely deaf ears at the doctor's office, where physicians thought he was losing weight on purpose. (As we address in chapter 8, gluten intolerance is sometimes mistaken for an eating disorder because they share certain symptoms.) Spear tried to gain weight by eating more—upward of 4,000 calories per day. But as he soon found out, and as many other athletes in this book have experienced, he was suffering from malabsorption. He wasn't getting the nutrients from the foods he was eating.

At last, he was diagnosed with celiac disease in 2004 at age fifteen. Once gluten-free, he felt better than he had his whole life. It had a huge impact on his performance as a fencer. Fencing, like tennis in some regards, is a sport that requires balance, excellent hand-eye coordination, both endurance and explosive forms of physical fitness, and also great chess-like mental stamina. Free of gluten, the 2010 graduate of Columbia University was ready to finally fence to his full potential.

And what a potential it has been: named to the USA's Junior World Championship Teams in 2007 and 2008; NCAA Individual National Champion in 2008; first team All American.

He travels regularly to exotic cities such as Moscow, Madrid, Athens, Warsaw, and Budapest for competitions. Most recently, he was named to the U.S. Senior World Championship Team in 2011. It was the culmination of a stellar year for Spear that involved a number of strong results at the highest levels of national and international competition: thirty-eighth at the World University Games, twenty-fourth at the Madrid World Cup, sixth at the

USA Fencing National Championships, and team gold at the Pan American Championships.

As of mid-December 2011, Spear was ranked fourth in the country for senior men's sabre by USA Fencing. Now, as of this writing, he's a London 2012 hopeful with a realistic shot at representing the United States in the Olympics—thanks, in part, to his gluten-free edge.[12]

FAVORITE GLUTEN-FREE FOODS: chicken or fish with rice or potato, rice and beans, rice pasta, carrots, apples, dried fruit, nuts

HOW DO YOU LIKE YOUR TONIC? WATER VERSUS SPORTS DRINKS

All sports drinks—water and electrolyte beverages included—can be classified as falling into one of three groups: isotonic, hypotonic, and hypertonic. All are rated according to their carbohydrate concentration.[13]

Isotonic beverages have roughly the same carb concentration as human blood. They typically contain 4 to 8 percent carbohydrates, and because they match your blood, offer ideal uptake rates of fluids, carbohydrates, and electrolytes. Most, but not all, commercial sports drinks fall into this category.

Hypotonic beverages are less concentrated than blood. They typically contain 3 percent or less carbohydrates. Water is a classic example of a hypotonic beverage. They're fine for basic rehydration, but *not* for carbohydrate and electrolyte replenishment.

Hypertonic beverages are more concentrated than blood. They typically contain more than 8 percent carbohydrates. Because of their higher concentration, hypertonic fluids spend more time in your stomach before moving to the small intestine, causing gastrointestinal discomfort and delayed uptake of fluids, carbs, and electrolytes. They're generally not recommended for sports hydration, except in instances where they're used as a recovery beverage following activity, especially if you're not as concerned with rehydration and want to focus mostly on restoring glycogen and electrolytes.[14]

CALCULATING THE CARBOHYDRATE CONCENTRATION IN YOUR SPORTS DRINK

DIVIDE THE TOTAL grams of carbs per serving by the serving size in milliliters, and multiply by 100. For example, classic Gatorade contains 14 grams of total carbs in an 8-ounce (240 ml) serving of sports drink.

$$(14 / 240) \times 100 = 5.8\% \text{ carbs}$$

As expected, this value—5.8 percent carbs—places Gatorade right in the middle of the isotonic sports drink window of 4 to 8 percent carbohydrates.

GENERAL GUIDELINES: MATCHING YOUR BEVERAGE TO YOUR SPORT

So what should you drink to coax maximum performance out of your body? It depends in large part on the duration of your sport. Follow these basic guidelines.[15]

If your sport lasts . . .

- *Less than 1 hour*: Water and sports drinks are equally good options. Your primary concern is maintaining hydration.
- *1 to 3 hours:* Choose an isotonic sports drink with 4 to 8 percent carbohydrates for maximum fluid absorption and glycogen replenishment.
- *More than 3 hours:* Choose an isotonic sports drink that also includes high levels of sodium and other electrolytes to avoid the dangers of hyponatremia.

Whether you opt for a carb-only or carb-plus-electrolyte sports drink, it's important to choose an option that matches your replacement needs. For example, don't fall into the trap of buying a canister of commercial sports drink powder and thinking that you can just add a few extra scoops beyond the manufacturer's specifications to an 8-ounce serving of water in the hopes of boosting its carbohydrate or electrolyte content. Doing so will just create a hypertonic solution, which won't be very agreeable to your system. Do your research and choose a formulation that's right for you.

Also keep in mind that companies today offer a variety of delivery options: ready-to-drink beverages, powders you mix yourself with water, and pills or caplets that dissolve in a bottle of water. Don't be afraid to experiment until you find a hydration plan that works well for you.

The overwhelming majority of sports drinks on the market are gluten-free (though there are some rare exceptions). Gatorade, Powerade, Hammer Nutrition HEED, First Endurance's Electrolyte Fuel System (EFS) Drink, and a long list of others are all gluten-free. Always read the labels, and check with the company if you're unsure.

ADDITIONAL CONSIDERATIONS

Hydration is affected by other factors, as well. Be sure to consider the following as you formulate a hydration plan.

WEATHER: HOT AND HUMID VERSUS COLD AND DRY

Although people tend to think most about the dangers of dehydration during hot weather when they are sweating profusely, dehydration is also a concern for cold-weather athletes, who still lose fluids and electrolytes through perspiration, as well as water vapor through exhalation. No matter what your sport, and no matter what climate you're in, hydration should remain central to your fitness plan.

FOOD AS HYDRATION?

Food contains water. And as you might guess, some foods have more water in them than other foods, sometimes by a wide margin. Processed foods—both glutenous and gluten-free—such as cakes, cookies, and snack foods, have almost no water content. By comparison, many raw vegetables and fruits contain over 90 percent water, including cucumbers, lettuce, Swiss chard, bean sprouts, celery, cantaloupe, watermelon, and berries. They offer up some valuable phytonutrients, and they also count as additional hydration. Those wedges of oranges so common at halftime during youth league soccer games? They provide some energy in the form of sugars in the orange, but they're also helping to rehydrate the players.

THE GREAT (NON)DEBATE: SIP VERSUS GULP

Should you frequently sip your beverage of choice, or take big swigs from time to time? There's no debate here: Those fluids will move more quickly and smoothly from your stomach to your small intestine and then get taken up into your body if you sip along the way. Don't slam your stomach with lots of fluid all at once.

DIETARY SOURCES VERSUS PILL POPPING

While part of this chapter has focused on carbohydrate and electrolyte replacement through fluids and rehydration, don't forget the virtues of natural dietary sources of these nutrients as well. Elsewhere in this book we've gone into great detail about great gluten-free sources of carbohydrates. For electrolytes, and especially sodium, you can look to salty foods such as salted gluten-free pretzels, pickles, bacon, or salt potatoes. (For more, see the boxes on dietary sources of sodium and potassium on pages 164 and 165.) Plus, dietary sources of sodium can have the added benefit of making you thirsty, which encourages drinking fluids to satiate the thirst and rehydrate—this is good since exercise can suppress thirst, prompting you not to take in all the fluids you need to replace sweat losses.

And, if dietary sources of carbs and electrolytes aren't your thing, a number of companies make pills that you can take, usually in combination with isotonic or even hypotonic fluids such as water. Pro triathlete Tyler Stewart has found that formula works for her. "I'm not a huge fan of electrolyte drinks," she says. "I've had stomach issues with a lot of beverage mixes." Plus, "I'm a huge sweater," she adds. "I find that electrolyte pills and water are what works best for my body."

ATHLETE INSIGHT

Tyler Stewart

PROFESSIONAL TRIATHLETE

Born: 1978 • Lives: California • Gluten-Free Since: 2007

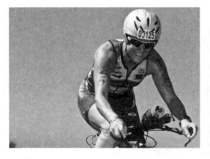

LIKE FELLOW PRO triathlete Amanda Lovato, Stewart grew up riding horses competitively. "The horse was the athlete; I was just the rider," she jokes. After attending Trinity College in Connecticut, she ended up in San Francisco. Stewart went to the gym three or four days per week, lifted some weights, and took spin classes—"general calorie-burning exercises," she says. She did her first triathlon in 2003 as a dare.

In just her second triathlon ever, she qualified for Kona and the Ironman World Championships. Kona was her first actual Ironman, and she placed sixth. Then in 2005 *and* 2006, Stewart was the overall women's amateur champion at Kona. She went pro after that.

In 2007, Stewart was named USAT Rookie of the Year. Today, she's tallied many wins, and more podium finishes than you can count. Winning the Ironman Coeur d'Alene in 2009 and setting a new course record in the process stands out as a particularly memorable moment for her. More recently, at Ironman Texas in 2011, she clocked the fastest women's Ironman bike split of all time.[16]

FAVORITE GLUTEN-FREE FOODS: Food for Life gluten-free English muffins with peanut butter, honey, and a banana; fruit; veggies; hummus; for lunch, a salad with salmon, chicken, or steak; for an afternoon snack, an almond milk yogurt; for dinner, potatoes or rice with vegetables and again chicken, fish, or steak

Like many athletes, she's still after the elusive "perfect solution," she says. "I have yet to have an Ironman race where nutrition didn't become an issue." This, from one of the best Ironman triathletes around.

INDIVIDUALITY (AGAIN)

This brings us back, once again, to the topic of individuality. Athletes have great variability in their need for rehydration, carbohydrate replenishment, and electrolyte replacement. Your personal biology and diet, your perspiration rate, and your level of exertion and energy expenditure will all influence what your body needs to keep going.

Some people prefer to get everything they need through fluids. Some find their stomach feels better with some easily digested solid foods. Some prefer fluids in combination with energy gels or energy chews. And some show a preference of formulated energy drinks, whereas others gravitate toward whole natural sources (bananas, oranges, sandwiches, etc.).

We said it in chapter 6, regarding finding your personal perfect ratio of carbs to protein to fat, and we'll say it here, this time in reference to your preferred mode of hydration and the carb and electrolyte replenishment that goes along with it: Take time to find your sweet spot.

SMOOTHIES AND JUICING

While we're talking about this nexus of hydration and nutrition, it seems an opportune time to talk about smoothies and juicing. They can play roles in hydration and nutrition, and depending on what ingredients you use, in recovery (see chapter 6) and cleanses (see chapter 9).

SMOOTHIES: PULVERIZED PLANT POWER FOR PEAK PERFORMANCE

Smoothies are the perfect way to get lots of raw vegetables and fruit into your diet with minimal effort. Even if you aren't fond of green things in their natural form (think spinach, Swiss chard, beet greens), by blending up green smoothies, you'll be providing your body with high-quality vitamins, minerals, enzymes, fiber, chlorophyll, and a big dose of nourishing plant chemicals—all in the form of an enlightened, tasty drink.

It doesn't take much to unleash the sustaining and healing power of plants when you pulverize the ingredients into a form of liquid nutrition. Your blender does half the digestive work (the "chewing," if you will); all your body has to do is ship out those restorative building blocks to your bazillions of hardworking cells. Start the day, fuel a workout, or speed up recovery time with a fresh mix of whole-food goodness. Easy to make, easy to digest, and easy to adjust according to individual needs and preferences, smoothies should be on every busy athlete's menu.

FUN FACT

THE BODY OF an average adult is made of up nearly one hundred trillion cells in the form of about two hundred different cell types. Nourish them well.

SMOOTHIE MAKING 101

If you're going to become a smoothie addict, you need a good blender— one with a high-speed motor powerful enough to propel a small car (okay, that might be a slight exaggeration, but you get the idea . . .). These appliances can be expensive, but they're worth the investment. Raw beet chunks, celery, broccoli stalks, nuts, and seeds aren't easy to conquer with a wimpy blender. You want your smoothie to have a liquid consistency; that way your body can kick back, relax, and assimilate the nutrients with ease.

By making your own smoothies from scratch with whole foods, there's little chance of gluten sneaking in. There are no cryptic labels to read or chemical-sounding words to decipher. Unprocessed (preferably organic), real food is naturally gluten-free and contains health-enhancing attributes that packaged food lacks. When you eat the whole food, you benefit from the synergistic combination of all the phytonutrients. Many nutrients team up with others present in the same plant to deliver more antioxidant power than they would on their own. They work together, making the total effect greater than the sum of the parts. Rather than rely on supplements with over-the-top health claims, go for the real thing.

Vegetables should take center stage in creating your smoothies. They're loaded with vitamins, minerals, and an assortment of natural chemicals that give the plants their intense colors and provide us with enhanced healing power. Blending also retains every piece of the plant, so you get a big hit of fiber with your liquid.

Rotate your smoothie ingredients to receive a wide variety of hard-working compounds. Each plant has its own special substances that help fight disease and boost immune function. Along with all the good stuff, some plants also contain small quantities of toxins (such as naturally occurring alkaloids in leafy greens and the nightshade family; e.g., white potatoes, tomatoes, or peppers). These normally aren't a problem, but if you continually eat the same thing over and over, you might react to the substance. Some plants contain antinutrients, which can interfere with digestion or disrupt the absorption of nutrients (for example, oxalates found in leafy greens, such as spinach, bind to calcium and lower its absorption). Alternate among spinach, kale, chard, beet greens, romaine lettuce, mustard greens, and radicchio—be creative and shuffle it up for a nourishing mix of superstar ingredients.

SMOOTHIE-MAKING TIPS

- Use two to three vegetables per each piece of fruit.
- Choose organic if possible. Peel fruit that is not organic.
- Use coconut water, filtered water, nut milks, or green tea as the liquid, rather than high-calorie fruit juices.
- Stalks of collard greens, chard, kale, and mustard greens have a slightly bitter taste. Stalks of beet greens, spinach, baby chard, and dandelion greens are mild.
- Add a protein choice, such as ground hemp or chia seeds.
- Cut ripe bananas into chunks. Place on a small, parchment paper–lined tray and freeze. Place the

frozen chunks in a plastic bag, store in the freezer, and use as needed.

- Sweeten smoothies by adding soaked and pitted dates or prunes to the mix. Use the soaking water as well. A tablespoon of honey, agave nectar, maple syrup, or coconut sugar will also do the trick. Alternatively, ¼ teaspoon of powdered stevia or a drop of liquid stevia will work, too.
- A scoop of Greek yogurt adds creaminess.
- Freeze any extra in small ice cube trays. Let thaw and add to new smoothies, keep frozen and use as smoothie ice cubes in new smoothies, or freeze them with wooden tongue depressor sticks or something similar to make into frozen smoothie pops.

JUICING

Juicing is essentially making a smoothie without the fiber. With the fiber removed, you get a direct shot of easy-to-assimilate nutrition. Smoothies provide a more balanced and complete "meal" because fiber is an essential, health-promoting substance, but there are times when juicing is a great option. If you've been sick or have digestive problems, juicing gives you plenty of nourishment when you can't tolerate the fiber.

Unless you're using easy-to-juice citrus fruits such as oranges, grapefruit, lemons, and limes, you'll want to look into buying a good juicer. Like a good blender, these can be expensive.

JUICING TIP

DON'T DISCARD THE fiber. Instead, save it and add it to meatloaf, veggie burgers, or even to baked goods (in small quantities) to boost the fiber content.

ATHLETE INSIGHT

Kendra Nielsen
AMATEUR TRIATHLETE
Born: 1979 • Lives: California • Gluten-Free Since: 2009

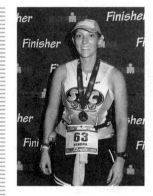

WHILE A LAW student, Kendra Nielsen had unexplained weight and hair loss (at the time she attributed it to the stress of law school) and elevated liver enzymes. Later, she developed a skin rash on her elbows and knees that would come and go. A new primary care doctor tested all her patients, including Nielsen, for gluten sensitivity. Test results came back positive. "The doctor suggested I go try going gluten-free for a few months," Nielsen says. "Looking back, she probably knew it was a problem for me, but didn't want to freak me out." Follow-up testing confirmed celiac disease.

"The first few months after going gluten-free, I felt like I had a lot more energy. My asthma got a lot better," she says. Her iron-deficiency anemia resolved, too. Meanwhile, Nielsen got into open-water swimming, running, cycling, and triathlons, building her way up to half Ironman distances with aspirations for more. In fact, she received her celiac diagnosis mere weeks before her first full Ironman. She successfully finished Ironman Florida and has her sights set on new sporting adventures. "I like doing challenges that I don't really know if I can do. . . . The idea of trying is really exciting," she says.

FAVORITE GLUTEN-FREE FOODS: sweet potatoes; Lundberg gluten-free rice pasta, with a bit of Earth Balance and sometimes Parmesan cheese and some greens; hot gluten-free cereal or gluten-free cream of buckwheat with sliced apples for breakfast ("smells like banana bread"); Larabar cashew cookie bar; Hammer Nutrition HEED sports drink

NEED TO KNOW

- Depending on age, sex, percent body fat, and other factors, your body is 40 to 70 percent water by weight.
- Body fluid is divided between intracellular (about two thirds) and extracellular (about one third).
- The balance of water and electrolytes (such as sodium, chloride, and potassium) in the body is crucial for health and performance.
- Dehydration is the result of fluid loss and can have disastrous effects on health and performance.
- Dehydration via sweat results in unequal losses of water and electrolytes, resulting in electrolyte imbalances and loss of fluid from both intra- and extracellular regions.
- Dehydration via gluten-induced (or other) diarrhea causes equal losses of water and electrolytes, resulting in loss of extracellular fluid only.
- Hydration and rehydration play three important roles: fluid replacement, carbohydrate/glucose/glycogen replenishment, and electrolyte replenishment.
- Hyponatremia is a potentially life-threatening condition associated with elevated water intake and plummeting electrolyte concentrations.
- Isotonic sports drinks contain 4 to 8 percent carbohydrates, and are ideal for maximum fluid, carb, and electrolyte uptake. Water is hypotonic.
- As duration of your sport increases, carbohydrate and electrolyte replacement become increasingly important. For shorter duration sports, water and sports drinks may serve equally well for hydration.
- Smoothies and juices (vegetable- and fruit-based drinks with and without the fiber, respectively) are great ways to naturally get fluids *plus* nutrition.

8

Getting Personal: Sport-, Gender-, and Age-Specific Advice

W E'VE SPENT MUCH of this book building a case for the gluten-free edge, adding detail as we go along—why gluten is bad, why gluten-free is good, how your body recruits energy, how gluten-free food is the foundation for your body's fuel, and how you can tweak your gluten-free nutrition to make it high-octane, high-performance stuff. Now, it's time to get specific, with advice tailored to your sport, your gender (special concerns for female athletes), and your age (special concerns for older athletes). Plus, we address that nagging problem that will rear its ugly head from time to time for gluten-free athletes with gluten intolerance (hopefully not too often): what to do when you've been "glutened"—accidentally exposed to gluten.

BACKCOUNTRY RECREATION (SKIING, HIKING, MOUNTAINEERING, BACKPACKING)

Skiing Magazine is one of the marquee publications of the ski world. For a snowsports athlete, landing a photo within its pages, let alone on the cover, is often considered a career highlight. Such a notch in a skier's belt can validate a career built on snow . . . or even launch one. Pick up a copy of the November 2011 issue, for example, and you'll see a stunning shot of a skier somewhere in the mountains near Snowbird, Utah. Save for a silver helmet, rainbow reflective goggles, and the pink arms and chest of the person's jacket, the skier is hidden behind a spray of deep powder. That person is professional freeskier Angeli VanLaanen. She's equally at home in the park and pipe or shredding a big mountain line, and as you might guess, she's gluten-free—diagnosed with gluten sensitivity nearly one year earlier, around January 2011.

For athletes like VanLaanen, maintaining the gluten-free diet takes on additional considerations in the backcountry, whether high on a mountain, deep in a canyon, or in the forests somewhere in between. Skiing, hiking, mountaineering, backpacking, rock or ice climbing, sea kayaking, whitewater paddling—they all have at least one thing in common: You're carrying your gluten-free nutrition in a pack on your back (or the cargo space of your boat). That means the food has to be portable. Unless you're out during winter, it also has to get by without the benefit of refrigeration. Both size and weight of the food are issues, because you're limited by how much you can (or want) to carry. You face the dilemma of how much of that food should be fresh and ready to eat, versus how much should be dehydrated and require water, boiling, and or cooking to make it into a meal. And of course, you're tasked with appropriately fueling your body, sometimes under adverse weather conditions, for many hours—or even days—on end.

Just ask gluten-free climber, mountaineer, and snowboarder extraordinaire Michelle Smith (whose husband, Jason, coincidentally works at *Freeskier Magazine*, in which VanLaanen has also appeared). The resident of Jackson Hole, Wyoming, has the Teton Mountains as her backyard and playground, where she pushes herself to extremes. "I climb and snowboard peaks in the Tetons. I'm in the mountains pushing myself for sometimes ten to twenty hours at a time," she says. "And I'm out there doing it in all kinds of harsh conditions and weather." These are no casual Sunday afternoon hikes; we're talking ski mountaineering on exposed, heart-pounding, technical terrain. None of it would be possible without her previous diagnosis of gluten intolerance and her switch to the gluten-free diet.

But what does it take to fuel "peak" performance in the backcountry?

Backcountry recreation is a different beast than other sports. You have to sustain low to moderate intensity all day long. It takes the right kinds of fuel, and a lot of it, to do it right. Unfortunately, many athletes don't fuel up properly. For example, elite backcountry athletes that compete in endurance adventure races such as Primal Quest—in which there might be legs of the race involving whitewater paddling, canyoneer-ing, trekking, mountain biking, and rappelling—typically perform at about 50 percent of their VO$_2$ max. That's not terribly intense, but as any such racer will tell you, keeping up that kind of exertion for as long as they do takes its toll. They tend to undereat, resulting in a negative energy balance, and decreases in body mass and percentage of body fat. Their diet and body fat oxidation just can't keep up with the exertion.[1]

Here the campfire metaphor is more than apt. You want to base your backcountry nutrition on the principle of "twigs, sticks, and logs" (see page 146). High-fiber, complex carbs mixed with some high-quality, healthy fats are your sticks and logs. They'll help you handle long hours on the trail, and are digested slowly and help maintain consistent blood sugar levels so you don't bonk when you need to pick up the pace if threatening clouds are moving in. Brown rice, quinoa, teff, oatmeal, buckwheat pancakes, nuts, seeds, shredded coconut, jerky, and even fresh fruit—such as apples—with peanut butter make excellent choices. (A wide range of companies also offer a growing list of trail- and athlete-ready snack, protein, and energy bars to suit your tastes and needs.)

Twigs play a role, too. Say you've been plodding along at a moderate intensity for several miles. You check your topographical map and sud-denly realize you have a substantial climb ahead. You need a quick fix in the form of simple sugars—something that is quickly digested. Your work-ing muscles need energy ASAP. Look to choices such as gluten-free jelly beans, dried fruit, a piece of chocolate, a shot of honey, or even a gluten-free energy gel or energy chew (more on those later in this chapter).

At the end of a long day, you need to replenish carbs to restore glyco-gen levels so you can start all over again the next day. You also need protein to repair muscles and connective tissue you break down during long hikes, and fat to help you sleep through the night, especially if it's cold.

And if you're out for several days, you're in it for the long haul. Al-though some ready-made backcountry meals are gluten-free, many— even most—aren't. If you're serious about gluten-free wilderness wandering, you might want to consider investing in a dehydrator, which will enable you to make all your own meals—lightweight, full of nour-ishment, and always gluten-free.

ATHLETE INSIGHT

Angeli VanLaanen

PROFESSIONAL FREESKIER

Born: 1985 • Lives: Utah • Gluten-Free Since: 2011

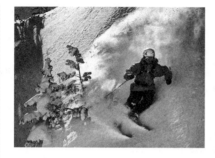

"I'VE ALWAYS BEEN an athlete for as long as I can remember," says Angeli VanLaanen. In the beginning, her chosen sport was ballet. It was all-consuming, so much so that she felt like she was missing out on family ski trips to Mount Baker in Washington. "My feet were so damaged from performances, I couldn't even put ski boots on initially," she recalls.

After trying other sports, including soccer and aikido, she found her way back into skiing (this time with more cooperative feet). When her older brother moved to Colorado to attend college, she followed, skiing the park and pipe in Breckenridge. In many ways it was the classic mountain town ski bum lifestyle. Then, "someone suggested that I compete, that I could win some money," VanLaanen explains.

Her first competition was the U.S. Open in 2006. She made it to the finals before getting injured. Even so, it was enough for her to head to SnowSports Industries America, the premier trade show for the ski and snowboarding industry, and land her first sponsors. Later that same season, having healed from the U.S. Open injury, she won her first comp—the halfpipe event at the Vermont Open. "That's really when I feel like I arrived," she says. "In one weekend I made $6,000 or something. It was quite outrageous for my life at that point." The win also resulted in her first photos and write-up in *Freeskier*.

Meanwhile, she'd been battling underlying health problems for several years without knowing the cause. As it would turn out, there were two unrelated issues going on: gluten sensitivity and chronic Lyme disease. She didn't know that at first, and so when she initially dabbled with a gluten-free diet, she didn't see the huge improvement she was hoping for. And so "I'd go back to eating gluten," she says.

Between fall 2009 and winter 2010–2011, doctors got her Lyme disease under control and she decided to cut out gluten for good. This time, it paid off. "The main thing I noticed was that I don't feel sluggish and tired after eating," VanLaanen says. "There's no feeling of heaviness in my stomach. My digestive system is way smoother."

Now, she's coaching another athlete, appearing in photo shoots, and working on a film project. She may ski downhill, but with her Lyme disease continually improving and the gluten out of her system, things are looking up.

FAVORITE GLUTEN-FREE FOODS: acorn and spaghetti squash, sweet potatoes, unsweetened almond milk ("the water of my life"), Pamela's Baking & Pancake Mix, Tinkyada brown rice pasta, fruits and veggies, gluten-free oatmeal, agave nectar and stevia (for sweetening)

TRAIL TIP

ALTHOUGH MANY BACKCOUNTRY athletes prefer to carry dehydrated fruit, some opt for fresh fruit. If going the fresh route, peel oranges ahead of time at home, saving both space and weight in your pack. Carry them in a lightweight zip-top plastic bag, which can later double as a garbage bag for tissues, energy/protein bar wrappers, and other waste. If you don't mind a little oxidation, you can also slice apples ahead of time to avoid lugging around the apple cores. Apple slices pair great with peanut butter or a nut butter, providing an excellent combination of carbs, fats, and protein.

Michelle Smith

CLIMBER, MOUNTAINEER, BIG-MOUNTAIN SNOWBOARDER

Born: 1980 • Lives: Wyoming • Gluten-Free Since: Circa 2000

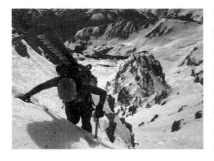

MICHELLE SMITH was once a top Division I collegiate distance runner. She was at James Madison University on scholarship. At the NCAA women's cross country championship fall meet in 1998, she was named Rookie of the Year. She ran in two more championships, in 1999 and 2000. But by then, the wheels were coming off the wagon.

Nagging issues, some related directly to food, were undermining her health. "My body seemed to have trouble absorbing the food I was eating," she says. "I always felt starving even though I was eating as much as I could. The food seemed to pass right through me. I couldn't understand why at the time—I was eating supposedly easy-to-digest foods like bread, pasta, and cereal."

Her health began to deteriorate. "I felt worse each day," she says, "but as a stubborn college runner, I was adamant about keeping up with my 60- to 80-miles-per-week training regimen, even though I felt terrible." She thought she could push through the pain. She couldn't.

Smith's weight dropped. She became light-headed and fainted often. She couldn't recover from training session to training session, or race to race. Then came chronic fatigue, followed by a particularly long-lived case of mono—weeks turned into months— followed by sleeping as much as twelve hours per day by the end of her junior year. Just as she seemed to be reaching her peak, her college running career was over.

An alternative medicine doctor listened to her progression of symptoms and told her to try giving up gluten. To her shock, "gluten" was in some 90 percent of her diet. "I thought he was crazy," she remembers. "But since I was determined to get my health and life back, I listened to him. I started to eat lots of rice, vegetables, fruits, nuts, and meat. After a few weeks I started to actually feel a little better. I reintroduced gluten into my diet as a test and my body completely rejected it like I had severe food poisoning. I couldn't believe it."

She graduated from JMU and moved to Colorado, looking for a fresh start. "After a year out West on the gluten-free diet I felt healthy and strong again. I then started my new life pursuing sports in the mountains."

FAVORITE GLUTEN-FREE FOODS: Peanut butter and Nutella balls, gummy bears, trail mix (fruit and nuts), chia seeds, almond butter, quinoa pasta

ENDURANCE SPORTS

Running, cycling, triathlon, and other endurance sports share some nutritional similarities (twigs, sticks, and logs) with backcountry sports. But because they are often highly competitive—either against other athletes or against a personal record—they are frequently defined by higher intensity that's maintained over a time frame ranging from moderate to long (a few hours in the case of a marathon or sprint triathlon, to half a day or more in the case of an Ironman, to a day or more in the case of a 100-mile ultramarathon).

Here, we address a few issues unique to the endurance sports scenario.

FIT WITH FAT

As we previously noted in chapters 3, 4, and 6, endurance athletes depend primarily on two aerobic pathways for their energy during a race—carbohydrate oxidation and fat oxidation. We described in chapter 3 how, per gram, fat provides more than twice as much energy as carbohydrates but burns more slowly, making it an excellent energy pathway for endurance athletes.

While targeted training (see chapter 10) and gradual muscle glycogen depletion can "teach" your body to burn fat better, did you know that you can also improve your body's fat-burning ability by eating more fat? It's true. Athletes with high-fat diets have better fat oxidation than do those with lower-fat, higher-carb diets. This is consistent with studies that found that higher-carb diets tended to favor carbohydrate oxidation, and that low-glycemic-index carbs maintained fat oxidation rates better than high-glycemic-index carbs do.

If you want to improve your fat oxidation, however, a high-fat diet is hardly a silver bullet. It comes with caveats, so don't discount your carbs and protein! For example, you still need to worry about rebuilding and repairing your muscles (which requires protein) and replenishing and maintaining liver and muscle glycogen stores (which requires carbohydrates), including during periods of intense training. Plus, researchers are finding that high-fat diets may give rise to other physiological concerns for athletes, such as increased heart rate and higher perceived exertion.

For these reasons, endurance athletes experimenting with a high-fat diet are practicing a technique known as *diet periodization*. During training, they eat a well-balanced diet of carbohydrates, proteins, and healthy fats. Then, two weeks before a major event, they switch to a high-fat diet to turn on the body's super-fat-burning mode. Finally, one, two, or possibly three days before the event, they switch to a high-carb diet to make sure that their tanks are topped off with glycogen.[2] (Switching to the high-carb diet sooner than three days prior to the event seems to negate the fat-burning effect of the high-fat diet.)

Warning: Some athletes are taking a low-carb, high-fat diet to an extreme, inducing a state of nutritional ketosis. During ketosis, the body circulates elevated levels of ketones, the result of breaking down fat for energy. While the carbohydrate scarcity (and glucose and insulin control) associated with a ketogenic diet can be an effective strategy for managing certain metabolic conditions, such as diabetes, it is inappropriate for most athletes because of impaired carbohydrate oxidation and diminished muscle glycogen.[3]

FORCE THE FOOD IN

During-activity nutrition is perhaps more important for endurance athletes than for any other athletes. The relatively high intensity and exceptionally long duration of the effort place incredible demands on the body. Without replenishing fluids, glycogen, and electrolytes, your body's going to quit before you reach the finish line.

Here's the catch-22, though—you need to eat, but if you push your body hard enough for long enough, you may find yourself not wanting to eat. You may lose your appetite, begin to feel nauseous, start farting more, or feel as if you need to use the restroom, any of which could suppress your desire to eat and discourage you from maintaining proper race nutrition. This is all normal; it's part of the game. Intense exercise affects your gut, even without gluten hurting the system.

But there's a secret successful endurance athletes already know: You must force yourself to eat what you intellectually know your body needs, *not* what your body may be feeling in the moment. It can be difficult at times to distinguish between when it's appropriate to listen to the feedback your body is giving you and when you need to override the system and force the nutrition in. The athletes that do keep the food going in—sometimes despite a possible temporary increase in undesirable gut systems and discomfort—have been shown to perform better.[4]

Bottom line: You can't go the distance if you don't have the fuel in the tank, and going far enough will require refueling.

ENERGY GELS AND SPORT CHEWS

Carefully formulated energy gels and sport chews have found a loyal following among many endurance athletes, including gluten-free pro triathlete Amanda Lovato. They're compact, lightweight, and portable. And they're made of mostly simple carbs and some complex carbs that provide instant energy—carbs that are easily digested, quickly absorbed, and sent to your muscles where they're needed.

Many companies make both gels and chews in a variety of flavors: First Endurance (EFS Liquid Shots), Honey Stinger (Energy Gels and Organic Energy Chews), Clif (Shot Gels and Shot Bloks), GU Energy

Labs (Energy Gels, Roctane Ultra Endurance Energy Gels, and Chomps), Hammer Nutrition (Hammer Gels), Jelly Belly (Sport Beans), and others. As of this writing, all of the aforementioned options are free of gluten-containing ingredients. *Always* read the label to confirm a product's gluten-free status, and contact the company if you're unsure.

While some athletes prefer more natural, whole gluten-free foods, such energy gels and sport chews can and do have a place in endurance nutrition, even if you go back to the "natural stuff" for training and day-to-day living. "In a race, I need sugar available *now*," says pro triathlete Heather Wurtele, who uses First Endurance's EFS Liquid Shots. "I'm burning through calories like crazy. That's why I like the liquid shots of simple sugars. You may look at the ingredients and think, wow! The drinks and the gels and the energy bars are totally highly processed, but on a long training day or in a race, they give you what your muscles need. Outside of that, though, I'm compelled to eat the more natural, ultra-healthy stuff . . . real food."

ENERGY GELS AND SPORTS CHEWS TASTE TIP

SOME ATHLETES LOVE the taste of energy gels and sport chews. For some, they're only tasty in the heat of competition or intense training. And for some, they're simply too sweet, "different," or processed. If you do opt to use energy gels and sport chews, as many athletes do, for longer endurance events, consider balancing and rounding out your nutrition with savory items and solid foods. This can help make your race nutrition more palatable, and help to quiet an unsettled stomach that desires something substantial.

ATHLETE INSIGHT

Sarah-Jane Smith

PROFESSIONAL GOLFER

Born: 1984 • Lives: Australia • Gluten-Free Since: 2007

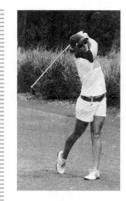

A VETERAN OF the Australian Ladies Professional Golf (ALPG), Futures, and Ladies Professional Golf Association (LPGA) tours, Australian Sarah-Jane Smith's golf career initially went for a bit of a roller-coaster ride because of gluten.

Celiac disease runs in her family. Her mother started experiencing symptoms in 2004 and was officially diagnosed one year later. Smith wondered if her own celiac disease would "turn on." By 2007, she had her answer: yes.

Smith had begun to experience digestive problems, bloating, abdominal pain. At first she tried to ignore the symptoms. She didn't want to admit she was following the same path as her mother. But after six months of particularly bad pain, she relented and went to see her doctor. "I was risking my health with permanent damage to my digestive tract," she said.

Meanwhile, her performance on the golf course had faltered. On the Futures tour—a sort of "minor league" ticket into the LPGA—her ranking dropped from tenth to twenty-seventh to twenty-ninth from 2005 to 2007.

Following her doctor's advice, and her mom's example, Smith went gluten-free. "I was shocked at what an impact that had on me," she told *Celebrity Health Minute*. "In addition to the pain and bloating subsiding, I couldn't believe how much more energy I had."

The LPGA noted that the dietary change "contributed to her success on the course," including two runner-up finishes in the

2008 Futures Tour. In short order, Smith earned her LPGA card, where she now competes at the highest levels of pro golf.

Her 2011 season included a Top 10 finish at the LPGA Founders Cup, plus a berth in the U.S. Women's Open and more than a dozen other major tournaments. She also serves as an ambassador for the National Foundation for Celiac Awareness as one of the organization's Athletes for Awareness.[5]

FAVORITE GLUTEN-FREE FOODS: gluten-free bread, gluten-free energy bars, fresh fruit, nuts, rice cakes with peanut butter

LIFESTYLE SPORTS

Fitness activities such as yoga, swimming, golf, tennis, and even dancing—while sometimes competitive—are sports in which we hope to participate throughout our lifetime as part of an active lifestyle that can (hopefully) last into our twilight years. Successfully making that happen means minimizing inflammation, maintaining good digestion, maximizing recovery, and a long list of other goals. This is where a whole-foods, gluten-free diet comes in. As we've said time and again, getting gluten out of your system and your diet can pay great dividends, including in the long term. (On that note, pay particular attention to the "For Older Athletes" section later in this chapter.)

It's about optimizing every system in the body, a goal that involves not only diet, but activity as well.

Yoga is a great example of that process in action. Yes, your muscles, joints, and connective tissue will benefit from regular yoga practice, but so will your digestive system, circulation, balance, and mental focus. As board-certified internal medicine specialist Timothy McCall says in his book *Yoga as Medicine: The Yogic Prescription for Health and Healing*, "Yoga is medicine, but it's slow medicine. Don't expect overnight cures with yoga (although for many people it does start to yield benefits right away). One major difference between yoga and many other approaches to healing is that yoga builds on itself, becoming more effective over time."

ATHLETE INSIGHT

Taro Smith

YOGI, CYCLIST, PHYSIOLOGIST

Born: 1972 • Lives: Colorado • Gluten-Free Since: Circa 2005

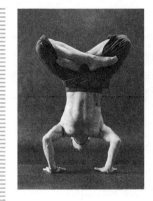

HIGHLIGHTS: TARO SMITH wears many hats: Bike shop owner. Committed yogi. Physiologist. Fierce mountain bike competitor. Podium finisher as a master's racer at the National Mountain Bike Championships. Trained as a physiologist, he became curious about his own occasional subpar performances in races and wondered if it was tied to his carb choices. "I was often lethargic and bloated during races," he says. Was there a connection with wheat and gluten? "One day I randomly skipped my ritual prerace day pasta feed for a zero-carb, high-protein meal and had my best race ever," he says. Once totally gluten-free, Smith felt even better. His body today feels "more normal by abstaining" from gluten.

FAVORITE GLUTEN-FREE FOODS: rice, potatoes, Udi's Cranberry Gluten Free Granola

The same is true for food. A sound gluten-free nutrition plan builds on itself. It is slow medicine, and sometimes in the case of a gluten-intolerant athlete who's been sick on gluten and is suddenly healthy without gluten, it can be quick medicine of sorts, too.

Taro Smith knows well this intersection of food and active lifestyle, and, in his case, yoga. He holds a PhD in physiology and has conducted extensive research in exercise physiology, aging, and immunology. After a brief stint as a big-mountain skier and several years of bike racing, he now owns two bicycle shops in Boulder, Colorado, and co-owns a yoga media and education company. He understands the mix of ingredients necessary to stay in the game, so to speak, no matter what your age or activity.

A committed yoga practice is part of his formula, and so is a predominantly whole-foods, gluten-free diet. He discovered that he had a wheat sensitivity after a visit to an allergist, confirming what he already suspected. He began correlating bike race results and his experience in yoga class with whether he had eaten wheat or not. "Eating wheat translated to feeling bloated, sluggish, and having low energy. I couldn't wait for yoga class to be over because I felt heavy," he says. He's no longer racing bikes, but his yoga practice is in high gear—both on and off the mat.

TEAM SPORTS

From New Orleans Saints star quarterback Drew Brees[6]—the MVP of Super Bowl XLIV and *Sports Illustrated*'s 2010 Sportsman of the Year— to Florida State University quarterback Clint Trickett,[7] athletes in team sports are going gluten-free by design and by diagnosis. The list grows longer each week, it seems: Raúl Ibáñez from the New York Yankees,[8] Kyle Korver from the Chicago Bulls, Jay Beagle and teammate Karl Alzner from the Washington Capitals, and Taylor Mokate from the U.S. men's rugby national team.

You'll find them in every team sport—soccer, lacrosse, football, basketball, baseball, rugby, and more. The hallmark of team sports is that you're, well, working as part of a team. Other players are depending on you, and you're depending on them. The success of a team is a collective effort. That effort extends beyond the field, and beyond the locker room. It's also a matter of what happens in the kitchen, in the cafeteria, in the restaurant.

FEELINGS OF ISOLATION

At first, going gluten-free—especially if it's due to a medical diagnosis, not done by choice—can feel isolating. You may look around and see all of your teammates eating one shared meal, while you're eating another

ATHLETE INSIGHT

Elyse Sparkes

CERTIFIED PERSONAL TRAINER, YOGA INSTRUCTOR, LINDY HOP DANCER

Born: 1982 • Lives: New York • Gluten-Free Since: 2002

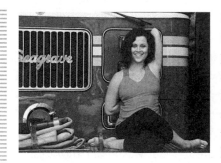

HIGHLIGHTS: AS A child, Elyse Sparkes had dermatitis herpetiformis (a gluten-related skin rash). That didn't stop her from dancing ballet, modern, and jazz. Around puberty, though, "digestive stuff started happening," she says—gassiness, bloating, constipation, "and really low energy."

She went to the dance conservatory at SUNY Purchase for college. She also went to a gastroenterologist. "I decided to really commit to being gluten-free and see how it felt. I was so much better that I never went back," she says today.

Since then, Sparkes has become a certified personal trainer and certified yoga instructor. She has also has dabbled in martial arts, CrossFit training, yoga, and, most recently, Lindy Hop dancing. "I like to be moving a lot," she jokes. Sparkes recently began cohosting events with the New York City Celiac Meetup Group—yoga classes first, followed by a trip to a local restaurant with a gluten-free menu.

FAVORITE GLUTEN-FREE FOODS: chicken, turkey, eggs, fish, beans, vegetables, quinoa, brown rice

prepared especially for you (whether made by your own hands or someone else's). Hopefully this book helps to show you that you're not alone. Even if no one else on your team is gluten-free, you're part of a large and varied family of athletes thriving without gluten.

In addition, remember that every athlete—gluten-free or not—eats to maximize his or her own performance. Any athlete has to put the right fuel in the tank. For you, that fuel is gluten-free. If that's how you perform best, or if that's what you need to do for medical reasons, that's all you—or anyone—needs to know.

Nevertheless, although some team bonding happens on the field and during team dinners, much of it also happens during social time together during the week and on the weekends. When being gluten-free restricts your ability to participate in those events, or at least *how* you participate in those events, it can be frustrating, even difficult.

Collegiate lacrosse player Kristen Taylor initially felt that way. Shortly after her celiac disease diagnosis in the midst of health troubles and her sophomore year at the University of North Carolina, Taylor found herself crying in her dorm room. "I felt so weird crying over food," she says in retrospect. "It wasn't about the food. It was about the lifestyle . . . going out to eat with teammates."

FEEDING THE "FAMILY"

The challenge with team sports, at least from a nutrition perspective, is feeding so many mouths. Buffets rule the day. It's all about one big team dinner, often pasta, sometimes pizza. It's too often easier to do one thing for all. But such an approach isn't especially effective if you have dietary restrictions. You're left in the lurch. "A lot of foods get laid out in bulk when you travel with a team of twenty-six girls," Taylor says.

Being gluten-free doesn't have to pose a challenge in a team environment, however.

In the cafeteria of the NFL's Jacksonville Jaguars, nutritionist Anita Nall Richesson was committed to accommodating her gluten-free players. "I've brought in options," she explains. "There's gluten-free bread, gluten-free English muffins, rice noodles. There's always potato and protein and lots of vegetables and rice. I always make sure there's an option." Plus, she notes, having those options available for the rest of the team may subtly enable other gluten-eating players to slowly make the transition to gluten-free, too. It's a sort of soft sell, "instead of heavy-fisting everyone into turning gluten-free," she says.

ATHLETE INSIGHT

Anita Nall Richesson

FORMER OLYMPIC MEDALIST SWIMMER AND NUTRITIONIST TO THE
JACKSONVILLE JAGUARS (NFL)

Born: 1976 • Lives: Florida • Gluten-Free Since: 2007

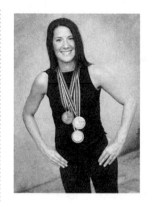

ANITA NALL RICHESSON came from a swimming family. Although she never had any diagnosed food sensitivities, she was always sick . . . with ear infections, sinus infections, common colds, the flu. "Doctors chalked it up to the swimming," she says. As a child she bounced from one antibiotic to another. Meanwhile, she noticed that other swimmers didn't get sick the way she did—one week sick, plus another to recover. "I distinctly thought, 'This is not right,'" she says today.

In a sort of last-ditch effort at regaining her health, Richesson had her tonsils removed the year before the 1992 Olympics—surgery in October, U.S. Olympic trials the following March. Incredibly, she made the squad as the youngest swimmer on the U.S. women's team, at age fifteen. In the process, she set two then–world records. At the Olympics in Barcelona that summer, Richesson swam for the cycle, bringing home gold, silver, and bronze medals.

From that peak, things fell off drastically. "After the Olympics my body shut down. It's like I did what I needed to do," she says. That following year, she got really sick. Her pediatrician suspected meningitis. "My body was never the same," Richesson explains. "From that point on I struggled to train, to swim. It was frustrating, because I knew what I was capable of."

Her swimming career fell apart. In 1998, she eventually saw a doctor who suggested she eliminate dairy. "I finally felt a slight change in my health," she says. "It was this realization that, my gosh, what I'm eating could be affecting my health." Since then, her life has been a long progression of eliminating certain trigger foods, which for her includes gluten. "The best thing I can describe now is that I have control over my body and these illnesses." She's once again healthy.

Most recently, Richesson has applied her nutrition knowledge and holistic approach to the Jacksonville Jaguars NFL football team, where a number of players found improved performance and better health by sticking to a gluten-free diet based on whole, nutrient dense foods.[9]

FAVORITE GLUTEN-FREE FOODS: gluten-free, dairy-free, egg-free, low-sugar spiced bread (containing brown rice, sorghum, and tapioca flours with molasses and spices); vegetable salads; quinoa salads; a lot of greens; potatoes; protein; some maple syrup and brown rice syrup in foods for sweets

For Allen Lim (formerly the physiologist for teams Garmin and Radio-Shack) and the more modest but still significant needs of a pro cycling team—compared to the army that is an NFL pro football team—there is a certain pragmatism to catering to the gluten-free side of the team. "If two or three out of nine guys are doing better gluten-free and for the others it doesn't matter, it's easier for us from a practical perspective to cook gluten-free, rather than make separate dishes," he says.

FENDING FOR YOURSELF

During times and in environments where the team meal isn't gluten-free, some athletes find it easier to bring their own food—to fend for themselves rather than worry whether every meal has been properly prepared gluten-free or whether there's gluten cross-contamination. (If you're very sensitive, you might react if the same knife was used to cut your gluten-free sandwich that was just used to cut twenty-five other sandwiches made with wheat bread.) Staying truly gluten-free can require a constant vigilance, and a constant education of coaches, teammates, restaurant chefs, and so on, until they all get up to speed. That vigilance—and the worry that can go along with it—uses up mental energy better used on the field of play. As an athlete, you have enough things to worry about. The possibility of gluten in your food shouldn't be one of them.

"Some teammates caught on right away. They were really conscientious," says Kristen Taylor. "With others, it's not that they didn't care. They just didn't understand it. There's a learning curve. Or they didn't know how sensitive I was. A lot of times it came down to, rather than fighting the battle, wondering if the food was gluten-free or not, I would just bring my own food."

"I don't really talk about it a lot," Korver of the Chicago Bulls says. Other teammates do their thing; he does his. And that works.

FINDING SUPPORT

One of the great things—of many—about team sports is the camaraderie. When you're gluten-free, a mutually caring team can become an instant support network. For Taylor, coaches at UNC made sure home games and practices had the gluten-free food she needed. They made sure the team ate at restaurants with gluten-free options when on the road. The athletic department reimbursed her for extra gluten-free foods she bought to supplement the team meals. And as awareness spread throughout the team, players' parents joined in, too, for tailgate meals and other foods they contributed to the team effort. "So many different families would bring gluten-free options," Taylor says. "They went out of their way. They would check every ingredient. Everyone was so worried and careful."

Kelsey Holbert, a soccer player at the University of Wisconsin–Milwaukee, had a similar experience. "Everyone here has made being gluten-free a lot easier than it otherwise could be," she says.

Andie Cozzarelli, who has suspected celiac disease, finds the same thing as a cross country runner at NC State. "The team is so supportive," she says. "At our weekly team dinner, they always get a gluten-free option so I can come and enjoy it." (Her coaches also call ahead to find restaurants with gluten-free menu options, and she packs some of her own lunch food—such as gluten-free bread and snacks.)

Alex Borsuk

ROCK CLIMBER, BACKPACKER, FORMER COLLEGIATE RUNNER
Born: 1988 • Lives: Ohio • Gluten-Free Since: 2010

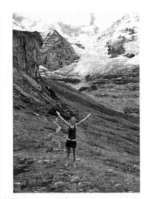

ALEX BORSUK played soccer her whole life, from age five straight through high school. As a freshman at Ohio University, however, she decided to try distance running and made the team as a walk-on. But as her freshman year transitioned into her sophomore year, Borsuk started experiencing symptoms that not only impacted her health, but also had a detrimental effect on her performance.

"This was a D-I school, and I was running well. But after a while, my runs were four, five, six minutes slower than they usually were. That's a big deal in a 5K," she says. "It was depressing. No matter how hard I trained, I couldn't do well at all."

The problems didn't stop there. She developed low potassium. She became anemic "no matter how much iron I was taking," she says. She started developing stress fractures. And she lost "a ton of weight."

Borsuk was eventually hospitalized briefly. After that, still without answers as to what was causing her health problems, she made the difficult decision in her junior year to quit the team. "I lost my best friendships," she says, "or at least they weren't as strong as they used to be."

She lost another thing she loved as well: the outdoors. A passionate rock climber and wilderness backpacker, Borsuk would spend vacations climbing at the Red River and New River gorges, or hiking and backpacking in Arizona, Utah, California, and beyond. Now she found herself too weak to climb and too fatigued to do anything more than short hiking trips, which left her exhausted.

Then came the explanation she'd been seeking: celiac disease.

Her story then followed a familiar pattern: "Within a few weeks of being gluten-free I was running better." Now she's back to climbing, back to backpacking, and studying medical dietetics as a grad student at Ohio State University.

FAVORITE GLUTEN-FREE FOODS: home-baked gluten-free bread; gluten-free pizza ("I think it tastes better than regular pizza, with its good thin crust"); rice; quinoa; chia seeds; natural, whole foods

Teams also have another reason for being supportive: They're interested in seeing one another at their best, working toward the common goal of victory over an opponent. Teams want each player to have an edge. If gaining that edge means that you have to go gluten-free, then go gluten-free. "Whatever makes you feel and play your best," says Jay Beagle, of the Washington Capitals.

FOR WOMEN

Some female athletes are beset by a trio of challenges known as the *Female Athlete Triad*—disordered eating (which usually takes the form of restricted dieting and inadequate calorie/energy intake), osteoporosis (bone density loss), and amenorrhea (cessation of the menstrual cycle).[10] Although the full triad hardly affects all female athletes, many will experience at least one component of the trio. What does any of this have to do with gluten?

Gluten intolerance—and celiac disease in particular—in women often evidences as many of the same symptoms. The sudden and extreme weight loss and frequent trips to the bathroom that often come with celiac disease can appear, to the outside observer, to be an eating disorder. (In fact, in chapter 2 we wrote about a female collegiate volleyball player whose coaches and team physicians thought she had an eating disorder. They later learned it was celiac disease.) These women do not have an eating disorder; they're experiencing nutrient malabsorption and malnutrition—but the end result is similar: inadequate calorie uptake. Celiac disease, because of calcium and vitamin D malabsorption issues, is often associated with bone density loss and osteoporosis. (We addressed that issue in chapter 5.) And celiac disease is also associated with amenorrhea and other reproductive challenges.

And so, gluten intolerance can appear to be the Female Athlete Triad, and as such may not be properly diagnosed. And for athletes genuinely experiencing the Triad, gluten intolerance can be a compounding factor that makes an existing problem even worse. Heck, even without the Female Athlete Triad or gluten intolerance, disordered eating and bone density issues can be problems within certain circles of the female population.

What's a female athlete to do? Most important—and as you might have guessed we'd say—go gluten-free. There are specific reasons why.

First, going gluten-free will improve digestion and intestinal absorption of nutrients, especially if you're gluten intolerant. This can help the disordered eating and inadequate-calorie-intake issues. It's not an eating disorder and it's not your fault if you're not absorbing the nutrients from the food you're eating to try to stay healthy and fuel your athletic performance.

Second, athletic amenorrhea seems to be associated with multiple factors: low estrogen levels, decreased bone mass, and insufficient calorie/ energy intake. If you can improve gluten-induced amenorrhea, bone density issues, and nutrient deficiencies, you can also theoretically help the athletic amenorrhea.

And third, there's the issue of osteoporosis. Like amenorrhea, decreased bone density is the result of multiple factors, including insufficient exercise that generates a force or "load" on bones; decreased estrogen (which plays a role in maintaining healthy bone tissue in women); and, in athletes with gluten intolerance, decreased absorption of calcium and vitamin D. The National Osteoporosis Foundation includes calcium and vitamin D deficiencies as possible contributors to bone loss in women, alongside hormone imbalances, gastrointestinal disorders, and autoimmune disorders (including celiac disease by name).

In combination with appropriate exercise, a gluten-free diet rich in natural sources of calcium and vitamin D can help to (a) improve digestion and nutrient absorption, (b) provide sufficient calorie intake, (c) provide sufficient calcium and vitamin D to hold steady or even reverse bone density loss, and (d) restore menstruation and reproductive function.

FOR OLDER ATHLETES

When we hear the word *aging*, we automatically think of older people, but the truth is, we start aging at birth when we choke, sputter, and take our first screeching breath announcing our arrival into the world. Functional and structural changes occur in the body throughout life, but once maturity is reached at age twenty to twenty-five years, growth stops, and by thirty, age-related changes can become noticeable. The key word there is *can* (not *will*): For active people with healthy lifestyle habits, many of these changes aren't inevitable. But first, we have to make sure we don't have underlying medical conditions sabotaging our hard work and good intentions. Yes, we're still talking about gluten.

As Dr. Alessio Fasano, director of the University of Maryland's Center for Celiac Research, says, "You're never too old to develop celiac disease." What we used to think of as a rare "failure to thrive" disease of childhood is currently being redefined. "You cannot grow out of it, but you might grow into it," says Fasano.

People with a genetic predisposition to celiac disease can develop it at any age, but that doesn't mean you're home free if you don't have the genetic marker. It also doesn't mean you're home free if you've been able to tolerate gluten for fifty, sixty, even seventy years. As we've mentioned throughout the book, gluten is a stubborn protein, and gluten intolerance is tricky to diagnose in the older population, as many of the symptoms can also be signs typically associated with aging—and can "turn on" at any time, even in older age if you've "safely" eaten gluten all your life.

Let's take a quick look at the numbers—the "graying of America" numbers. According to 2010 U.S. Census Bureau data, America's fifty and older population will reach one hundred million in 2012. Now, let's factor in a 2008 Finnish study that found the rate of celiac disease in people over age fifty to be almost two and a half times higher than in the general population. A recent study by Fasano and his colleagues found similar results. We have an aging population, an increased prevalence of adult-onset celiac disease, and rapidly rising rates of gluten intolerance.

The reasons for the sharp increases in gluten intolerance among older adults is unclear, but the amount of gluten ingested, the increased

gluten content in foods, stress, changes in age-related intestinal function, intestinal bacteria alterations over time, and environmental stressors all take a toll on the immune system. Aging adults are prime
candidates for problems with gluten, so if you're an older athlete looking for an edge, eliminating gluten might be a good place to start.

What else happens as we age? Changes in body composition occur.
Lean muscle decreases and body fat increases. As these ratios shift, resting metabolic rate declines—so do strength, power, and reaction time.
We also don't recover as quickly after a strenuous workout and are more
prone to free radical damage to cells. Our joints, ligaments, and tendons
aren't as flexible and are more prone to injury. Cardiac output declines.
There's less blood pumped with each beat of the heart (stroke volume)
making aerobic exercise more difficult. After age twenty-five, VO_2
max—discussed in chapters 3 and 10—drops steadily. By age fifty-five,
VO_2 max is almost 30 percent below scores reported for twenty-year-
olds.[11] We also don't recover or bounce back as quickly after long bike
ride or a day of skiing.

That's the downside to aging, but if you're middle-aged or beyond and
have an active lifestyle, many of these age-related changes might not apply
to you—at least not to that degree. Here's the good news: If you're reading
this book, you're already interested in exercise and nutrition. You're on the
right track. Research is accumulating that shows an active lifestyle, along
with a diet of nutrient-dense, whole foods, is more of a determinant of
aerobic capacity and overall health than is chronological age.

Although a reduction in muscle mass and an increase in fat tissue are
the norm with aging, they aren't inevitable. It takes some effort, but
with regular cardiovascular exercise, some type of strength training,
yoga, controlled energy intake (it's that "calories in vs. calories out"
thing), and eating the right kinds of foods, older athletes can maintain
lean muscle tissue and fat ratios of athletes half their age. There's just
not as much room for error as there is at age twenty.

No matter what your age, strength training can increase muscular
strength and power. Whether you take a yoga class with lots of downward-
facing dog poses, arm balances, and inversions, or begin a weight-training
program, it's possible to gain muscle mass at any age. For example, one
series of studies showed that untrained men between ages seventy-three

and ninety-four achieved significant improvements in strength and balance after just ten weeks of strength training, and that eight weeks of endurance training resulted in an increase in VO$_2$ max in fifty-five- to seventy-year-olds.[12] A wide variety of studies show how well older men and women respond to vigorous exercise, with rapid improvements well into the ninth decade of life. The human body is impressive in its ability to regenerate—as long as we're providing building blocks while eliminating roadblocks. We also know strength training protects against osteoporosis. Cardiac health can be enhanced, and functional losses can be reduced with proper training and nutrition as well. Many of the cardiovascular changes that take place as we age are the result of lack of use and poor lifestyle choices, rather than aging. You've heard it before—use it or lose it!

Flexibility can also be maintained or increased at any time of life. Being aware of proper hydration and participating in a flexibility program can help prevent injuries and protect joints, muscles, and connective tissue. You're never too old to make positive changes in your health.

But first, it's worth taking a close look at some typical signs and symptoms of aging. Don't accept that "it's just part of getting old" if you have joint pain, irritable bowel syndrome, anemia, osteoporosis, unexplained neurological problems (e.g., balance problems, dizziness, or numbness and tingling in extremities). Sure, life takes a toll on the body, but don't let something like gluten add fuel to the fire and undermine your hard work. The digestive system is our barrier to the outside world, our protection against environmental hazards. Older adults have simply been exposed to more wear and tear on the digestive system and may have lower levels of gastric enzymes that break down food. Dietary choices play a huge role in our ability to minimize inflammation and utilize the nutrients we take in. This is especially true for older athletes, who need to make the most of the potential energy in food to synthesize ATP for cellular energy, boost recovery time, and protect against age-related diseases. Don't let gluten get in the way.

ON THE ROAD

Maintaining a gluten-free diet at home is one thing, with the comfort of your own kitchen, familiar supermarkets, and local restaurants. But keeping up the gluten-free diet when you're on the road can be quite another matter, especially if you're traveling farther afield for a big race or game.

Follow these strategies that have worked for many of the athletes profiled throughout this book:

- **SEEK OUT RESTAURANTS WITH GLUTEN-FREE MENUS.** National chains such as Outback Steakhouse and P. F. Chang's China Bistro are popular with athletes. They offer gluten-free menus, consistently trained staff who are knowledgeable about gluten-free issues and cross-contamination concerns in the kitchen, meals that combine hearty and lean proteins with complex carbs (great for night-before dinners), and have locations throughout the country. There are a growing number of excellent resources for finding gluten-free restaurants, including the Gluten-Free Restaurant Awareness Program, AllergyEats, Find Me Gluten Free, GREAT Gluten-Free Kitchens, and Triumph Dining, to name a few.

- **GIVE YOURSELF TIME TO SHOP.** Plan time into your travel schedule to visit a local Whole Foods Market or other supermarket that stocks naturally gluten-free and specialty gluten-free foods. From fresh fruits to gluten-free breads, load up on your favorite go-to gluten-free items.

- **KEEP A KITCHEN IN YOUR CORNER.** Seek out hotels, condo rentals, and other locations that offer kitchenettes or full kitchens. That way, you can cook your own meals and not be reliant on finding a restaurant with a gluten-free menu (and you can avoid the risk of gluten cross-contamination). If you're especially sensitive to gluten, consider washing pots, pans, and dishes before you use them. You don't know what a previous guest cooked, or how well everything has been washed.

- **BRING A GOODIE BAG.** If you're unsure about location restaurant and supermarket options where you're traveling, don't risk it. Bring your favorite gluten-free foods from home. Pack them in the car, in your checked baggage, or as a carry-on in the airplane. You've trained hard. Don't sabotage your nutrition at the last minute by leaving the gluten equation to chance.

- **PLAN AHEAD**. Whether it's researching restaurant options, or local supermarkets, or lodging options with kitchenettes, be the master of your own gluten-free destiny. Play the odds in Las Vegas—not with your gluten-free nutrition.

YOU'VE BEEN GLUTENED! NOW WHAT?

In June 2011 pro cyclist Greg Henderson—riding then for Team Sky—was in the Tour of Switzerland, the same year of the same multistage race won by gluten-free cyclist Levi Leipheimer (then with Team RadioShack). On the gluten-free diet, Leipheimer was at the top of his game, but because of accidental exposure to gluten, Henderson was at the bottom of his.

At breakfast one morning, Henderson was mistakenly served the wrong cereal, one that had gluten in it. It resulted in a devastating day on—and off—the bike for the Kiwi. The press kindly noted his need for "extra nature breaks." The gluten-intolerant community knew the real story—that Henderson was in a world of hurt. He finished the day as the second-to-last rider to cross the finish line, twenty-two long minutes back from the field.[13] His story shows the devastating effect gluten can have on a sensitive gluten-intolerant athlete.

It can be frustrating at best, catastrophic at worst. You try your best to adhere to a strict gluten-free diet. You read labels, eat whole naturally gluten-free foods, ask questions about the food being served to you, dine out judiciously and cautiously. But inevitably, somewhere along the way, you get zapped. What do you do?

Every athlete is different. Some hardly notice having been exposed to gluten; others feel like they've been hit by a freight train. The timing of your response can vary, too. Some feel it almost immediately; others feel it two days later. (Refer back to chapter 1 to review our list of possible signs and symptoms of gluten exposure.)

It will also matter whether you're a healthy athlete who's voluntarily gluten-free, in which case a random dose of gluten will probably be no big deal, or whether you're a gluten-intolerant athlete. And if you're gluten intolerant, how sensitive are you? How serious and severe are your reactions? Were you exposed to a low dose of gluten cross-contamination, or were you mistakenly served a heaping bowl of whole wheat pasta?

Depending on your answers to questions like these, you may be able to push through the gluten. Or you may miss a practice, a training session, or even a game or big race.

Among the four dozen athletes interviewed for this book, you'll find a wide range of reactions spanning the gamut from "That was no big deal as a one-time thing" to "Yikes! I don't want to do *that* again" to "That was totally devastating."

Consider these real-life examples, roughly ordered from less serious to more serious:

- **PRO HOCKEY PLAYER JAY BEAGLE:** He doesn't feel his body respond to one meal here or there. But if he's eaten gluten consistently, say, on a five-day road trip, "then I start to feel a difference," he says.
- **PRO BASKETBALL PLAYER KYLE KORVER:** As for Beagle, a stray meal here or there is no big deal. "I don't notice dramatic changes," he explains. But enough cheating on the gluten-free diet, and he might notice feeling sore or tired, which motivates him to get back on track for his next meals.
- **DOCTOR AND CROSSFIT PRACTITIONER PETER OSBORNE:** He feels it in his stomach and sometimes gets bloating and, less often, nausea. "My pants fit a lot tighter," he notes.
- **RECREATIONAL RUNNER KIMBERLY BOULDIN:** Gastrointestinal symptoms last for a day, maybe two, but it takes a good one to two weeks for her body to get fully back on track.
- **PRO TRIATHLETE CHRISTIE SYM:** "I've always gone on and competed, even if I know I'm contaminated," she says. In August 2011, Sym competed in the San Francisco Triathlon at Alcatraz. The day before the race she ate lunch at a diner and was sick and in pain within half an hour. On race day, she experienced stomach cramps on the bike, and "full-on diarrhea" during the run. But she was in second place chasing down first (she missed winning the race by thirty-five seconds) and pushed through the pain. "Yeah, it was a bit messy," she says. "But I don't like to let it stop me. It definitely affects me in a big way, but I don't want the disease to win."

- **OLYMPIAN AND DISTANCE RUNNING NATIONAL CHAMPION AMY YODER BEGLEY:** She was cross-contaminated during a flight en route to a meet. "That was the worst plane ride I've ever had," she recalls. Yoder Begley was doubled over in pain, two days out from a race. "You deal with it and you go on," she says. "I've had races with food poisoning before. It's the same deal. Sometimes I actually run better, thinking I've got nothing to lose."
- **COLLEGIATE BASKETBALL PLAYER DIANA ROLNIAK:** "I've missed games because of it," she says. "I'm out of commission for two or three days."
- **COLLEGIATE LACROSSE PLAYER KRISTEN TAYLOR:** The team was on the road and had a "huge game the next day against Maryland," she says. Taylor was cross-contaminated at a restaurant. "I was up the entire night before the game, so terribly sick," she remembers. "How frustrating it was, and that it was beyond my control. I was completely run-down."
- **HIGH-ALTITUDE MOUNTAIN GUIDE AND SKI PATROLLER DAVE HAHN:** "In about three hours, I begin to sweat profusely, faint, and vomit," he says, "which usually solves the problem . . . but it isn't pretty."
- **COLLEGIATE CROSS COUNTRY RUNNER ANDIE COZZARELLI:** "I normally just push through it," she says. "I won't feel as well; my stomach won't feel good. I'll make sure I'm near a bathroom, in case I get sick. I'll have stomachaches, a headache, then go home and take a nap, try to sleep it off."
- **YOGA PRACTITIONER CLEA SHANNON:** She gets horrible stomach cramps and is uncomfortable for days. At first, she experiences digestive symptoms, but then it transitions to terrible fatigue.
- **PRO TRIATHLETE TYLER STEWART:** "My body reacts really quickly . . . within fifteen to twenty minutes," she says. "I get really bloated; I look like I'm pregnant." (Before going gluten-free, she could barely run for 3 miles without having to stop and go to the bathroom. "What is wrong with me?" she'd wonder.)
- **RECREATIONAL RUNNER MICHAEL DANKE:** Gluten exposure once disrupted his training for two weeks. He missed some training and dialed back the intensity on other training. "You

just don't want to do anything when you feel that sick. And when you do come back, you don't want to hit it that hard," he says. It ultimately affected his performance in an upcoming marathon, where he missed his target time.

- **AMATEUR COMPETITIVE CYCLIST ASHLEY DIVERONICA:** She loses energy and gets dehydrated. It typically takes a few days for her to feel normal, and up to a week to be truly back to 100 percent. She has missed races because of being sick from gluten. "I can tell if I've been cross-contaminated within minutes," she says. DiVeronica once mistakenly poured regular soy sauce (which contains wheat) over an otherwise gluten-free restaurant meal. "I got so sick," she remembers.

- **PRO TRIATHLETE TERRA CASTRO:** "I notice my immune system on a long-term basis. My body's fighting off what I've digested," she says. "And I get really tired, almost like chronic fatigue. The symptoms have gotten worse as I've gotten older. I get knife pains, or gas pains. Now I just stay away. The one bite is not worth it."

No matter how you slice it, getting glutened can be disappointing to an athlete. You may have to seriously adjust your expectations. If you feel up to it, by all means persevere through the pain. But if you have to take a pass and give your body time to recover, cut yourself some slack. In essence, you've just been poisoned. But unlike coming down with the flu or food poisoning—which are pretty much the by-product of bad luck and bad timing—gluten can trip you up at any time if you're not careful, and even if you are.

Plus, these days we're finding a growing list of "silent" symptoms. Some people with gluten intolerance have minimal gastrointestinal symptoms but experience anemia, osteoporosis, and other problems that affect their athletic performance. In such cases, you may not even realize you're being exposed to gluten, because your body is not giving you the kind of immediate feedback that a bout of postmeal stomach pain and diarrhea will.

Gluten may cause inflammation and other problems that may not be bad enough to prevent you from training or competing. Or you may feel like you came down with the flu, when in truth it's gluten, and you end up skipping a few training days and rest on the couch in the meantime. Some people with celiac disease may eventually go to the doctor and find that they have intestinal damage or elevated blood antibodies, even though they think they've been eating a proper gluten-free diet. For them, damage is occurring whether they feel and recognize it or not.

When it comes to gluten cross-contamination, it's important to remain vigilant. University of Wisconsin–Milwaukee soccer player Kelsey Holbert knows that lesson too well.

Gluten-free since the seventh grade, when she was diagnosed with celiac disease, Holbert had been feeling great. Then, in 2010, she started having "random stomach issues again," she explains: "I wasn't feeling that great." Holbert met with a specialist at the University of Chicago Celiac Disease Center. To her surprise, her gluten levels were high. "I had to be really super strict with my diet and get back to feeling good," she says. "Since then I've had no issues, which has been great. I feel a lot better. But it's a good reminder that you have to be really careful and keep checking in with how you're feeling."

CROSS-CONTAMINATION

IF YOU'RE VERY sensitive to gluten—for example, because of celiac disease—and need to be strictly gluten-free, remember to remain vigilant about cross-contamination. Has that jar of peanut butter had knives dipped in it that previously touched wheat bread? Was that pasta boiled in separate water from wheat pasta? Even minute amounts of gluten can cause big reactions in sensitive individuals. Don't let cross-contamination ruin a game, a race, or even a training session.

ATHLETE INSIGHT

Kelsey Holbert

COLLEGIATE SOCCER PLAYER, UNIVERSITY OF WISCONSIN–MILWAUKEE

Born: 1992 • Lives: Wisconsin • Gluten-Free Since: 2005

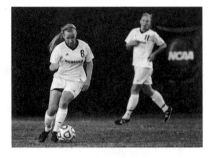

EVER SINCE SHE was little, Kelsey Holbert played soccer. In fact, before she was old enough to play in a league of her own, she played on the team of her older sister, who was four years old at the time.

In the fifth grade she started feeling sick, with mild stomachaches constantly. "I would complain almost every day after every meal," she says, "but it wasn't enough to keep me out of school or prevent me from doing things."

At first doctors diagnosed her with acid reflux, then stress, then IBS. But in the seventh grade, an intestinal biopsy confirmed a diagnosis of celiac disease. It wasn't a total surprise. Her grandmother had celiac, so she knew the genes ran in the family.

Within two weeks of going gluten-free, "I felt completely different and better," Holbert says. "I felt so much stronger. You don't realize how much pain you're in until you don't have that constant pain anymore."

As her body recovered into the eighth grade, Holbert got more serious about soccer and started thinking of playing at a more competitive level. She played for her high school team, but also for a highly competitive club team known as Windy City Pride, which won the U-17 U.S. Club National Championship during her senior year in 2010. That team was where she caught the eye of college recruiters. Holbert ultimately chose UWM.

Thanks to her earlier diagnosis and savvy with the gluten-free diet, her transition into life as a gluten-free college athlete at the University of Wisconsin–Milwaukee was smoother than for most. She worked with her coaches, athletic trainer (who's also gluten-free), team, the head of dining operations, and the school to ensure that her gluten-free needs would be met and that she could stay healthy.

But that's just the kind of leadership people have come to expect from Holbert. During high school she founded the Celiac Attack, an annual 3-on-3 soccer tournament that raises money for celiac disease research. The event draws 100 to 150 participants each year and has fund-raised for the National Foundation for Celiac Awareness and the University of Chicago Celiac Disease Center. In its first three years, from 2008 to 2010, the Celiac Attack tournament has raised nearly $10,000.

What's next for the rising young soccer star? Soccer, of course. But she also hopes to start an on-campus group for students with gluten intolerance.[14]

FAVORITE GLUTEN-FREE FOODS: Schär gluten-free pasta; Udi's Gluten Free bread; Luna protein bars; gluten-free pizza

RECOVERING FROM BEING GLUTENED

- **IF YOU DON'T FEEL LIKE EATING SOLID FOOD:** Don't. Let your body recover. Rest and drink fluids (coconut water is excellent). This is a good time for juicing. You'll get a big hit of antioxidants and healing phytochemicals without the fiber that can be too much for your gut while it's healing.
- **IF YOU DO FEEL LIKE EATING:** Choose unprocessed whole foods (brown rice, roasted vegetables, soups), or blend up a raw-foods smoothie.
- **REPLENISH FRIENDLY BACTERIA:** Take probiotics, drink kefir, and eat yogurt.
- **CONSIDER SUPPLEMENTING WITH HIGH-GRADE ESSENTIAL FATTY ACIDS (FISH OIL):** This supports the body's natural anti-inflammatory response. When allergens or antigens (gluten, in this case) are present and the immune system is triggered, fatty acids are released from cell membranes to assist in healing. It's part of the internal repair system.

- **PROTECT THE LINING OF THE GUT WITH THE AMINO ACID GLUTAMINE**: It's important fuel for intestinal immune cells. Prolonged strenuous exercise depletes glutamine levels. If you've been glutened *and* you train hard, you have two reasons to be deficient. Eat foods high in glutamine (raw spinach, raw cabbage, beets, parsley, beef, poultry, yogurt). Also see page 150 for a more comprehensive list of foods rich in glutamine.

NEED TO KNOW

- Athletes in backcountry sports such as hiking, skiing, and climbing have additional considerations to incorporate into their gluten-free nutrition plan: water availability, portability, weight and space constraints, and lack of refrigeration.
- Athletes in endurance sports such as triathlons, cycling, and ultramarathons should pay greater attention to the fat oxidation energy pathway and dietary fat intake. Gluten-free energy gels and chews can also serve as an effective source of formulated, portable nutrition during racing.
- Lifestyle sports such as yoga, tennis, and golf work in conjunction with gluten-free nutrition to yield long-term fitness, health, and quality of life.
- Team sports such as soccer, football, basketball, and lacrosse introduce group dynamics to the gluten-free equation. A gluten-free athlete may feel isolated from his or her team, or supported by coaches and teammates. Safely eating gluten-free in a group environment can pose an added challenge.
- For women, the Female Athlete Triad—disordered eating/calorie intake, osteoporosis, and amenorrhea—can resemble serious forms of gluten intolerance, such as celiac disease. A gluten-free diet can help to resolve such symptoms.

- For older individuals, you are never too old to develop gluten intolerance, and it's never too late to regain your health with a gluten-free diet.
- Successfully eating gluten-free when traveling involves several strategies: finding restaurants with gluten-free menus and knowledgeable kitchen staff and servers, taking time to shop for gluten-free foods at your destination, packing gluten-free foods from home, staying in hotels or other places with kitchenettes where you can prepare some of your own meals, and keeping constant vigil to beware gluten cross-contamination.
- Cross-contamination from gluten can range from inconsequential for some athletes to devastating for others. Whether you persevere and train or compete, or sit out and take time for your body to recover, is up to you. If needed, give your body time to heal, and know that such occasional setbacks, though disappointing and frustrating, are temporary bumps in the road, which any athlete—gluten-free or otherwise—faces from time to time.

9

Time for a Tune-up

I F WE KEEP the "your body is a high-performance engine" metaphor going, it's time to talk about giving it a seasonal tune-up. And by *tune-up*, we mean a sports detox cleanse.

Before you make any assumptions based on our use of the term *detox cleanse*, read on. It's probably not what you think. We're not talking about your celebrity fad "I need to lose weight fast before I walk the red carpet" detox cleanses. We're talking about a sports-oriented detox cleanse that—when done right and timed appropriately—can leave your body feeling recharged and ready to tackle the next cycle of training and competition.

Think about your car's engine. You put in good fuel, some high-quality motor oil. But you still get buildup in the engine that will gradually and slowly degrade its performance. And so, from time to time, you flush the system and replace the fluids to keep it running optimally. A sports detox cleanse does a similar thing for your body.

Detox cleanses come in many shapes and sizes. Most claim to help remove toxins from your body, and many tout their effectiveness for weight loss. Let us be very clear about this: We do *not* advocate deprivation-type cleanses that severely restrict calorie and nutrient intake. Some such cleanses take the form of liquid-only cleanses that consist of drinking large amounts of solutions containing a very limited number of ingredients. That's not something you want to be doing as an athlete. In fact, that runs counter to pretty much everything else we've said in this book about sound gluten-free sports nutrition and getting the calories and the macro- and micronutrients you need as an athlete.

We advocate a healthier type of detox cleanse for athletes, one you should undertake in the off-season, rather than during training or com- petition. Such a cleanse reduces your body's load of inflammatory foods (such as gluten) and other dietary stressors (such as alkaloids, which can negatively impact digestion and nerve-muscle function in high concentrations or sensitive individuals), helps to recalibrate your taste buds (and your taste for salty and sweet foods), and restarts your system, in a sense, in preparation for the next round of training and competition.

Done properly, a sports detox cleanse is characterized by (a) proper timing, and (b) proper nutrition. Cleanses, especially ones that involve fasting or other forms of restricted calorie intake, can have a negative impact on performance during training and competition.[1] Your body won't be getting the fuel it needs for performance and recovery. That's why we recommend planning a sports detox cleanse for your off-season, when there is less demand on your body and you're in a transition pe- riod from one season to the next.

On the other hand, a good cleanse during the off-season can boost lean tissue development, muscle formation, tissue repair, organ health, bone strength, and energy levels.[2]

As you'll see, you can also think about a sports detox diet as a kind of elimination/reintroduction diet. In our 14-day cleanse, you'll temporar- ily remove certain foods from your diet. Gluten, of course, is always a no-no. If you're an athlete who's committed to the gluten-free diet, think of the cleanse as a tune-up. If you're a gluten-eating athlete, think of our 14-day gluten-free cleanse as a trial run to see how your body feels when you get the gluten out of your system—and just as important, how it feels when you bring the gluten back at the end of the fourteen days (if you choose to).

Adam Korzun, a high-performance dietitian for the U.S. Ski and Snowboard team, knows the value of a sports detox cleanse firsthand. Also a chef, Korzun teaches cooking workshops and stresses the impor- tance of taking personal responsibility for individual nutrition needs.

ATHLETE INSIGHT

Clea Shannon

YOGA INSTRUCTOR, NUTRITION/WELLNESS COACH, FORMER COLLEGIATE
LACROSSE PLAYER

Born: 1973 • Lives: California • Gluten-Free Since: 2004

CLEA SHANNON was a gymnast in high school, a college athlete who played lacrosse for Stanford, and later worked for Nike in Oregon. Along the way, though, she began developing problems with chronic fatigue, her skin, swelling around the ankles, general bloating, and some abnormal blood tests. At first doctors thought it was cancer. Then a rheumatologist settled on lupus as the cause of her problems.

But the lupus didn't explain all of her symptoms, and Shannon was wary of some of the steroid medication doctors were proposing. And so she started talking with naturopaths about her options for treating the lupus through food. For the first time, gluten as a trigger entered the conversation. Shannon tried an elimination diet.

"When I took everything out and then reintroduced gluten, alarms went off," she says. An intestinal biopsy confirmed it: celiac disease. That was in 2004.

"They basically handed me a list of things I couldn't eat and shoved me out the door," Shannon says. She had some false starts in those first months on the gluten-free diet, eating crackers that were wheat-free, not gluten-free, and not realizing that wheat is an ingredient in most soy sauces. As she researched the diet further, more and more she found herself eating primarily vegetables and fruits and what she called "plain simple food."

Eventually, she became focused on a gluten-free, whole-foods diet. "It transformed the way I ate," she says. It transformed her health, too. Shannon's symptoms resolved. "It made me feel so much more connected with my body in so many ways," she reflects. "It encouraged me down a path of evaluating, considering, building awareness for what I put in my body."

She was transforming professionally as well. At the Nike facilities in Oregon, Shannon had started taking yoga classes as a hobby. That led to becoming a yoga teacher. When she later moved to Southern California, she hosted stroller strides and group fitness classes for moms and babies. For a time she ran a yoga studio. Now she's coaching clients and pursuing certification as a holistic health coach.

None of it would have happened without her diagnosis and the gluten-free diet, she says. She wouldn't have had the health or the energy for it. "At first, the diagnosis was overwhelming. I thought it would be a struggle. I didn't think I'd be able to do things. But wow! Look at all these things I can do," she says, fresh off running the NYC Marathon in fall 2011. "Our whole family is thriving and we're gluten-free. It doesn't need to hold you back at all."

FAVORITE GLUTEN-FREE FOODS: "lots of fresh smoothies with berries, a little apple juice, kale"; some gluten-free oatmeal on occasion; quinoa; tuna; hummus; egg whites; lots of vegetables, usually steamed or sautéed; Udi's gluten-free whole-grain bread and bagels ("nothing like having a bagel once in a while with almond butter in the morning")

If Korzun sees athletes with a questionable energy drink or junk food, he tests them on it. "I ask if they can pronounce and explain the benefit of every ingredient in the list," he says. "If they can, I'm okay with their choice." He knows the havoc gluten can wreak for certain athletes.

Although there are no athletes with diagnosed celiac disease currently on the U.S. team, a few over time have been sensitive to gluten. Korzun also requests full celiac blood test panels when he suspects an athlete has gluten intolerance. A gluten-free sports detox cleanse is another litmus test Korzun uses to evaluate his athletes. "When I'm suspicious of gluten,

I end up doing a lot with elimination/reintroduction diets," he explains. In fact, he plans a sports detox cleanse for all of his athletes at the end of each winter season.

The cleanse helps to strengthen the digestive system, boost immune function, and enhance the removal of metabolic waste. And for Korzun, it helps to identify which athletes benefit most from the gluten-free edge.

Our version of a cleanse is all about wholesome, nourishing foods. As we said earlier, we're not into deprivation. The last time we checked, our cars' engines didn't run better on fumes. Instead, you'll be focusing on fresh vegetables, fruits, nuts, seeds, certain grains, and, if desired, some animal-based proteins. What you won't be eating are things such as gluten, refined sugar, and alcohol. Here's how to do it:

THE 14-DAY GLUTEN-FREE SPORTS DETOX CLEANSE

For two weeks, you'll base your diet on a range of nourishing foods, mostly plant based, while eliminating certain other foods from your nutrition plan. Don't stray too far from your typical meal schedule. However, eat smaller amounts. Eat when you're hungry. And eat only until you're no longer hungry, as opposed to eating until you feel full.

Then, at the end of the two weeks, gradually add back in the eliminated foods to see how your body responds to them. Reintroduce one food every three to five days. If you add two or more foods back to your diet at once—say, corn, tomatoes, and cow's milk—and react to one of them, you won't know which one caused the reaction. In this sense, reintroducing foods after a select elimination cleanse is like introducing new foods to a baby for the first time: one at a time to watch for a reaction.

WHAT TO EXPECT

During the first few days, don't be surprised if you initially feel worse before feeling better. You may experience headaches, fatigue, dizziness, abnormal bowel movements, food cravings, or general crankiness, especially if you are sensitive to gluten. (On the other hand, with gluten out of your system you may suddenly feel positively fabulous.) Hang in there! Those unpleasant symptoms will subside. You'll soon start feeling better—with more mental clarity, more bodily vitality, and a calmer digestive system.

TIPS FOR SUCCESS

- Make sure your family and friends are supportive. It's often best to have someone to share the process with—someone to whine to on occasion.
- Try to exercise daily. Yoga is perfect. Sweat, twist, and bend to wring out and eliminate toxins. Don't try to do too much; let your body rest and repair. Now's not the time to be running a marathon.
- Plan to prepare most of your own food. It's hard to find healthy, allergen-free, cleansing food while on the go. Plan ahead. Make sure you have snacks and meals ready ahead of time so you don't cave in and grab something unhealthy while out and about. Cut up veggies and fruit and keep a stash in the fridge. Prepare brown rice and quinoa ahead of time to mix with sautéed vegetables.
- Keep a journal of how you're feeling. Make note of symptoms like fatigue, headache, sinus problems, achy joints, rashes, puffy eyes, dark circles under the eyes, upset stomach, gas, bloating, or increased heart rate. This is especially beneficial as you reintroduce foods after the cleanse. See if you can associate symptoms with certain foods. (Remember, reintroduce eliminated foods to your diet one at a time.)
- Drink lots of filtered water to help hydrate and flush out the system.
- Check out the section on Smoothies and Juicing in chapter 7 for great ideas on making shakes that are compatible with a sports detox cleanse.

FOOD CATEGORIES TO AVOID

- Gluten
- Refined sugar
- Caffeine
- Yeast
- Alcohol
- Dairy
- Nightshades

ATHLETE INSIGHT

Amy Ippoliti

YOGA TEACHER AND ENTREPRENEUR

Born: 1969 • Lives: Colorado • Gluten-Free Since: 2006

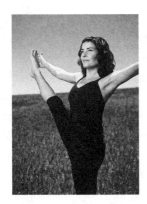

WHEN GLOBE-TROTTING YOGA teacher Amy Ippoliti asks people to "turn up your volume and live like you mean it," they do it. Her empowered spirit and joyful enthusiasm are contagious. Ten minutes spent with Ippoliti and you're inspired to eat better, live better, and take better care of the environment. You might even start meditating and drinking green juice.

Between her roles as a faculty member at the Omega Institute in New York and the Kripalu Center for Yoga & Health in Massachusetts, and creating and teaching advanced yoga programs around the world, Ippoliti travels extensively. What's her secret to staying healthy and radiating boundless energy despite a hectic travel schedule that would otherwise exhaust the best of us? Radical self-care, a positive attitude, and a gluten-free, whole-foods diet.

Medical testing years ago revealed a sensitivity to gluten, corn, and a few other foods for Ippoliti. "I've always kept those test results in mind when making food choices," she says.

Sticking to a gluten-free diet gets complicated on the road. "In the USA and Asia it is really easy," she says. "Italy, on the other hand, is really tough. They live on pasta, bread, and gluten!" Not one to be deterred, Ippoliti has been known to pull packages of gluten-free pasta out of her bag and kindly ask chefs to substitute it in her meals. "They are usually very sweet about it," she says.

As someone who has been gluten-free on and off for the past nineteen years, Amy took it seriously in 2006 and found an immediate improvement in her strength and energy. "I would say

I am stronger and more powerful eating gluten-free. And I have way less slumpiness during the postlunch time of the day! Almost none, actually," she says cheerfully.

Demonstrating difficult yoga poses, holding arm balances and handstands for minutes on end, and sharing her vast knowledge of yoga therapy with other yoga teachers could take a toll on her body if she's not careful. So what happens if Amy gets zapped with gluten, despite her best intentions? "I get zits, my lean mass decreases, and I get lethargic," she says. For a woman who's been featured on the cover of *Yoga Journal* and *Fit Yoga*, looking and feeling her best is important.

Choosing nutritious, naturally gluten-free, whole foods is a way of life for Amy. She has a performance-based career and knows the value of nourishing food and an occasional cleanse. Rather than fill up on refined foods, sugar, and prepackaged gluten-free products, Amy advises her students to "reach for green veggies, seaweed snacks, nuts, seeds, jicama, peppers, sprouts, avocados, grapefruits, and everything coconut. Drink lots more pure, alkaline water and watch your health benefits increase radically."

FAVORITE GLUTEN-FREE FOODS: jicama, Tinkyada gluten-free pasta, "gobs of coconuts, avocados, and veggies"

FOODS TO AVOID

- Gluten grains (wheat, barley, rye, triticale, spelt, einkorn, and emmer)
- Breads, baked goods, basically anything made with flour
- Processed foods and candy (even if gluten-free)
- Corn products (even though they're gluten-free)
- Beer, wine, spirits
- Soda pop
- Coffee and black tea
- Cow's milk, regular butter, cow's yogurt, most dairy cheese
- Nightshades: Potatoes (white, red, purple), tomatoes, tomatillos, sweet and spicy peppers, paprika, cayenne

- Most chocolate (see the following list for exceptions)
- Most soy foods and products (tofu, edamame, soy milk, protein bars with soy protein)

FOODS TO ENJOY (ORGANIC WHENEVER POSSIBLE)

- Gluten-free grains (brown rice, wild rice, quinoa, amaranth, gluten-free oats, teff, buckwheat, millet)
- Fresh fruit (apples, pears, peaches, bananas, berries, grapes, cherries, mangoes, figs, plums, apricots)
- Lemons and limes (add to herbal teas and filtered water; squeeze on steamed veggies and salads)
- Dried fruit, unsulfured, no sugar added (dates, raisins, figs, apricots, cherries, cranberries, prunes)
- Fresh vegetables other than nightshades (lettuce, spinach, kale, celery, cucumber, peas, collard greens, beet greens, burdock root, asparagus, bok choy, cabbage, broccoli, cauliflower, Brussels sprouts, chard, beets, carrots, daikon radish, parsnips, sweet potatoes, yams, onions, garlic, cilantro, leeks, avocados, squash)
- Legumes other than soy (lentils, chickpeas, adzuki beans, navy beans, mung beans, and peanuts and peanut butter)
- Natural sweeteners in limited amounts; for example, over oatmeal or in herbal tea (honey, blackstrap molasses, maple syrup, agave nectar, stevia)
- Healthy fats (coconut oil, olive oil, ghee/clarified butter)
- Seeds and seed butters (pumpkin, flax, chia, sesame, sunflower, hemp)
- Nuts and nut butters (pecans, almonds, walnuts, cashews)
- Sea vegetables (hijiki, wakame, nori, kombu, arame, kelp, dulse flakes)
- Herbs and spices (such as cinnamon added to smoothies, yogurt, or porridge)
- Cacao powder (preferable) and dark chocolate (beware of sugar, as well as dairy and soy ingredients in many chocolates)
- Gluten-free tamari (wheat-free soy sauce), apple cider vinegar, vegetable broth
- Coconut milk, coconut water

- Herbal tea
- Goat yogurt, goat kefir
- Raw, less processed, organic cheeses (in small amounts)
- Animal protein, if desired (pastured eggs, organic grass-fed bison or beef, wild-caught salmon, lamb)

As you can see, we've kept our promise! This cleanse is not at all about deprivation. You have lots of great food options. But we've steered you toward nourishing, whole, nutrient-dense foods and away from processed foods and foods with inflammatory and other undesirable characteristics.

NEED TO KNOW

- For athletes, we do *not* advocate celebrity fad cleanses or fasts that severely restrict calorie intake and nutrition.
- A sports detox cleanse is based upon proper timing (in the off-season or preseason) and proper nutrition.
- Undertaking a sports cleanse is like getting a seasonal tune-up for your athletic engine, which aids muscle recovery, energy levels, organ health, and other factors that support good athletic performance.
- Our version of a sports cleanse is an elimination diet that avoids gluten, refined sugar, processed foods, caffeine, dairy, nightshades, and other food groups that can place a load on the body. It incorporates primarily fresh plant-based foods rich in antioxidants and other healing properties.

10

No Train, No Gain:
Training and Exercise Strategies to Complement Nutrition

ALTHOUGH *The Gluten-Free Edge* is primarily about gluten-free nutrition for athletes and anyone interested in living an active gluten-free lifestyle, we'd be remiss if we didn't address the training component. Good gluten-free nutrition can only get you so far. It's one part of a larger program, which includes training.

Whether you're interested in training to win Olympic gold or for lifestyle fitness, a well-rounded exercise routine should accomplish several goals:

- Improve cardiovascular health
- Improve strength and power
- Improve endurance and stamina
- Raise metabolism
- Maintain or improve flexibility
- Maintain or improve bone density (through load-bearing strength exercises, high-impact sports, or both)
- Raise lactate threshold
- Raise VO_2 max

These goals are accomplished through a range of training strategies. Entire books (and many of them, at that) have been written on sport-specific training protocols. Here, we offer overarching principles and strategies that you can apply to any sport and any athletic goal. Our advice combines personal experience, tried-and-true exercise and training principles, and the latest, updated peer-reviewed research.

FITNESS FACTORS

When we talk about training, we're talking about building strength, increasing explosive power, building endurance and long-term stamina, raising aerobic capacity, maintaining flexibility, and fending off problems such as muscle fatigue and cramping. All of these are ways of contributing to what we're ultimately aiming for—not just fitness for fitness' sake, but for performing better in your chosen sport, and for living a healthier, active, gluten-free life.

As a general rule, we can divide exercises into two major categories: aerobic (which helps with cardiovascular health, fat burning, endurance, and aerobic capacity) and anaerobic (which builds speed, strength, and power). As you'll see, some techniques, such as interval training, combine the best of both of these worlds.

But before we dive into specific training protocols and how they can positively impact your performance, let's first talk about two important terms that come up regularly in the athletic world: your VO_2 max and your lactate threshold.

The VO_2 max is a measure of your body's peak capacity to transport and use oxygen during exercise. If you think back to chapter 3, the VO_2 max is the theoretical dividing line between your aerobic (oxygen-based) and anaerobic (oxygen-deprived) energy pathways. If you're performing at or above your VO_2 max, your body can't get more oxygen to your muscles any faster than it's already doing. That will leave you with an oxygen deficit, which will force you to rely on anaerobic energy pathways. Your VO_2 max basically says how hard you can push in a sustained effort, and as such it's a major predictor of peak athletic performance.

Part of your VO_2 max comes down to genetics. Some people are born with a naturally high value. But you can also raise your VO_2 max, sometimes significantly, through the right kinds of training. A higher VO_2 max means you can get more oxygen to your muscles faster, and that means better athletic performance and a larger aerobic zone.

ATHLETE INSIGHT

Kim Bouldin

RECREATIONAL RUNNER

Born: 1973 • Lives: Ohio • Gluten-Free Since: 2006

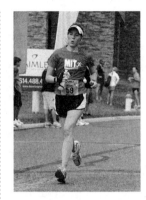

KIM BOULDIN experienced on-and-off stomach trouble after having her son in 1996. The problems got worse after having her daughter in 2002: bloating, pain, and a back-and-forth between constipation and occasional diarrhea. "At first, I couldn't figure it out," she says. Then Bouldin received a positive celiac disease diagnosis on her birthday in 2006. Ironically, Bouldin had been eating a lot of whole wheat, whole-grain pasta, and cereal as part of a "healthier" diet.

"I went gluten-free, and within twenty-four hours, I noticed a huge difference. It was like, 'Oh my gosh. This is what's been bothering me all these years.' I had figured it out," she recalls. "It was a welcome change."

She got into running as a fluke. Bouldin grew up going to her dad's races, "standing in the rain watching," she says. "Who does this? Why is this fun?" But in 2008, she decided she needed to get fit, and so she joined a gym. Bouldin started on the elliptical machines, then moved to a treadmill. "I loved it," she says. Then she wondered, "If I can run, can I do a 5K? And then, can I do a half marathon? And then, can I do a marathon? Now, if I don't run, it feels like I'm missing something."

FAVORITE GLUTEN-FREE FOODS: brown rice; quinoa; lean protein such as chicken; a lot of salads and rice bowls; for breakfast, a huge fruit salad, plus gluten-free oatmeal or rice cakes with almond butter and jelly; tons of green salad ("at least two per day"); bison burgers and spinach or kale for iron; cottage cheese for calcium;

brown rice tortilla wraps; beans; plus, "a sweet tooth for ice cream
. . . Hey, there's protein in that, and calcium, too."

In practice, though, there's a second limiting factor on your performance: your lactate threshold. It's the level of exertion at which lactic acid begins to build up in your muscles and blood faster than it can be dealt with. Normally, under aerobic conditions, lactic acid in your muscles has a relatively low concentration and stays that way, as long as you're within the aerobic zone. The lactic acid is basically a flat line. But as you approach (and exceed) your lactate threshold, anaerobic energy pathways kick in and lactic acid begins to build up rapidly, inhibiting your performance before you've ever reached your VO_2 max.

In an ideal scenario, your VO_2 max and your lactate threshold would directly overlap. In the real world, that's not the case. In untrained individuals, in fact, there can be quite a large difference between the level of exertion that hits your lactate threshold and the level of exertion that theoretically corresponds with your VO_2 max. As with the VO_2 max, however, there's good news: Through training you can raise your lactate threshold, too. In elite, well-trained athletes, their lactate threshold and VO_2 max, while still not identical, are much closer together, enabling those athletes to maintain higher levels of sustained output.

So how do you train properly to improve your lactate threshold and VO_2 max (not to mention all the other athletic factors we just mentioned)?

MEASURING ATHLETIC OUTPUT

We're about to describe three major training protocols, which differ both in their relative intensity and in their duration. And so we need ways to talk about that intensity . . . we need ways to measure your athletic output. There are many ways to do so, including:

- **HEART RATE MONITORS:** measure your heart rate in real time as beats per minute
- **PERCEIVED EXERTION:** a subjective experience of how hard you *feel* like you're pushing; surprisingly accurate

- **STOPWATCH**: allows you to measure time, splits, and (if you know distances covered) pace
- **GPS WATCHES**: record route, pace, distance, time, and other information; often used in conjunction with computer software, mobile apps, or websites
- **WATT METERS**: measure power or work output; common in cycling

Each method has its merits. Since training zones and VO_2 max and lactate threshold are often expressed as a percent of your max heart rate or max exertion, for the three training protocols that follow, we follow that convention. As a general rule (the specifics will vary by individual athlete), the lactate threshold is usually in the realm of 85 percent output, while your VO_2 max is usually in the 95 to 100 percent range.

CALCULATING YOUR MAX HEART RATE, LACTATE THRESHOLD, AND VO_2 MAX

THERE ARE MANY ways to calculate these values. The simplest ones are often a straightforward formula based only on your age. More complex methods may take into account your age, sex, height, weight, and/or resting heart rate. Even more complex methods involve performing an exertion test (often walking or running a prescribed distance and/or for a prescribed amount of time) and then recording factors such as your time and heart rate. The most complex methods involve getting your values tested at a sports medicine lab. As you might expect, the simpler the method, the more general and less accurate the results.

LONG SLOW DISTANCE TRAINING

As its name implies, long slow distance (LSD) training involves exercising at a reduced intensity for a greater duration of time and distance, putting in high mileage (or the equivalent, if you're not a cyclist or runner) at typically 50 to 70 percent output.[1] This type of training offers a number of benefits.

For one, it's commonly employed in endurance training as a way to improve fat oxidation. LSD training keeps you comfortably within your aerobic range for long periods of time, while also slowly depleting muscle glycogen. This is ideal for entering the fat-burning zone, the fat-oxidation energy pathway that many endurance athletes like to optimize.

LSD training can improve muscle power, oxygen uptake, stamina, and overall performance.[2] It can also increase your VO_2 max.[3] And it can even help boost your power at a given VO_2 max, through more efficient use of existing oxygen and aerobic energy pathways.[4] LSD training can likewise improve your lactate threshold, though not necessarily to the degree that tempo training or interval training do (we describe them in the next two sections).[5]

Because of its lower intensity, LSD training can be a good choice for novice athletes. For the same reason, it's also popular with older athletes.[6] The cumulative effect (and sheer effectiveness) of LSD training helps to explain why older athletes often make great endurance athletes well into their "mature" years. Although older athletes typically have a lower VO_2 max than do their younger counterparts, they have trained to increase their lactate threshold and more efficiently use oxygen, allowing them to work closer to their VO_2 max, while younger athletes perform at a lower percentage of their VO_2 max, because of their lactate threshold and other limiting factors.[7]

LSD training is also good for building an aerobic base among younger and experienced athletes alike, especially in the off-season or early training season before switching to higher-intensity modes of training to build performance.[8] It can be part of an overall training plan that includes other strategies, and it can be part of a general lifestyle fitness plan, too.

All of this said, LSD training is not for every athlete. For example, while some ultraendurance athletes swear by it, taking pride in their unbelievably high weekly running mileage, others have been very successful with much lower training volume. As researchers have found, training volume isn't everything. One set of researchers found a training correlation in athletes' performance in a twenty-four-hour ultraendurance run, not with training volume, but with personal best marathon time.[9] With LSD training, it's not about just putting in any old miles, and as many of them as you can, however you'd like. There's also something to be said for making those miles count by adding quality to volume in the training equation.

In addition, too much LSD training can be detrimental to athletes in power and sprint sports. It may not be appropriate for them because it causes changes and physiological adaptations that are great for endurance and overall fitness, but not so much for other sports.[10]

HOW SLOW IS SLOW ENOUGH IN LONG SLOW DISTANCE?

FOR THE UNINITIATED, long slow distance training may have *slow* in its name, but it's not nearly as slow as some people think. Believe us, you'll still be working and sweating. It's only slow in the sense that you're staying in your aerobic zone and below your lactate threshold. If you train with a technology tool such as a heart rate monitor, you can lock in your pace for 60 or 70 percent of your max. But if you don't, how hard or easy should you push? Use this measure: You want to be working for it, but you should be able to maintain a conversation with a training partner without getting out of breath or panting. Train solo without a partner and don't want to have a conversation with yourself to judge your pace? No problem. Just dial in your "perpetual pace," the rate at which you're putting in an honest effort but still feel like you could keep going and going. No matter what measure you use, LSD training should still make you work. Walking can be a good exercise for some people, but it's not long slow distance training.

TEMPO TRAINING

Tempo training involves training at or near your lactate threshold (about 85 percent output), also known as your *anaerobic* or *aerobic threshold.* Tempo training is frequently in the 75 to 85 percent output range; the closer you can stay to your threshold the better. Maintaining such a level of intensity—where your body has to continually work to keep up with lactic acid levels, trains your body to better and more efficiently deal with it. This can help you raise your lactate threshold and improve your aerobic capacity by closing the gap with your VO$_2$ max, enabling you to maintain higher levels of exertion without the detrimental performance effects of lactic acid buildup. And you don't necessarily get this same beneficial effect from doing only higher intensity exercise that pushes you beyond your lactate threshold.[11]

INTERVAL TRAINING

Interval training (IT), sometimes known as *polarized training,* involves rapidly cycling between anaerobic and aerobic output. You may do fifteen seconds on, fifteen seconds off; or one minute on, one minute off; or another sequence. Regardless, interval training involves a short period of work near your limit (90 to 100 percent output), followed by a period of active recovery below your lactate threshold (85 percent output) where you dial back the intensity to between 70 and 80 percent output.[12] At the end of the short recovery period, you immediately begin another cycle. This toggling between the two levels of exertion is what provides the benefit.

IT can yield overall improved performance, better recovery from lactic acid buildup,[13] improved heart and muscle power,[14] and improved endurance.[15] And like other training strategies, interval training increases your VO$_2$ max. In fact, it does so better than either LSD or tempo training.[16]

One of the difficult things about IT is that it's tough. Many training protocols emphasize either high volume (such as LSD) or high intensity. IT combines both. It will yield great benefits for your athletic performance, but will really make you work for it.

IT may be especially useful for well-trained athletes who've already benefited from easier methods of training, as a way to squeak extra percentages out of their performance.[17] For example, some elite athletes who already have a high VO$_2$ max through training have only been able to elevate their VO$_2$ max further through IT.

ATHLETE INSIGHT

Carrie Willoughby

U.S. PARALYMPIC SWIMMER, ASPIRING PARALYMPIC CYCLIST

Born: 1977 • Lives: Colorado • Gluten-Free Since: 2005

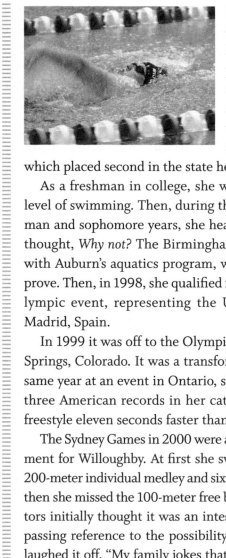

LEGALLY BLIND WITH 20/400 corrected vision, Carrie Willoughby didn't discover her passion for athletics until high school in the mid-1990s, when she was part of the swim team that won the state championship in her junior year, and which placed second in the state her senior year.

As a freshman in college, she was exposed to a more serious level of swimming. Then, during the summer between her freshman and sophomore years, she heard about the Paralympics and thought, *Why not?* The Birmingham, Alabama, native joined up with Auburn's aquatics program, which really helped her to improve. Then, in 1998, she qualified for her first international Paralympic event, representing the United States at an event in Madrid, Spain.

In 1999 it was off to the Olympic Training Center in Colorado Springs, Colorado. It was a transformative experience. Later that same year at an event in Ontario, she came out of the water with three American records in her category, including a 200-meter freestyle eleven seconds faster than her previous best.

The Sydney Games in 2000 were at once a thrill and a disappointment for Willoughby. At first she swam well, taking eighth in the 200-meter individual medley and sixth in the 50-meter freestyle. But then she missed the 100-meter free because she was sick. Most doctors initially thought it was an intestinal virus. When one made a passing reference to the possibility of a food allergy, Willoughby laughed it off. "My family jokes that there's single-size, family-size, and Carrie-size portions of foods," she jokes. "The idea of my being allergic to food, I snickered at it. Have you seen me eat?"

But back at home after Sydney, her health continued to spiral downward. Willoughby persevered with her swimming anyway, becoming a Home Depot–sponsored athlete in 2002. During the run-up to the 2004 Athens Games, though, the bottom dropped out.

She had unexpected training struggles one day, with sharp pains that felt as if they were coming from her bones, rather than her muscles. It turned out her iron levels were very low. Willoughby started supplements, but less than a year later, more problems surfaced, this time with low energy and vitamin D malabsorption.

Finally, in March 2005, almost five years after she first got sick at the Sydney Games, doctors had an answer: celiac disease. She could begin the road to recovery on a gluten-free diet. "Ever since going gluten-free, the positive changes have been dramatic," she says.

Willoughby returned to the pool, this time looking ahead to Beijing in 2008. She became the first alternate, having missed making the team by one second. Willoughby entered one last race—the International Blind Sports Association Pan-American Games in 2009. Then she hung up her goggles.

Her sporting days aren't over, however. With her celiac disease symptoms behind her on the gluten-free diet, Willoughby has found renewed athletic motivation in velodrome cycling on a tandem bike with a sighted copilot. In a way she's doing her part, not just for her own athletic aspirations, but for those of others. Like pro triathlete Desirée Ficker, Willoughby is a mentor for Team Gluten-Free, raising money to help send gluten-intolerant children to gluten-free summer camps.

FAVORITE GLUTEN-FREE FOODS: eggs; Udi's Gluten Free Bagels with Peanut Butter & Co. White Chocolate Peanut Butter; Gluten-Free Pantry muffin mix with peanut butter and chocolate chips or bananas and pecans; for lunch, often a large salad with barbecued chicken and a bowl of rice with gluten-free mushroom soup over it; for dinner, something light, such as a piece of chicken and half a can of corn; for snacks, yogurt, fruit, muffins

Finally, depending on your goals, interval training may not be appropriate, at least on its own. For example, ultraendurance athletes interested in maximizing their fat-oxidation energy pathways will do well to use IT judiciously in combination with other strategies, as it relies on anaerobic and carbohydrate oxidation pathways primarily.

PERSONALIZING FOR YOUR SPORT

At the end of the day, there are a number of similarities between LSD, LT, and IT strategies. For example, all can help increase both your VO_2 max and your lactate threshold.[18] What you choose for your training will come down to your sport and how you're best served by the attributes of each training protocol.

And of course you're not limited to one or another. You can combine strategies, or transition from one to the next in a periodization schedule (more on that to come).

FAT BURNING AND WEIGHT LOSS, REVISITED

Earlier in this book, we addressed the issue of whether the gluten-free diet should be thought of as a weight-loss diet. Let's recap:

- It will matter whether you traded a glutenous diet for (a) a healthy, nourishing, whole-foods, gluten-free diet or (b) a gluten-free junk food diet.
- On the gluten-free diet, your body's recovery from gluten-induced inflammation and bloating and your improved digestion and absorption can yield unexpected weight changes—loss or gain.
- Weight maintenance partly comes down to calories consumed versus calories absorbed versus calories burned.
- Different energy pathways (ATP-PCr, anaerobic glycolysis, carbohydrate oxidation, and fat oxidation) contribute differently to calorie burning and fat loss.
- Your activity level combined with your balance of dietary carbs, proteins, and healthy fats, plus the balance of low- versus high-glycemic-index carbs (not to mention glucose tolerance, insulin

sensitivity, and insulin resistance) influence which energy pathways predominate and how your body uses and stores food energy.

Now that you understand several training protocols, including LSD,
we can add an exercise perspective and example to the weight-management
and fat-burning issue. Studies have shown that the human body is good
at oxidizing fat across a range of exertion levels. Some suggest that 50
to 70 percent output yields the best fat burning. Others suggest that as
you get closer to your lactate threshold, fat-burning peaks around 75
percent output. These findings would seem to emphasize LSD or light
tempo training to put your body into fat-burning mode.

Other factors come into play, too. For example, fat oxidation tends to
kick into higher gear as glycogen levels get depleted. You can reach that
point in one of two ways—by exercising for longer duration, so that you
deplete muscle glycogen further, or by exercising first thing early in the
morning (before breakfast, even), when your body's glycogen stores are
naturally low following the overnight fast.[19]

With these factors in mind, let's consider a hypothetical scenario familiar to many people. Say you've been going to the gym five days per
week after work. Each time you go, you hop on one of the elliptical
machines, tune in to your favorite half-hour sitcom, put the machine
into fat-burning mode, do your thing, and head home. But the weight
never seems to melt away. What gives? Shouldn't that be enough to
make a difference?

It might not be, and here's a reason why. If you keep all other variables constant (diet, sleep, etc.), you're never actually getting your
body into fat-burning mode. Think of it this way: You go to the gym
after work, when you've already had a few meals and snacks under
your belt throughout the day, raising your muscle glycogen levels.
When you start the elliptical—plugging in your height, weight, and
age—and engage fat-burning mode, it keeps you at a relatively modest
intensity, in the theoretical fat-burning zone. However, if you stop
after thirty minutes, you haven't even come close to exercising for the
forty-five minutes to an hour or more it normally takes to decrease
muscle glycogen levels sufficiently to engage your fat-oxidation pathway. The moment you stepped off the machine was right when you were

ATHLETE INSIGHT

Ryann Fraser

TRIATHLETE, CYCLIST, MODEL

Born: 1989 • Lives: New York • Gluten-Free Since: 2010

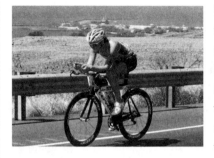

RYANN FRASER had been so tired for so long, she didn't realize she wasn't fully awake. But then, while on a photo shoot during the first two weeks of January 2010, she met another young woman who was gluten-free and raving about how great it was. On a whim Fraser decided to try the diet . . . for no particular reason. Within two days, "I felt like a different person," she says. "I had so much energy that I'd never even experienced before. What is this?"

In fact, she felt *so* much better off gluten that she figured something was wrong when she was on it. She tried eating gluten again, to see what would happen. Her body revolted. Blood tests revealed antibodies, and in March 2010, she was diagnosed with celiac disease.

What's so remarkable about her story is how well she managed to perform before getting diagnosed. Between the ages of six and ten, Fraser lost her hair to alopecia. "When I was seven, I wanted to train for the Olympics," she says. Instead, she eventually set her sights on another goal: "I always told people I'd do an Ironman when I turned eighteen." It wasn't entirely unreasonable—her father runs Ironman Canada.

During training when she was seventeen, "I knew something was abnormal. I kept going to the doctor exhausted," she says. "I assumed I was wearing myself down." It turns out she was severely anemic. Yet, taking supplements and "eating steak every day for the entire summer" did little to budge her iron levels. "It was mysterious at the time, but explained in retrospect by celiac disease now," she says.

Fraser finished Ironman Canada and quickly followed it up with an even more impressive accomplishment: In 2009 she was the youngest finisher at the Ironman World Championship in Kona, Hawaii.[20]

Most recently, Fraser teamed up with fellow gluten-free athlete and celiac Carrie Willoughby for a 200-mile tandem bike ride. It served as a dual fund-raiser for the Challenged Athletes Foundation and the Celiac Disease Foundation. "I got involved with CDF because I really felt like there needed to be a lot more education about celiac disease. I didn't like that some people don't take it seriously. When you say you can't have gluten, it's not a trivial thing," Fraser says.

Bottom line, though: "I've never looked at it as a negative thing. I feel so much better; I'm healthy this way. If all I have to do to be this healthy is change my diet, I'll take it."

FAVORITE GLUTEN-FREE FOODS: Luna protein bars, Udi's Gluten Free Bread, treats from Tu-Lu's Gluten-Free Bakery, pancakes made with Pamela's Baking & Pancake Mix, Bob's Red Mill Gluten-Free Cornbread Mix, Custom Choice cereal, Clif Shot Bloks, Honey Stinger gels, Udi's Gluten Free Bagels with peanut butter

going to start reaping benefits in the fat-burning department. Of course, the machine didn't tell you that.

To get more weight-management and fat-burning potential out of shorter workouts, consider going the route of interval training, or at least pumping up the intensity of your workout. As one set of researchers showed recently, you'll not only burn more calories during the workout itself; your body will also burn more calories for up to fourteen hours following that workout. They didn't observe the same effect with low-intensity exercise.[21] How intense is intense enough? If you're sweating, your body temp is up, and your heart's beating faster, then you're in the right neighborhood. By these measures, LSD, tempo, and interval training all qualify.

In part, it comes down to a difference between taking the time to turn on your body's fat-burning pathway, and kicking the overall calorie burn into higher gear. Both can be part of an effective weight-management and fat-loss strategy . . . if used correctly.

PERIODIZATION

As any athlete will tell you, it can be hard—if not impossible—to be at your best all the time. You'll have off days, off weeks, even off months or off seasons. That's why many athletes employ what's known as *periodization training* to reach their peak performance just in time for a major race or a big game. Just as with the training protocols we already mentioned, periodization training can get very sport specific. In general, follow these guidelines:

- Following a rest or recovery period, start by building an aerobic endurance base during the early part of your training season. This is a great time to do some LSD. (Long slow distance. Not the other kind.)
- As your training season progresses, shift into higher-intensity modes of training designed to build power, more endurance, and a higher lactate threshold and VO$_2$ max.
- Once you're in the heart of competition season, employ training tapers, good nutrition management, and proper recovery to keep your body in top form.

Although there are myriad ways to construct a periodization training program, consider this basic sequence from pro freeskier Pip Hunt. During her summer off-season, she focuses on maintaining baseline fitness through "play"—trail running, mountain biking, and stand-up paddling, plus CrossFit routines three times per week. Then, from September through the start of the ski season in November, she adds strength training to get her body ready for competition season. By competition time, she shifts again, scaling back her training to focus on maintaining her strength and fitness and optimizing recovery following each competition.

STRENGTH TRAINING

While we've been talking a lot about aerobic forms of training, don't forget about the importance of strength training. Strength and power are not just for bodybuilders and sprinters. They have a place in team sports and endurance sports. And they have a place for anyone living an active lifestyle because of their beneficial influence on bone density (as do high-impact sports such as running) and offsetting the potential for osteoporosis (the gluten-intolerant community, take note!). Plus, strength training can also increase your lactate threshold.[22]

Here are a few strength-training techniques you can try:

- **ISOLATION TRAINING** — The typical gym experience you probably think of with free weights and machines. It includes exercises such as bicep curls and tricep extensions that very particularly focus on one specific muscle group at the exclusion of others.
- **FUNCTIONAL TRAINING** — Includes the currently popular Cross-Fit protocol. It uses large-scale, everyday, whole-body motions that call upon multiple muscle groups for balance, coordination, strength, and endurance. This arguably translates better to everyday fitness and sports.
- **PILATES AND WEIGHT-BEARING YOGA POSES** — These are great for improving strength *and* maintaining or improving flexibility and balance.

As you might guess, these options just scratch the surface.

STRETCHING AND FLEXIBILITY

Don't forget about the importance of maintaining flexibility. Muscles, tendons, and ligaments can get tight over time, especially with exercise. This can impact your range of motion and performance, and can also cause pain. From static to dynamic stretches, from yoga to Pilates, there are lots of ways to stretch. Just don't forget to do it in the first place! And don't do it before your exercise or event, which has been shown to decrease performance. Save the stretching for later. Instead, warm up your muscles with some light exercises.

THE IMPORTANCE OF BALANCE

Finally, a note about balance. Just as we've talked before about maintaining good balance in your gluten-free diet, so, too, is it important that you maintain good balance in your training. One of the easiest things for athletes to do is overtrain. You see someone out biking or running during one of your rest days, and you decide you want to go out, too. Or you fall into the trap of thinking that if you can just squeeze in one more training day, one more workout, it will make you that much stronger or faster.

Nothing could be further from the truth. Overtraining in athletes can lead to a number of problems that will undermine your health and performance, rather than help it: lack of recovery, immune suppression, chronic fatigue, and stress fractures, to name a few.[23]

Yet, many athletes show signs of addiction to exercise.[24] The reasons are many. They may be hooked on the desirable psychological states associated with things such as the runner's high. They may feel guilt or anxiety about missing a workout. They may be competitive and want to gain an edge on other competitors. Or—gasp!—they may simply love their sport or find exercise fun and therapeutic.

But it's crucially important to give your body—and your mind—the time it needs to recover from workouts and competitions. You'll be a better, happier, and healthier athlete because of it. And contrary to what you might think, it's not the elite professional athletes that tend to have the biggest problem with overtraining. They know what their body needs, and as professionals, they can devote themselves to proper cycles of training, competition, and recovery.

The greater problem with overtraining and lack of recovery is among working professionals who are also athletes. Maybe you're among them. We are. You're trying to squeeze lots of training into the margins of your day, worked in around a full-time job, quality time with family, sleep, and other demands on your time.[25]

Tyler Stewart knows the problem well. As both a professional elite triathlete and the owner of a busy, successful business in San Francisco, she was often working eighty hours per week and training twenty to twenty-five hours per week. "Working a full-time job and being a professional athlete, my body always seemed super taxed," she says. "I felt like I wasn't recovering. I wasn't bouncing back." Going gluten-free helped her energy and her recovery, but so did finding some semblance of balance in her busy life.

It's not always easy, but strive to find that balance.

That includes getting enough sleep at night. Many athletes get too little of it, and it can have consequences for your body and your performance.[26] Sleep is a time when your body rebuilds muscles and you recharge your system. On the flip side, getting less sleep and spending more time awake each day and night is associated with heightened snacking (especially after eight p.m.), increased calorie intake, hormone changes, and higher risk for weight gain and other negative changes—all because you skip out on a few needed hours of sleep. You train hard and you eat right. Don't slide backward by overtraining or losing sleep.

And with that, your introduction to the gluten-free edge is complete. It's time to put the knowledge into action! It's time to experience the gluten-free edge firsthand.

NEED TO KNOW

- Training provides a variety of benefits for heart health, muscle strength, bone density, building stamina or endurance, maintaining flexibility, and much more.
- Aerobic exercise targets cardio and endurance factors, whereas anaerobic exercise emphasizes speed, strength, and power.
- Heart rate monitors, perceived exertion, stopwatches, GPS watches, and watt meters are just a few of the tools—technological and otherwise—you can use to measure your output.
- The VO_2 max is a measure of your peak ability to transport and use oxygen. It is a major predictor of maximum athletic output, and appropriate training can raise its value.

- The lactate threshold is the level of exertion at which lactic acid builds up in your muscles and bloodstream faster than it can be dealt with. It is a second limiting factor on athletic performance, and training can also raise it.

- Long slow distance (LSD) training involves high mileage, moderate intensity (50 to 70 percent max) exercise. It helps build an aerobic endurance base, raise the lactate threshold, and improve the efficiency of your fat oxidation energy pathway.

- Tempo training (TT) involves exercise at or near your lactate threshold, typically 85 percent max. It is a good way to raise your lactate threshold, as well as VO_2 max.

- Interval training (IT) involves alternating between exerting above and below your lactate threshold, with relatively brief periods of intense exertion (90 to 100 percent) followed by brief periods of active rest (70 to 80 percent). It is excellent for raising your lactate threshold and VO_2 max, but it is an intense form of training.

- Periodization involves modifying the focus and balance of your training to emphasize different aspects (aerobic base, increased power, overall fitness), depending on the seasonal timing (off-season, preseason, active training, competition season).

- The importance of balance—appropriate rest and recovery days, getting enough sleep, and so on—cannot be overemphasized. Resist the temptation to overtrain.

11

On Your Mark, Get Set, Cook!

Flavorful, Nutrient-Dense Recipes

O N THE PAGES that follow you'll find a unique collection of more than fifty recipes. They're built upon the same sound gluten-free nutrition principles we've written about extensively in this book: whole, fresh foods; complex carbs; lean protein; healthy fats; and natural sources of calcium, iron, electrolytes, vitamins, antioxidants, anti-inflammatory compounds, and other micronutrients. The athletes we interviewed and profiled inspired many of these recipes.

Considering that time is at a premium for athletes (balancing work, family life, and training), we've included recipes that are fairly straight-forward and don't require long hours in the kitchen. They're geared toward fueling an active lifestyle, reducing inflammation, and support-ing recovery.

We also include a range of recipes—everything from trail food to high-octane smoothies to power breakfasts to hearty dinners, and even a few gourmet desserts.

The gluten-free diet is not about deprivation; it's about thriving on naturally gluten-free, nutritionally complete, whole foods, and enjoying the ever-expanding whole-grain and flour alternatives to wheat, barley, and rye. Recognizing the important connection between gluten-free nutrition and sports performance and how your body responds to dif-ferent foods is vital for good health, but enjoying that food is what will make the transition long lasting, delicious, and satisfying.

NUTRITIONAL COMPARISON OF INDIVIDUAL GLUTEN-FREE FLOURS AND STARCHES

FLOUR OR STARCH (¼ CUP)	CALORIES	FAT (G)	CARB (G)	PROTEIN (G)	FIBER (G)	CALCIUM (MG)	IRON (MG)
Almond Meal	162	14	6	6	3	69	1
Amaranth Flour	112	2	20	4	3	46	2
Arrowroot Starch	114	0	28	0	1	4	0
Brown Rice Flour	144	1	31	3	2	13	1
Buckwheat Flour	100	1	21	4	4	12	1
Coconut Flour	124	4	17	5	11	14	3
Corn Flour	106	1	22	2	4	2	1
Cornstarch	120	0	28	0	0	0	0
Garbanzo Bean (Chickpea) Flour	109	2	18	6	5	32	2
Hazelnut Meal Flour	176	17	5	4	3	32	1
Mesquite Meal Flour	136	0	31	3	10	63	2
Millet Flour	113	1	22	3	4	2	1

FLOUR OR STARCH (¼ CUP)	CALORIES	FAT (G)	CARB (G)	PROTEIN (G)	FIBER (G)	CALCIUM (MG)	IRON (MG)
Oat Flour	156	3	27	7	4	22	2
Potato Flour	119	0	27	3	2	11	6
Potato Starch	110	0	27	0	0	17	0
Quinoa Flour	106	2	18	4	2	14	1
Sorghum Flour	115	1	25	4	3	10	2
Soy Flour	109	5	9	9	1	52	2
Tapioca Flour	100	0	26	0	0	4	0
Teff Flour	113	1	22	4	4	41	17
White Rice Flour	146	1	32	2	1	4	0
Whole Wheat	110	1	23	4	4	0	6

All information was obtained from Bob's Red Mill, unless otherwise noted. The nutrient composition for mesquite was obtained from Peter Felker at Casa de Fruta. The nutrient composition for soy flour was obtained from the U.S. Soyfoods Directory. Values have been rounded to the nearest g or mg.

Good nutrition should be an integrated part of every athlete's life-style. Preparing your own meals from wholesome ingredients supports that process. Taking control of your nutrition means taking an interest in cooking. No gimmicks, no magic formulas, and no costly supplements required—these recipes are based on nutrient-dense foods for active people. They're the extra edge you need, so turn the page and start cooking!

THE RECIPES

BREAKFASTS
Backcountry Muesli
Banana-Nut Muffins
Buckwheat-Banana Pancakes with Pecans
Chocolate-Beet Muffins
Old-Fashioned Oatmeal
Scrambled Omelet
Teff Power Porridge

SMOOTHIES
Apple-Ginger-Beet Green Smoothie
Beet Endurance Smoothie
Cherry-Cabbage Recovery Smoothie
Orange–Green Tea Smoothie

ON THE GO: SNACKS AND TRAIL FOOD
Cranberry-Almond Energy Bars
Fudge Power Balls
Gorp
Granola-Style Energy Bars
Kale Chips
Spicy Lime Tortilla Chips
Spicy Pepitas
Tamari Bison Jerky with a Kick

SALADS AND SAVORY DIPS

Hummus

Mixed Green Salad with Grapefruit and Avocado

Quinoa Salad with Vinaigrette

Raw Kale Salad with Jicama and Cranberries

Roasted Beet and Spinach Salad

Salmon Salad

Toasted Garlic Guacamole

LUNCHES AND DINNERS

Beans and Greens

Bison Chili with Beans

Chicken Tikka Masala

Classic Lasagna with a Twist

Fried Rice

Gourmet Grilled Cheese Sandwich

Hearty Beef Stew

High Country Hash

Lentil Dal over Rice

Macaroni and Cheese

Poached Eggs on a Bed of Chard

Vegetable Frittata

Veggie Pizzas

Power Pizza

Quinoa–Sweet Potato Veggie Burgers

Roasted Brussels Sprouts and Cipollini Onions

Roasted Salmon and Asparagus

Spinach and Chickpeas

Spinach Pesto

Stuffed Peppers

Sweet and Spicy Moroccan Stew

Turkey Burgers and Sweet Potato Fries

Turkey Meatballs and Spaghetti

Turkey-Quinoa Meatloaf

Twice-Baked Potatoes

DESSERTS

Apple-Pecan Crumble

Cacao Fondue Dip

Sweet Potato–Walnut Cupcakes

NOTE: See page 311 for metric conversion charts.

Artisan Gluten-Free Flour Blend

MAKES ABOUT 3 CUPS

There are a wide variety of all-purpose gluten-free flour blends (see page 97 for a nutritional comparison of several commercial blends). Some are store-bought; others you mix up yourself based on a recipe. We're big fans of this blend, a cornerstone of the baking recipes found in Artisanal Gluten-Free Cooking *and* Artisanal Gluten-Free Cupcakes.

1¼ cups (156 g) brown rice flour
¾ cup (88 g) sorghum flour
⅔ cup (84 g) cornstarch
¼ cup (37 g) potato starch
1 tablespoon plus 1 teaspoon potato flour
1 teaspoon xanthan gum

Combine all the ingredients and store in an airtight container in the refrigerator.

Backcountry Muesli

MAKES 4 CUPS (ABOUT 8 SERVINGS)

Start the day off right with a big bowl of turbocharged muesli, and you'll hike farther, climb higher, and last longer. This muesli is perfect for extended backpacking trips.

½ cup chopped almonds
1 cup unsweetened coconut flakes
½ cup instant brown rice baby cereal
½ cup quinoa flakes
⅓ cup turbinado sugar
¼ cup ground flaxseeds
¼ teaspoon sea salt
⅓ cup dried cranberries
⅓ cup raisins
Milk, nondairy milk, or yogurt, optional

1. Preheat the oven to 300°F. Cover a baking sheet with parchment paper. Spread the almonds over one half of the baking sheet. Place on the center rack of the oven and toast for 6 minutes, until the almonds just begin to brown.

2. Remove from the oven and add the coconut to the other half of the baking sheet. Toast the almonds and coconut for another 6 to 8 minutes, until both are golden brown. Watch carefully, as the coconut burns easily. Remove from the oven and set aside to cool.

3. Place the rest of the ingredients in a large bowl and stir to mix well. Add the toasted nuts and coconut and stir to blend. Place in a large plastic bag. Store in the refrigerator.

4. To eat at home, place ½ cup of muesli in a bowl. Bring water to a boil, pour ½ cup over the muesli, stir well, cover, and let sit for 2 to 3 minutes. Drizzle with a little milk or yogurt and enjoy!

ON THE TRAIL

To make your muesli breakfast on the trail, put ½ cup of muesli in your camp bowl. Pour ½ cup of boiling water over it and stir well. You may want to add more water, depending the consistency you desire. Cover and let sit for 2 to 3 minutes.

NOTE: If you want to increase the calories for backpacking, add additional nuts, dried fruit, or powdered milk to the mixture.

PER SERVING (½ cup): 235 calories; 13 g fat; 27 g carbohydrate; 5 g protein; 5 g fiber

Banana-Nut Muffins

MAKES 12 MUFFINS

The balanced flavors of banana, nuts, and spices make these muffins a great option before a big workout or competition.

> **3 large or 4 medium bananas**
> **1 large egg**
> **⅔ cup sugar**
> **¼ cup (½ stick) butter, melted**
> **1 teaspoon gluten-free pure vanilla extract**
> **1½ cups all-purpose gluten-free flour mix (see page 252)**
> **1 teaspoon xanthan gum**
> **1½ teaspoons gluten-free baking powder**
> **¼ teaspoon baking soda**
> **1 teaspoon ground cinnamon**
> **½ cup chopped pecans**

1. Preheat the oven to 350°F. Spray one 12-cup muffin tin with non-stick cooking spray. Place paper liners in the greased muffins cups if desired.

2. Mash the bananas in a large mixing bowl until mostly smooth with a few large lumps. (Using the paddle attachment of a stand mixer is great for this.) Mix in the egg, sugar, melted butter, and vanilla.

3. In a separate bowl, combine the flour, xanthan gun, baking powder, baking soda, and cinnamon, whisking to combine.

4. Add the dry ingredients to the banana mixture and, using a stand mixer or handheld electric mixer, mix at low speed to combine, about 10 seconds. Scrape down the sides of the bowl and mix at high speed for 5 seconds, until the batter is thoroughly blended.

5. Stir in the pecans.

6. Scoop the batter into the prepared muffin cups.

7. Bake for 20 to 25 minutes, until the muffins are golden brown on top and spring back when lightly pressed.

8. Let the muffins cool for 5 minutes in the tin before transferring to a wire rack to cool completely.

PER SERVING (1 muffin): 197 calories; 8 g fat; 31 g carbohydrate; 3 g protein; 3 g fiber

—Adapted from *Artisanal Gluten-Free Cooking*, 2nd Ed.

Buckwheat-Banana Pancakes with Pecans

MAKES ABOUT SIXTEEN 4-INCH-DIAMETER PANCAKES

Despite its confusing name, buckwheat is not wheat. It's also not a cereal grain; it's a seed-containing fruit related to rhubarb. Naturally gluten-free, incredibly tasty, and a good source of high-quality protein, fiber, and powerful antioxidants, buckwheat is perfect for the athlete's table.

1 cup buckwheat flour
½ cup brown rice flour
1½ teaspoons gluten-free baking powder
½ teaspoon baking soda
¼ teaspoon sea salt
1 large egg
1¾ cups rice milk
1 tablespoon olive oil
1 ripe banana, well mashed (about ⅓ cup)
¼ cup chopped pecans
Oil for the skillet

1. Whisk together the flours, baking powder, baking soda, and salt in a medium bowl.

2. Beat the egg for 15 seconds on medium speed in a stand mixer. You can also use a handheld mixer. Add the rice milk, tablespoon of olive oil, and banana and beat for about 30 seconds longer.

3. Add the dry ingredients and mix on low speed until well blended, about 30 seconds.

4. Stir in the pecans.

5. Preheat and lightly oil a skillet.

6. Pour about ⅓ cup of batter onto the skillet for each pancake. These hearty pancakes take longer to cook than regular ones do, so don't flip too soon. Cook until the edges are well set before flipping, about 4 minutes on each side. Repeat with the remaining batter.

PER SERVING (4 pancakes): 373 calories; 14 g fat; 57 g carbohydrate; 9 g protein; 6 g fiber

Chocolate-Beet Muffins

MAKES 12 MUFFINS

Rich, moist, and not too sweet, these muffins could also qualify for cupcake status if you slice them in two, put them in a bowl, and top them with vanilla ice cream. Either way, they're a healthy surprise.

> 1¾ cups Pamela's Baking & Pancake Mix, or another all-purpose,
> 　　gluten-free baking mix (see page 252)
> ¾ cup unsweetened cacao powder
> ¼ cup coconut oil, melted
> 2 large eggs
> ⅔ cup pure maple syrup (see note, page 267)
> 1 teaspoon gluten-free pure vanilla extract
> 1 cup cooked and pureed beets (about 3 medium beets; see note)

1. Preheat the oven to 350°F. Line 12 muffin cups with paper liners.

2. Whisk together the baking mix and cacao powder in a medium bowl.

3. Place the melted coconut oil, eggs, maple syrup, and vanilla in a stand mixer. (You can also use a handheld mixer.) Beat on high speed for about 30 seconds.

4. Add the beets and mix on low speed for another 15 to 30 seconds, until well blended.

5. Add the dry ingredients to the wet ingredients and mix until blended.

6. Fill the prepared muffin cups two thirds full. Place on the center rack of the oven. Bake for 20 to 22 minutes, until a toothpick inserted into the center of a muffin comes out clean.

7. Remove from the tins and let cool on a wire rack. Store in the refrigerator.

NOTE: Roast or steam the beets, let cool, and puree. You can prepare the beets ahead of time and store in the refrigerator for 2 to 3 days.

PER SERVING (1 muffin): 184 calories; 8 g fat; 28 g carbohydrate; 4 g protein; 3 g fiber

Old-Fashioned Oatmeal

MAKES 2 SERVINGS

Eat better, feel better, perform better. Your grandmother was right. Sweetened with honey, molasses, or maple syrup, this powerhouse oatmeal makes a great prerace breakfast. Optional add-ins may include gluten-free pure vanilla extract, ground cinnamon, nuts, raisins, dates, prunes, cranberries, tart cherries, dried apricots, chopped apple, or blueberries. Be creative.

> 1¾ cups water or rice milk
> Pinch of salt
> 1 cup certified gluten-free rolled oats (such as Bob's Red Mill; see note)
> Add-ins of choice, optional
> Sweetener of choice
> Whole milk or rice, coconut, or almond milk

In a medium pot, bring the water and salt to a low boil. Slowly add the oatmeal and stir. Stir in any desired add-ins. Turn down the heat and simmer, stirring occasionally, until the oats are tender and the oatmeal is thick, about 5 minutes or according to the package directions. Serve with your desired sweetener and milk.

NOTE: Oats, as part of the gluten-free diet, are somewhat controversial. Recent research indicates that pure, uncontaminated oats used in moderation are safe for most people with celiac disease. One study did show that a small number of people with celiac disease displayed a negative response to oats. Oats are a power-packed addition to the gluten-free diet, especially for athletes. If you're not used to the high fiber content in oats, start with small servings (¼ cup uncooked) two or three times a week and build from there. The reaction some people have to oats can be attributed to the sudden increase in fiber rather than the oat peptides. Check with your health-care provider if you have questions about including oats in your diet.

Like most ingredients, not all oats are created equal. Make sure the oats you purchase are tested and certified as gluten-free. Scientists at Montana State University have selected a high-protein variety of oats (20 to 22 percent protein) that a group of local farmers are growing and processing in an entirely gluten-free facility (Montana Gluten Free Processors, or MGFP). Their oats test to less than 2 parts per million (ppm) of gluten. The general industry standard is 20 ppm. The nutrition facts for this recipe were calculated using ½ cup of uncooked MGFP oats.

PER SERVING (½ cup, oats only): 150 calories; 3 g fat; 26 g carbohydrate; 7 g protein; 5 g fiber

Scrambled Omelet

MAKES 2 SERVINGS

This one-skillet wonder is quick and easy, and offers up a great blend of carbs, protein, and fat, plus some sodium, thanks to the potato, eggs, and bacon. Feel free to jazz it up with additional vegetables as well.

3 strips bacon
3 tablespoons olive oil
1 large russet potato, shredded and squeezed of excess moisture
½ green bell pepper, seeded and diced small
½ onion, diced small
4 eggs
Salt and freshly ground black pepper

1. In a large skillet, cook the bacon until crispy. Crumble and set aside. Discard the bacon fat.

2. Heat 2 tablespoons of the oil in the same skillet over medium-high heat. Add the potato and cook, turning occasionally, until semisoft and beginning to turn golden brown in places, about 10 minutes.

3. Move the potato to the outside edge of the pan. In the center of the pan, add the remaining 1 tablespoon of oil. Place the pepper and onion in the pan and cook, stirring occasionally, until soft. Add the crumbled bacon.

4. Whisk the eggs with salt and pepper in a bowl. Pour over the potato, bacon, and vegetables and scramble until the eggs are cooked, about 3 minutes. Serve hot.

PER SERVING: 566 calories; 35 g fat; 42 g carbohydrate; 22 g protein; 4 g fiber

—Adapted from *Artisanal Gluten-Free Cooking*, 2nd Ed.

Teff Power Porridge

MAKES 2 LARGE SERVINGS

Teff, native to Africa, is one of the smallest grains in the world. It's also one of the most nutritious. Rich in carbohydrates, protein, fiber, iron, calcium, and an assortment of other nutrients needed for an active lifestyle, this porridge will definitely get you going first thing in the morning.

2 cups water
Pinch of salt, optional
½ cup uncooked teff
½ teaspoon ground cinnamon
1 small apple, cored and diced (about 1 cup; see note)
¼ cup chopped walnuts
¼ cup raisins
½ teaspoon gluten-free pure vanilla extract
Milk
Honey or pure maple syrup (see note, page 267)

1. Bring the water and salt, if using, to a boil in a medium saucepan over medium-high heat. Slowly stir in the teff, followed by the cinnamon, apple, walnuts, raisins, and vanilla. Stir well, as the grain can clump together.

2. Turn down the heat to low, cover, and cook, stirring occasionally, until the teff grains are tender, about 20 minutes. Remove from the heat and let sit for 2 to 3 minutes. Top with milk and honey or maple syrup.

NOTE: Also peel the apple if it's not organic.

PER SERVING: 365 calories; 11 g fat; 61 g carbohydrate; 10 g protein; 7 g fiber

▶ **NUTRITION BONUS:** good source of iron

|||||||||||||||||||||||||||||||||||||| **SMOOTHIES** ||||||||||||||||||||||||||||||||||||||||||

Apple-Ginger-Beet Green Smoothie

MAKES ABOUT 3 CUPS (2 LARGE SERVINGS)

Ginger has a spicy, wake-up-call quality to it. It's also full of health-promoting goodness, so be adventurous and whip up this smoothie to help kick-start your day. You won't be disappointed.

> 2 cups well-washed, coarsely chopped beet greens
> 2 cups coconut water
> 1 green apple, cored and chopped (see note on page 308)
> 1 carrot, chopped
> 1 ripe banana, peeled
> 2 tablespoons ground chia seeds
> 1 tablespoon ground flaxseeds
> 1 tablespoon honey
> One ½-inch piece fresh ginger

Place all the ingredients in a blender and blend until smooth.

NOTE: Research shows ginger contains anti-inflammatory compounds and helps alleviate gastrointestinal distress.

PER SERVING: 339 calories; 8 g fat; 65 g carbohydrate; 7 g protein; 15 g fiber

Beet Endurance Smoothie

MAKES ABOUT 3½ CUPS (2 SERVINGS)

Hit the ground running (literally) with this high-octane blend of powerful nutrients. Studies show beet juice enhances tolerance to exercise and helps send oxygen to working muscles. Who knew the underappreciated and much maligned beet had so much going for it? Beets should be a staple on every athlete's shopping list.

2 cups coarsely chopped spinach
2 cups filtered water
¼ cup frozen blueberries
1 small raw beet, trimmed and chopped (about ⅓ cup)
1 pear, cored and chopped
1 stalk celery, chopped
2 tablespoons ground chia seeds

Place all the ingredients in a blender and blend until smooth.

NOTE: If you don't have a powerful blender, grate the beets and chop the celery into small pieces. This is also good with a dollop of Greek yogurt added to the mixture.

PER SERVING: 165 calories; 5 g fat; 30 g carbohydrate; 4 g protein; 11 g fiber

Cherry-Cabbage Recovery Smoothie

MAKES ABOUT 4 CUPS (2 LARGE SERVINGS)

Add healing power to your post-workout meal with this antioxidant-rich, immune-boosting smoothie. Research suggests eating tart cherries after an intense workout speeds muscle recovery. Cabbage contains nutrients that help maintain a healthy digestive tract. Don't panic; Napa cabbage is a sweet and tasty beginner cabbage. You won't even know it's there.

4 large Napa cabbage leaves, chopped coarsely
2 cups coconut water
½ cup fresh or frozen pitted cherries (10 to 12 cherries)
½ cup vanilla goat yogurt
2 tablespoons ground chia seeds
1 teaspoon ground cinnamon

Place all the ingredients in a blender and blend until smooth.

NOTE: Vanilla goat yogurt is excellent in smoothies.

PER SERVING: 269 calories; 8 g fat; 44 g carbohydrate; 9 g protein; 11 g fiber

Orange–Green Tea Smoothie

The health benefits of green tea have been touted in dozens of research papers. This smoothie is a perfect way to get a big dose of immunity-boosting goodness before the day even starts. Make a jar of green tea and keep it in the refrigerator for smoothie making.

2 cups chilled brewed green tea
4 Medjool dates, pitted and chopped
2 cups mixed leafy greens
1 orange, peeled and chopped
⅔ cup chopped cucumber
1 stalk celery, chopped
2 tablespoons raw shelled hemp seeds, ground
2 tablespoons pumpkin seeds, ground

1. Soak the dates in the green tea while preparing the rest of the ingredients.

2. Place all the ingredients in a blender and blend until smooth.

NOTE: A coffee grinder is perfect for grinding seeds and nuts for smoothies. Unless you have a powerful blender, grind the measured seeds before adding them to the smoothie.

PER SERVING: 340 calories; 12 g fat; 54 g carbohydrate; 11 g protein; 8 g fiber

▶ **NUTRITION BONUS:** good source of vitamin C and magnesium

IIIIIIIIIIII **ON THE GO: SNACKS AND TRAIL FOOD** IIIIIIIIIIII

Cranberry-Almond Energy Bars

MAKES 12 BARS

Plain energy bars are nice, but throwing in some high-powered chia seeds, sweet dates, and antioxidant-rich cranberries make these tart little treats extra good. Wrap them individually and freeze. These bars taste great frozen; no need to let them thaw.

> **1½ cups unsweetened coconut flakes**
> **1 cup almond meal**
> **½ cup frozen cranberries**
> **2 tablespoons honey**
> **6 Medjool dates, pitted and chopped coarsely**
> **2 tablespoons ground chia seeds**
> **2 teaspoons ground cinnamon**

1. Preheat the oven to 300°F. Line a small baking sheet with parchment paper. Spread the coconut flakes over the parchment paper and place the baking sheet on the center rack of the oven. Toast for 5 to 8 minutes, until lightly browned. Watch carefully, as the coconut burns easily, and shake the pan occasionally to ensure even toasting. Remove from the oven.

2. Place the coconut and the remaining ingredients in a food processor and pulse until well mixed, 1 to 2 minutes. The mixture will resemble a smooth ball of dough.

3. Reline the baking sheet with a new piece of parchment paper. Transfer the mixture to the prepared baking sheet. Cover with another piece of parchment paper and, using a rolling pin, roll into a ¼- to ½-inch-thick rectangle. If you don't have a rolling pin, shape it with your hands. Refrigerate until well chilled, then cut into bars. Wrap individually in plastic wrap and freeze.

PER SERVING: 187 calories; 12 g fat; 19 g carbohydrate; 3 g protein; 5 g fiber

Fudge Power Balls

MAKES 18 BALLS

Yes, fudge can be a healthy indulgence! The key to enjoying these dense, chocolaty power balls is to freeze them first and eat them later. They're perfect straight from the freezer.

1 cup pecans
¾ cup unsweetened cacao powder
10 Medjool dates, pitted and chopped into small pieces
¾ cup almond butter
¼ cup orange juice, apple juice, coconut water, or plain water
2 tablespoons honey
½ teaspoon gluten-free pure vanilla extract
½ to ⅔ cup unsweetened shredded coconut

1. Pulse the pecans in a food processor until finely ground. Add the cacao powder and pulse until well mixed.

2. Add the dates, almond butter, orange juice, honey, and vanilla and pulse until all the ingredients are mixed together and a dough ball forms.

3. Line a small baking sheet with parchment paper. Roll the dough into golf-ball-size balls, roll in the coconut to cover, and place on the prepared baking sheet. Place the baking sheet in the refrigerator until the balls are well chilled. Remove and store the balls in a plastic container in the freezer. (When ready to eat, there's no reason to wait for them to thaw; they can be enjoyed straight from the freezer.)

PER SERVING (1 power ball): 180 calories; 13 g fat; 18 g carbohydrate; 3 g protein; 4 g fiber

Gorp

If you've been around hiking and backpacking long enough, you'll recognize gorp as old-school trail mix. Gorp was originally an acronym for "good old raisins and peanuts." This powerful gorp is the new-school, gourmet version, with whole nuts, seeds, and coconut. It will keep you going all day. It's perfect stowed in a backpack or briefcase, or served with milk and fresh fruit as a breakfast granola.

2 cups gluten-free crispy brown rice cereal
2 cups unsweetened coconut flakes
2 cups whole almonds
1 cup walnut halves
1 cup pecan halves
1 cup pumpkin seeds
1 cup sunflower seeds
⅓ cup almond butter
⅓ cup honey
¼ cup pure maple syrup (see note)
1 teaspoon gluten-free pure vanilla extract
1 teaspoon ground cinnamon
¼ teaspoon sea salt
1 cup raisins

1. Preheat the oven to 300°F. Position two oven racks in the center of the oven. Grease two baking sheets.

2. Place the cereal, coconut, almonds, walnuts, pecans, pumpkin seeds, and sunflower seeds in a large bowl.

3. Place the almond butter, honey, maple syrup, vanilla, cinnamon, and salt in a medium saucepan over medium heat. Bring to a slow boil, whisking continually, and cook for about 1 minute. Remove from the heat.

4. Drizzle the warm wet mixture over the dry mixture and gently stir to incorporate. Make sure the sauce coats the dry ingredients evenly.

5. Spread out evenly in a single layer on the prepared baking sheets.

6. Bake for 6 to 8 minutes, until beginning to brown. Remove, stir, and return to the oven, switching the positions of the baking sheets.

Bake for another 6 to 8 minutes, remove, stir, and switch again. Bake until golden brown. The total baking time should be about 20 minutes. Watch carefully, as the gorp can overbrown quickly.

7. Add the raisins. Let the mixture cool completely before storing in an airtight container for up to 1 week.

NOTE: Grade B maple syrup is thicker and richer, but any grade will work.

PER SERVING (½ cup): 335 calories; 25 g fat; 23 g carbohydrate; 9 g protein; 4 g fiber

Granola-Style Energy Bars

MAKES 16 BARS

There's another side to energy bars—the homemade side. Stash these delicious treats in your backpack or pack them in a school lunch. Either way, they'll be a hit.

¼ cup almond meal
2 tablespoons raw shelled hemp seeds
1 teaspoon ground cinnamon
¼ teaspoon salt
1 cup pecans
1 cup almonds
1 cup unsulfured dried apricots (about 6 ounces), chopped into chunks
¼ cup certified gluten-free rolled oats (such as Bob's Red Mill; see note, page 258)
½ cup chocolate chips
⅓ cup pure maple syrup (see note above)
1 large egg
1 tablespoon coconut oil, melted, plus some for the pan
1 teaspoon gluten-free pure vanilla extract

1. Preheat the oven to 350°F. Grease a 9-inch square baking pan.

2. Place the almond meal, hemp seeds, cinnamon, and salt in a food processor and pulse until well mixed.

3. Add the pecans, almonds, apricots, and oats and pulse several times, until the nuts are in small chunks but not completely ground. Add the chocolate chips and pulse a few times, leaving larger chunks.

4. In a bowl big enough to hold all the ingredients, whisk together the maple syrup, egg, melted coconut oil, and vanilla. Whisk for 1 minute to ensure the ingredients are well mixed.

5. Add the dry (pulsed) ingredients to the wet ingredients and mash together with a fork until well mixed. Use your hands if you have to.

6. Spread the mixture in the prepared pan. Cover with parchment paper and, using your hands, flatten evenly. You can also use a spatula to flatten the mixture.

7. Place on the center rack of the oven. Bake for 22 to 24 minutes, until golden brown. Remove from the oven and let cool. Place the pan in the refrigerator to chill before cutting into bars. Store in an airtight container in the refrigerator.

PER SERVING (1 bar): 206 calories; 14 g fat; 18 g carbohydrate; 5 g protein; 3 g fiber

Kale Chips

MAKES 1 MEDIUM BOWL OF KALE CHIPS

Bet you can't eat just one.

1 bunch kale
1 tablespoon olive oil
Optional seasonings: garlic salt, ground sesame seeds, crushed red pepper flakes, all-purpose herb seasoning
Kosher salt (larger-grain salt works best in this recipe)

1. Preheat the oven to 300°F.

2. Wash the kale and spin in a salad spinner to remove any moisture. Pat dry with a paper towel, remove the stalks (see note), and cut the leaves into large pieces (2 to 3 inches across).

3. Place the kale in large bowl. Drizzle with the olive oil and, with your hands, gently work the oil into the leaves. Sprinkle with your desired seasonings. A little extra kosher salt tastes great on these (just as with potato chips).

4. Spread the kale in a single layer on a large baking sheet.

5. Place the baking sheet on the center rack of the oven and bake for 15 to 20 minutes, until the kale is crispy but not overbrowned.

6. Serve immediately.

NOTE: Save the kale stalks for use in smoothies. They're packed with fiber and phytonutrients, but use them sparingly, as they can be overpowering and slightly bitter.

PER RECIPE: 220 calories; 15 g fat; 20 g carbohydrate; 7 g protein; 4 g fiber

Spicy Lime Tortilla Chips

MAKES 2 DOZEN CHIPS

These healthy tortilla chips are perfect for scooping up guacamole (page 277), hummus (page 272), or high-protein bean dip and make for a great post-workout snack.

Six 6-inch gluten-free 100% corn tortillas
Cold-pressed olive oil cooking spray
1 tablespoon freshly squeezed lime juice
½ teaspoon chili powder
Pinch of garlic powder
Sea salt

1. Preheat the oven to 375°F. Spray each side of the corn tortillas with olive oil and cut them into quarters. Arrange them in a single layer on a large baking sheet.

2. In a small bowl, whisk together the lime juice, chili powder, and garlic powder. Brush on the tortilla quarters. Sprinkle liberally with salt.

3. Place the baking sheet on center rack of the oven. Bake for about 15 minutes, or until crispy and golden brown. Watch carefully, as they can burn easily.

4. Serve immediately.

PER SERVING (12 chips): 196 calories; 6 g fat; 34 g carbohydrate; 4 g protein; 5 g fiber

Spicy Pepitas

MAKES 1 CUP

These pepitas are the spicy Spanish version of roasted pumpkin seeds. These treats are wonderful on their own or used as a topping for Southwest-style soups or salads.

1 cup large raw pumpkin seeds
1 teaspoon olive oil
1 teaspoon ground coriander
½ teaspoon sea salt
¼ teaspoon freshly ground black pepper
⅛ teaspoon cayenne pepper

1. Preheat the oven to 325°F.

2. In a small bowl, toss the pumpkin seeds with the olive oil. Spread in a single layer on a small baking sheet.

3. Place the baking sheet on the center rack of the oven and toast the seeds for 10 to 15 minutes. Shake the pan periodically to ensure even toasting. They burn easily, so watch closely.

4. Remove from the oven, place in a shallow bowl, and toss with the coriander, salt, black pepper, and cayenne. Serve warm.

PER SERVING (¼ cup): 197 calories; 17 g fat; 6 g carbohydrate; 9 g protein; 2 g fiber

▶ **NUTRITION BONUS:** good source of iron

Tamari Bison Jerky with a Kick

MAKES 6 SERVINGS

When it comes to making jerky, the leaner the meat, the better. Bison is perfect. It dehydrates well and makes for a great Lewis-and-Clark trail snack. Unless you have mad, ninja knife skills, ask your butcher to cut ⅛-inch strips for you. If you cut it yourself, partially freeze the meat first and cut against the grain. Also, note that this recipe requires a homestyle dehydrator with an adjustable thermostat and timer.

½ cup wheat-free tamari or gluten-free soy sauce
2 garlic cloves, minced
1 small shallot, minced
1 tablespoon agave nectar
1 tablespoon apple cider vinegar
½ teaspoon ground ginger
½ teaspoon crushed red pepper flakes
Freshly ground black pepper
1½ pounds bison meat, cut into ⅛-inch strips

1. Stir together all the ingredients except the meat in a medium bowl.

2. Place the meat and marinade mix in a zip-top plastic bag, press out the air, and zip the bag shut. Flip, toss, and slosh the bag, making sure the marinade completely covers all the meat pieces. Store in the refrigerator for 4 to 6 hours, turning occasionally, but don't overmarinate or it will be too salty.

3. Drain the strips and neatly arrange them on dehydrator trays. Do not overlap.

4. Dehydrate at 145° to 155°F for 8 to 12 hours, depending on your dehydrator. The strips should be chewy and leathery. Store in the refrigerator.

NOTE: Although *London broil* is a cooking method and not a cut of meat, many call a top round roast a "London broil." This is a good cut for jerky.

PER SERVING: 142 calories; 2 g fat; 3 g carbohydrate; 26 g protein; 0.5 g fiber

▶ **NUTRITION BONUS:** good source of B vitamins, iron, and zinc

IIIIIIIIIIIIIIIII **SALADS AND SAVORY DIPS** IIIIIIIIIIIIIIIII

Hummus

MAKES ABOUT 2 CUPS

Serve with crackers or fresh vegetables for a perfect midday snack.

One 15-ounce can chickpeas, with half of the liquid from the can
2 tablespoons tahini (sesame paste)
Juice of ½ large lemon
1 garlic clove
1 to 2 tablespoons olive oil
Salt

Place all the ingredients in a food processor and blend until smooth.

PER SERVING (¼ cup): 109 calories; 5 g fat; 13 g carbohydrate; 3 g protein; 3 g fiber

Mixed Green Salad with Grapefruit and Avocado

MAKES 4 SERVINGS

This salad is packed with antioxidant goodness. The blend of blueberries, avocado, and grapefruit makes for a nice mix of flavors.

DRESSING
2 teaspoons gluten-free Dijon mustard
2 tablespoons extra-virgin olive oil
1 to 2 tablespoons agave nectar
1 tablespoon apple cider vinegar

SALAD
6 cups mixed greens
1 grapefruit, peeled, seeded, sectioned, and chopped into large chunks
1 avocado, pitted and sliced

⅓ cup blueberries
⅓ cup chopped pecans
About ¼ cup crumbled feta cheese or shaved goat cheese
Currants or dried figs, optional
Sea salt and freshly ground black pepper

1. Make the dressing: First, place the mustard in a small bowl. (Starting with the mustard keeps the dressing from separating.) Add the olive oil, agave nectar, and vinegar. Whisk to blend well. Store in a small glass jar in the refrigerator and use for a general salad dressing. Shake before using.

2. Assemble the salad: Combine the greens, grapefruit, avocado, and blueberries in a large bowl. Drizzle with a small amount of dressing and toss. Sprinkle with the pecans and feta cheese. Add the currants or figs, if using. Season to taste with salt and pepper.

PER SERVING: 285 calories; 22 g fat; 21 g carbohydrate; 5 g protein; 7 g fiber (This analysis includes the entire allotment of dressing.)

▶ **NUTRITION BONUS:** good source of vitamin C

Quinoa Salad with Vinaigrette

MAKES 4 SERVINGS

The combination of quinoa, red bell pepper, and scallions makes for a bright and healthy salad. Serve as a side or over a bed of mixed greens for a complete meal.

1 cup uncooked quinoa, rinsed if necessary
2 cups water
¼ cup red wine vinegar
¼ cup olive oil
Salt and freshly ground black pepper
½ red bell pepper, seeded and diced small
3 scallions, sliced thinly

1. Combine the quinoa and water in a saucepan and bring to a boil. Turn down the heat, cover, and simmer for 15 to 20 minutes, until all the liquid is absorbed. The quinoa should be translucent and soft but not mushy. Refrigerate until cooled.

2. To make the vinaigrette, combine the vinegar and olive oil in a small bowl and season with salt and pepper. Whisk to blend well.

3. Mix together the cooled quinoa, bell pepper, scallions, and vinaigrette in a serving bowl. Serve chilled.

PER SERVING: 288 calories; 16 g fat; 31 g carbohydrate; 6 g protein; 3 g fiber

▶ **NUTRITION BONUS:** good source of iron

—Adapted from *Artisanal Gluten-Free Cooking*, 2nd Ed.

Raw Kale Salad with Jicama and Cranberries

MAKES 6 SERVINGS

Kale is at the top of the nutrition charts. It's low in calories and high in goodness. If you're new to raw kale, this is a good salad to start with.

1 bunch kale, stalks removed (see note), leaves finely chopped
2 tablespoons freshly squeezed lime juice
1 tablespoon olive oil
1 teaspoon agave nectar
¼ teaspoon salt
½ cup chopped pecans
½ cup jicama, cut into thin strips
½ cup dried cranberries

1. Place the kale in a large salad bowl.

2. In a small bowl, whisk together the lime juice, olive oil, agave nectar, and salt. Pour it over the kale and work it in with your hands.

3. Add the pecans, jicama, and cranberries. Toss to combine, then serve.

NOTE: Save the kale stalks for use in smoothies. They're packed with fiber and phytonutrients, but use them sparingly, as they can be overpowering and slightly bitter.

PER SERVING: 133 calories; 9 g fat; 14 g carbohydrate; 2 g protein; 3 g fiber

▶ **NUTRITION BONUS:** good source of vitamin A and vitamin C

Roasted Beet and Spinach Salad

SERVES 4 AS A SIDE SALAD

Pair this tasty salad with baked chicken and wild rice and you have every-thing you need to boost your immunity and fuel recovery. Beets and spinach provide a powerful blend of antioxidants.

SALAD
1 pound beets, rinsed and scrubbed
Olive oil
4 cups spinach leaves
½ cup chopped pecans
1 cup crumbled feta cheese or shaved goat cheese
Sea salt and freshly ground black pepper

DRESSING
1 tablespoon gluten-free Dijon mustard
3 tablespoons extra-virgin olive oil
2 tablespoons freshly squeezed lemon juice
1 tablespoon agave nectar
1 garlic clove, minced
1 tablespoon finely diced shallot

1. Preheat the oven to 400°F.

2. Prepare the salad: If the beets came with greens, trim the beet greens to about ½ inch from the root and save the greens for a healthy pizza topping. Drizzle the beets with a little olive oil, turn to coat well, and place in a shallow baking dish. Cover with tinfoil. Bake for 30 to 45 minutes, until tender when pierced with a sharp knife. The baking time depends on the size of the beets. Let cool to room temperature, then remove the stems and stringy roots. You can store them whole in the refrigerator for 3 to 4 days.

3. Prepare the dressing: First, place the mustard in a small bowl. (Starting with the mustard keeps the dressing from separating.) Add the olive oil and whisk well. Add the lemon juice and agave nectar and whisk again. Add the garlic and shallot and mix well.

4. Thinly slice the beets. Divide the spinach among four salad plates. Top each serving with sliced beets, chopped pecans, and feta cheese. Season with salt and pepper and drizzle with dressing (see note).

NOTE: It is unlikely that you'll use all of the dressing. Store the leftovers in a glass bottle. No need to refrigerate the dressing if you use it within a week.

PER SERVING: 374 calories; 30 g fat; 16 g carbohydrate; 12 g protein; 6 g fiber (This analysis includes the entire allotment of dressing.)

Salmon Salad

MAKES ABOUT 3 CUPS

The omega-3 concentration in salmon takes center stage, but there are other health-promoting benefits to salmon. Research shows salmon to have high levels of calcitonin, a substance that reduces joint inflammation. This salad not only tastes good, it's a great post-workout recovery meal.

½ **pound cooked salmon, flaked**
4 **scallions, sliced**
1 **stalk celery, chopped**
¼ **cup chopped zucchini**
¼ **cup chopped cucumber**
2 **tablespoons mayonnaise**
1 **teaspoon gluten-free Dijon mustard**
¼ **teaspoon sea salt**
Freshly ground black pepper
Lettuce or large Napa cabbage leaves

1. In a large bowl, gently toss together the salmon, scallions, celery, zucchini, and cucumber.

2. In a small bowl, whisk together the mayonnaise, mustard, salt, and pepper to taste.

3. Add the dressing to the salmon mixture and toss to coat.

4. Serve on a bed of lettuce or in large Napa cabbage leaves.

NOTE: This is also good with chopped bell peppers or jicama.

PER SERVING (1 cup): 131 calories; 4 g fat; 4 g carbohydrate; 19 g protein; 1 g fiber

▶ **NUTRITION BONUS:** very high in vitamin B_{12}, good source of selenium

Toasted Garlic Guacamole

MAKES ABOUT 1¼ CUPS

There's no need to feel guilty about eating guacamole when you make it yourself from nutrient-dense ingredients like this—especially if you serve it with homemade Spicy Lime Tortilla Chips (page 269). This is a powerhouse snack. Toast the garlic first for extra flavor.

2 whole garlic cloves, unpeeled
2 large avocados
2 tablespoons freshly squeezed lime juice
1 small tomato, chopped and drained
6 to 8 scallions (white and light green parts), finely chopped
(about 3 tablespoons)
1 jalapeño pepper, finely diced (about 3 tablespoons)
¼ cup coarsely chopped fresh cilantro
½ teaspoon crushed red pepper flakes
Sea salt

1. Place the unpeeled garlic in a small, dry skillet over medium heat. Toast for 10 to 12 minutes, turning often, until browned in spots. Set aside to cool.

2. Halve and pit the avocados. Scoop out the flesh and place in a medium bowl. Add the lime juice, tomato, scallions, jalapeño, cilantro, and pepper flakes.

3. Slip the garlic out of the skins and mince finely. Add it to the avo-cado mixture.

4. Add salt to taste and mash the guacamole with a fork. Taste and adjust the flavorings as you mash it; depending on your preferences, add more salt, lime juice, or pepper flakes.

PER SERVING (¼ cup): 126 calories; 10 g fat; 10 g carbohydrate; 2 g protein; 6 g fiber

IIIIIIIIIIIIIIIIIIIII **LUNCHES AND DINNERS** IIIIIIIIIIIIIIIIIIIIIIIIII

Beans and Greens

MAKES 4 SERVINGS

Chard is perfect for mixing with cannellini beans, but any hardy green will do. This makes for a nutrition-packed side dish. Or serve it over a bowl of brown rice for a full meal. It's even good for breakfast.

1 tablespoons olive oil
½ cup chopped onion
2 garlic cloves, minced
1 bunch chard (6 to 8 big leaves), stalks trimmed (see note, page 290), leaves rolled and cut into wide strips
¼ cup gluten-free chicken or vegetable stock, plus more if needed
One 15-ounce can cannellini beans, drained
Sea salt and freshly ground black pepper
¼ cup grated Parmesan

1. Heat the olive oil in a large skillet over medium-low heat. Add the onion and sauté for 4 to 5 minutes, until soft. Add the garlic and sauté for another 1 to 2 minutes.

2. Add the chard and toss with tongs to coat. Add the stock and beans, turn down the heat to low, and simmer just until the greens are slightly wilted and beans are warmed. The mixture should be moist but not wet. If you need more stock, add 1 or 2 tablespoons slowly. Season with salt and pepper to taste.

3. Sprinkle with the Parmesan and serve immediately.

PER SERVING: 258 calories; 8 g fat; 33 g carbohydrate; 16 g protein; 7 g fiber

▶ **NUTRITION BONUS:** good source of iron and magnesium

Bison Chili with Beans

MAKES 8 CUPS (ABOUT 6 SERVINGS)

This bison chili with beans is so versatile; you'll be making it often. Serve it in a bowl with grated cheese on top or over a gluten-free bun as a Sloppy Joe. You can even make tostadas and tacos with it. This recipe is a high-protein winner.

1 tablespoon vegetable oil
½ cup chopped onion
4 garlic cloves, minced
1 pound ground bison
Sea salt and freshly ground black pepper
Two 15-ounce cans pinto beans, drained and rinsed
One 15-ounce can fire-roasted diced tomatoes with green chiles
One 4-ounce can diced green chiles, hot or mild
One 15-ounce can plain (unseasoned) tomato sauce
1 to 2 tablespoons chili powder
Optional toppings: grated cheese, chopped lettuce, chopped
    avocado, sour cream

1. Heat the oil in a large pot over medium heat. Add the onion and sauté for 4 to 5 minutes, until soft. Add the garlic and sauté for another 1 to 2 minutes. Using a slotted spoon, transfer the onions and garlic to a small bowl and set aside.

2. Turn up the heat to medium-high and add the ground bison to the pot. Season with salt and pepper and cook, stirring often, until browned.

3. Add the beans, tomatoes with green chiles, green chiles, tomato sauce, and chili powder. Stir well. Turn down the heat and simmer for about 30 minutes, until thick.

4. Serve in bowls with the optional toppings.

NOTE: In addition to the chili powder, you can also experiment with spicing up your chili with ground cumin, oregano, coriander, garlic, and other herbs and spices. Or choose a ready-made (gluten-free) chili spice blend.

PER SERVING: 403 calories; 18 g fat; 39 g carbohydrate; 24 g protein; 8 g fiber

▶ **NUTRITION BONUS:** good source of B vitamins, iron, zinc, and selenium

Chicken Tikka Masala

MAKES 4 SERVINGS

The sweet and spicy flavors in this chicken dish work perfectly together. Served over basmati rice, this well-rounded dish will fill your tank with carbs, protein, and fat in roughly the 40:30:30 ratio popular with athletes.

3 boneless, skinless chicken breasts, cubed
Salt
1 tablespoon olive oil, plus some for the skillet
1 tablespoon butter
1 medium onion, sliced
1 large garlic clove, minced
1 tablespoon minced fresh ginger
½ teaspoon cayenne pepper, optional
2 teaspoons ground cumin
2 teaspoons paprika
1 teaspoon garam masala
1½ cups diced tomatoes, or one 14.5-ounce can no-salt-added diced
   tomatoes
1 cup heavy cream
½ cup gluten-free chicken stock
⅓ cup chopped fresh cilantro
2 cups cooked basmati rice

1. Season the chicken with salt. Heat a bit of olive oil in a large skillet over medium-high heat. Sauté the chicken until no longer pink, about 8 minutes, depending on the size of your cubes. Remove from the pan and set aside.

2. In the same skillet, over medium heat, melt the butter and the tablespoon of olive oil. Add the onion, garlic, and ginger and sauté until very soft, about 10 minutes.

3. Add the cayenne (if using), cumin, paprika, and garam masala and stir. Cook for 1 additional minute.

4. Add the tomatoes, cream, and stock. Using a handheld immersion blender, puree until smooth.

5. Simmer uncovered for 10 minutes. Add the chicken and simmer for an additional 10 to 20 minutes, or more. (The sauce becomes richer,

more flavorful, and thicker the longer you simmer it, but be careful, as simmering for too long will cause the sauce to separate.)

6. Add the cilantro just before serving. Serve over the rice.

PER SERVING: 700 calories; 41 g fat; 35 g carbohydrate; 49 g protein; 2 g fiber

—Adapted from *Artisanal Gluten-Free Cooking*, 2nd Ed.

Classic Lasagna with a Twist

MAKES 8 SERVINGS

Crunchy zucchini chunks make for a pleasant surprise in this classic lasagna dish. Serve with a spinach side salad for a power-packed meal.

One 10-ounce package gluten-free brown rice lasagna noodles (such as Tinkyada brand)
1 tablespoon olive oil
¾ cup chopped onion
4 garlic cloves, minced
1 pound grass-fed ground beef
Sea salt and freshly ground black pepper
1 medium zucchini, chopped in 1-inch cubes (about 2 cups)
Two 25-ounce jars gluten-free Italian herb pasta sauce
8 ounces mozzarella, shredded
8 ounces ricotta
⅓ cup shredded Parmesan

1. Preheat the oven to 350°F. Cook the pasta according to the package directions, then drain.

2. Heat the oil in a large pot over medium heat. Add the onion and sauté for 4 to 5 minutes, until soft. Add the garlic and sauté for another 1 to 2 minutes. Using a slotted spoon, remove the onion and garlic and set aside.

3. Add the ground beef to the pot and cook, stirring occasionally, until browned. Season with salt and pepper. Drain any excess grease if necessary.

4. Add the onion and garlic, zucchini, and pasta sauce to the ground beef and stir well.

5. In the bottom of a 9 × 13-inch baking dish, spread one third of the sauce. Arrange half of the pasta noodles side by side on top of the sauce. Spread one third of the sauce over the noodles and top with half of the mozzarella and ricotta. Repeat in the same order with the remaining noodles, sauce, and cheese. Sprinkle the top with the Parmesan.

6. Cover with tinfoil and place on the center rack of the oven. Bake for 30 minutes. Remove the foil and bake for another 15 minutes, until the cheese is bubbly and lightly browned.

7. Let the lasagna rest for 5 minutes before serving.

PER SERVING: 559 calories; 20 g fat; 61 g carbohydrate; 34 g protein; 3 g fiber

▶ **NUTRITION BONUS:** good source of B vitamins, iron, phosphorus, and zinc

Fried Rice

MAKES 4 SERVINGS

Sesame oil and tamari give this classic fried rice dish added kick. It's not only big in flavor—it packs nutritional punch as well.

4 tablespoons olive oil
1 tablespoon grated fresh ginger
2 garlic cloves, grated
1 chicken breast, julienned, or 4 to 6 ounces extra-firm tofu, diced small
1 large carrot, shredded
2 eggs
3 cups cooled cooked rice
5 tablespoons wheat-free tamari or gluten-free soy sauce
2 teaspoons sesame oil
5 scallions, chopped

1. Heat 2 tablespoons of the olive oil in a wok or large skillet over medium-high heat.

2. Add the ginger and garlic and stir-fry until fragrant, about 30 seconds.

3. Add the chicken and stir-fry for 1 minute.

4. Add the carrot and cook until the chicken is no longer pink and the carrot is soft.

5. Move the chicken and carrots to the perimeter, add the eggs to the center, and scramble until the eggs are nearly done.

6. Move the eggs to the perimeter, add the remaining 2 tablespoons of olive oil to the center, and heat for 1 minute.

7. Add the rice and stir-fry for a few minutes, until warm and any clumps have broken up.

8. Add the soy sauce, sesame oil, and scallions, toss all the ingredients together, and stir-fry for a few additional minutes, until the flavors have melded.

PER SERVING (with chicken): 458 calories; 24 g fat; 38 g carbohydrate; 23 g protein; 4 g fiber

—Adapted from *Artisanal Gluten-Free Cooking*, 2nd Ed.

Gourmet Grilled Cheese Sandwich

MAKES 1 SANDWICH

There are several good whole-grain, gluten-free breads on the market now, so there's no reason to do without an occasional grilled cheese sandwich. Here are some ideas to elevate the lowly grilled cheese to gourmet status.

> 2 tablespoons butter, or as needed
> 2 slices whole-grain gluten-free bread
> ½ Bosc pear, sliced thinly (or other firm pear; see note)
> 1 slice smoked Gouda

Melt the butter in a sauté pan over medium-low heat. Make sure the butter doesn't burn. Assemble the sandwich and grill in the sizzling butter until the first side is golden brown. Flip and grill the other side, adding more butter if needed.

Other options for gourmet grilled cheese sandwiches include:

- Cheddar, sliced peaches, and thinly sliced almonds
- Goat cheese, thinly sliced figs, and thinly sliced jicama
- Colby, roasted green chiles, and sliced tomatoes

NOTE: Bosc pears have a wonderful density that grills well. The texture is similar to a cross between a softer pear and an apple or jicama.

PER SERVING: 441 calories; 27 g fat; 36 g carbohydrate; 15 g protein; 4 g fiber

Hearty Beef Stew

MAKES 8 CUPS (ABOUT 6 SERVINGS)

There's nothing better after a day of skiing than a big serving of beef stew. Serve in a mug or over a chunk of gluten-free corn bread.

2 tablespoons vegetable oil
½ cup chopped onion
2 garlic cloves, minced
1 pound grass-fed beef stew meat
Sea salt and freshly ground black pepper
2 tablespoons brown rice flour or other gluten-free flour
4 cups gluten-free beef stock
½ cup tomato sauce
2 red potatoes, peeled and chopped into 1-inch cubes
2 stalks celery, chopped, leaves included
2 carrots, chopped
4 mushrooms, chopped (about ½ cup)
1 teaspoon all-purpose herb seasoning, such as Simply Organic All-
   Purpose Seasoning

1. Heat the oil in a large pot over medium heat. Add the onion and sauté for 4 to 5 minutes, until soft. Add the garlic and sauté for another 1 to 2 minutes. Using a slotted spoon, remove the onion and garlic and set aside.

2. Place the meat in the pan and cook, stirring occasionally, for 7 to 8 minutes, until browned on all sides. Season with salt and pepper. Add the flour and stir well to coat the meat.

3. Pour the beef stock and tomato sauce into the pot, add the onions and garlic, and stir well.

4. Stir in the potatoes, celery, carrots, mushrooms, and seasoning.

5. Turn down the heat to low and simmer for 2 hours, stirring occasionally.

PER SERVING: 256 calories; 8 g fat; 33 g carbohydrate; 13 g protein; 4 g fiber

▶ **NUTRITION BONUS:** good source of B vitamins, iron, and zinc

High Country Hash

MAKES FOUR 1-CUP SERVINGS OR TWO HEARTY 2-CUP SERVINGS

Savor every lingering bite of this updated version of old-style red flannel hash. Not only is this filling meal packed with a hefty dose of nourishment, it's big on comfort-food flavor.

2 medium golden beets, scrubbed, trimmed, and chopped into
    1-inch cubes (about 1 cup)
2 medium red potatoes, peeled and chopped into 1-inch cubes
    (about 2 cups)
1½ tablespoons olive oil
Sea salt and freshly ground black pepper
½ cup diced onion
½ cup diced celery
2 garlic cloves, minced
2 teaspoons all-purpose herb seasoning, such as Simply Organic
    All-Purpose Seasoning
3 cups chopped Swiss chard, spinach, or beet greens
¼ cup gluten-free chicken stock
2 to 4 poached eggs

1. Preheat the oven to 425°F. Lightly grease a baking sheet.
2. Place the beets and potatoes in a medium bowl. Drizzle 1½ teaspoons of the olive oil over them and stir to coat. Spread on the prepared baking sheet. Sprinkle with salt and pepper.
3. Place on the center rack of the oven. Bake for 30 minutes, until easily pierced with a sharp knife, checking once or twice and stirring if needed to ensure uniform roasting.
4. While the beets and potatoes are roasting, heat the remaining tablespoon of olive oil in a large skillet over medium-low heat. Add the

onion and celery and cook for 6 to 7 minutes, stirring often, until soft. Add the garlic and cook for another 2 minutes. Sprinkle the herb seasoning over the vegetables and stir well.

5. Turn down the heat to low, add the greens and chicken stock to the skillet, and cook for 1 or 2 more minutes. Add the roasted beets and potatoes, season with salt and pepper to taste, and stir well.

6. Top each serving with a poached egg, or 2 eggs for a hearty 2-cup serving.

PER SERVING (1 cup): 267 calories; 8 g fat; 42 g carbohydrate; 9 g protein; 6 g fiber

▶ **NUTRITION BONUS:** good source of vitamin C

Lentil Dal over Rice

MAKES 4 SERVINGS

Lentils should be in every athlete's pantry. They're packed with slow-burning complex carbohydrates and health-promoting nutrients. If you're not a lentil fan already, the layers of flavors in this dish will make you one. Serve over rice. This recipe makes a great option for carb-loading.

> **1 cup dried red lentils**
> **Olive oil**
> **1 small onion, diced**
> **1 garlic clove, minced**
> **2 teaspoons grated fresh ginger**
> **2 teaspoons curry powder**
> **¼ teaspoon ground cumin**
> **2 cups gluten-free chicken stock (see note)**
> **2 tablespoons chopped fresh cilantro**
> **1 tablespoon butter**
> **Salt and freshly ground black pepper**

1. Rinse the lentils under cold water.

2. Heat a bit of olive oil in a medium saucepan over medium-high heat. Add the onion and garlic and sauté until the onion is soft and translucent.

3. Add the ginger, curry powder, and cumin and sauté for 2 more minutes.

4. Stir the lentils, chicken stock, and cilantro and bring to a simmer. Turn down the heat to low, cover, and simmer for 20 minutes.

5. Add the butter and stir to mix well. Season with salt and pepper to taste.

NOTE: To make this dish vegetarian, substitute gluten-free vegetable stock for the chicken stock. To make it fully vegan, omit the butter or substitute Earth Balance Vegan Buttery Sticks (or something similar), olive oil, or another dairy-free, plant-based healthy fat.

PER SERVING (without rice): 251 calories; 5 g fat; 37 g carbohydrate; 15 g protein; 16 g fiber

▶ NUTRITION BONUS: low in calories, high in fiber and iron

—Adapted from *Artisanal Gluten-Free Cooking*, 2nd Ed.

Macaroni and Cheese

MAKES 6 SERVINGS

Sometimes there's nothing better than old-fashioned cheesy comfort food, especially when it's made with high-quality ingredients. This version of an old favorite uses organic whole-grain brown rice pasta and real Cheddar rather than refined white flour pasta and glow-in-the-dark cheese dust.

One 12-ounce package Tinkyada Organic Penne Brown Rice Pasta or
  other gluten-free pasta
2 tablespoons unsalted butter
2 tablespoons brown rice flour
1½ cups milk
8 ounces Cheddar (about 3 cups shredded)
1 cup shredded three-cheese blend (Parmesan, Romano, and Asiago)
1 tablespoon gluten-free Dijon mustard
Sea salt and freshly ground black pepper
4 slices hearty gluten-free bread, cut in ½-inch squares, optional

1. Cook the pasta as directed on the package and drain. Return the pasta to the pot. Preheat the oven to 350°F and move the oven rack to the center. Grease a shallow 10-inch square baking dish.

2. While the pasta cooks, melt the butter in a medium saucepan over low heat. Whisk in the brown rice flour until blended, and cook, whisking constantly, for about 2 minutes. Don't let it brown.

3. Slowly add the milk and whisk until the sauce is well blended. Add the Cheddar and continue whisking until the cheese is melted and the ingredients are mixed, 3 to 4 minutes. Add ½ cup of the three-cheese blend and the mustard. Whisk for another minute or two, until the cheese is completely melted and creamy. Watch it carefully and keep the heat on low.

4. Mix the cheese sauce with the pasta. Add salt and pepper to taste, stir, and pour into the prepared baking dish. Sprinkle with the remaining ½ cup of three-cheese blend and scatter the bread squares over the top. Bake for 30 minutes, until the top is nicely browned. Remove from the oven and let rest for 5 minutes before serving.

PER SERVING: 474 calories; 21 g fat; 53 g carbohydrate; 19 g protein; 1 g fiber

Poached Eggs on a Bed of Chard

MAKES 2 SERVINGS

Don't let the eggs fool you, this dish makes a perfect, easy-to-prepare, nutrient-dense, post-workout recovery dinner. You can also whip it up for breakfast and get a couple servings of vegetables in before the sun comes up.

> 1 tablespoon olive oil
> 4 cups chard, stalks removed (see note), leaves cut into strips
> 1 tomato, chopped
> 4 large eggs
> 2 to 4 slices whole-grain gluten-free bread, optional
> Sea salt and freshly ground black pepper

1. Heat the olive oil in a large skillet over low heat. Place the chard and tomato in the skillet and sauté for 5 to 8 minutes, or until chard is slightly wilted. Use tongs to mix for even cooking.

2. While the chard is cooking, poach the eggs in a pan of water and toast the bread, if using.

3. Using the tongs (or a slotted spoon to drain the moisture), layer the greens on the toast and top with the poached eggs. Season with salt and pepper to taste.

NOTE: Save the chard stalks for use in smoothies. They're packed with fiber and phytonutrients, but use them sparingly, as they can be over-powering and slightly bitter.

PER SERVING: 344 calories; 20 g fat; 26 g carbohydrate; 17 g protein; 3 g fiber

Vegetable Frittata

MAKES 6 SERVINGS

Nothing could be simpler than preparing and cooking your meal in the same skillet. This no-fuss, protein-rich meal can be served for breakfast or dinner.

2 tablespoons unsalted butter, plus more if needed
1 medium onion, chopped
2 garlic cloves, minced
2 cups chopped summer squash (zucchini, yellow, or mixed)
1 tomato, seeded and drained of liquid, chopped
1 ear of corn, boiled for 10 minutes, cooled, and kernels removed
    from cob, or ½ cup canned corn, drained and rinsed
2 teaspoons Italian seasoning
Sea salt and freshly ground black pepper
6 large eggs, beaten
½ cup shredded Parmesan

1. Preheat the oven to 375°F.

2. Melt the butter in a heavy, ovenproof skillet over low heat. Make sure the bottom and sides of the skillet are well coated with melted butter. If needed, add another tablespoon of butter to cook the vegetables.

3. Increase the heat to medium-low, add the onion, and sauté for about 5 minutes, stirring often. Add the garlic and sauté for another 1 to 2 minutes.

4. Mix in the squash and sauté for 5 more minutes. Add the tomato, corn, and Italian seasoning. Pour the eggs over the top and place the skillet on the center rack of the oven. Bake for 15 minutes.

4. Remove the skillet from the oven and sprinkle with the Parmesan. Return the skillet to the oven and bake for another 5 minutes. Lightly touch the center to make sure the mixture has set. Leftovers can be refrigerated and warmed or served at room temperature.

PER SERVING: 232 calories; 15 g fat; 11 g carbohydrate; 17 g protein; 2 g fiber

▶ **NUTRITION BONUS:** good source of selenium and phosphorus

Veggie Pizzas

MAKES 2 PIZZAS (4 SERVINGS, ½ PIZZA PER SERVING)

Homemade pizza crust is great, but sometimes you need a quick fix. Here are some fresh ideas for fast, easy, and healthful pizza. This recipe is for two different pizzas—one beet and one zucchini. To make two pizzas of one flavor, double the ingredient quantities listed for that flavor. Plus, don't be afraid to mix and match ingredients. It's hard to go wrong when you start with fresh vegetables, no matter what they are. Be creative!

1 package Udi's Gluten Free Pizza Crusts (2 crusts)
3 teaspoons olive oil
2 garlic cloves, minced

BEET PIZZA
½ cup thinly sliced raw beet rounds (1 medium beet, trimmed and
    sliced into thin rounds)
½ cup thinly sliced raw cauliflower florets
1½ cups coarsely chopped beet greens
4 ounces mozzarella, shredded

ZUCCHINI PIZZA
½ cup thinly sliced raw zucchini rounds (1 small zucchini)
1 tomato, sliced and drained
6 scallions (white and light green parts), cut lengthwise into 5- to
    6-inch pieces
4 ounces mozzarella, shredded

1. Preheat the oven to 375°F.

2. Brush 1½ teaspoons of olive oil on each pizza crust. Top each crust with 1 minced garlic clove.

3. Assemble the beet pizza: Place the sliced beet on one of the crusts, followed by the cauliflower and beet greens. Sprinkle with the 4 ounces of cheese.

4. Assemble the zucchini pizza: Place the zucchini rounds on the other crust, followed by the tomato and scallions. Sprinkle with the 4 ounces of cheese.

5. Place the pizzas on the center rack of the oven. Bake for 7 to 15 minutes, depending on the accuracy of your oven temperature and whether the crusts were frozen or not—follow the package directions.

6. Remove from the oven and let rest for a few minutes before slicing and serving.

NOTE: In addition to Udi's Gluten Free Pizza Crust, the Gluten Free Bistro, Venice Bakery, Schär, and many other companies now offer parbaked, ready-to-use gluten-free pizza crusts. If your local supermarket doesn't carry them (typically in the frozen foods section), they can also be ordered online.

PER SERVING (½ beet pizza): 425 calories; 19 g fat; 37 g carbohydrate; 21 g protein; 4 g fiber;

PER SERVING (½ zucchini pizza): 390 calories; 19 g fat; 35 g carbohydrate; 20 g protein; 3 g fiber

Power Pizza

MAKES 1 LARGE PIZZA, 8 SLICES

If you ask people who've recently gone gluten-free what they miss most, the answer is often, "Pizza!" No more. This recipe will satisfy your pizza cravings. Plus, it's packed with carbs, protein, and healthy fat in every bite.

PIZZA DOUGH
1 tablespoon sugar or honey
¾ cup warm water (about 115°F)
2¼ teaspoons (1 packet) active dry yeast
2 tablespoons olive oil, plus some for the pan
1⅓ cups plus 1 heaping tablespoon all-purpose gluten-free flour mix
   (see page 252)
1 teaspoon xanthan gum
1 teaspoon salt

DEEP-DISH TOPPING
8 ounces mozzarella, sliced thinly or shredded
One 14.5-ounce can San Marzano tomatoes, crushed or pureed
1 tablespoon dried oregano
1 scant tablespoon dried basil

1. Preheat the oven to 500°F.

2. Prepare the pizza dough: Dissolve the sugar in the warm water in a medium bowl, then stir in the yeast and let stand until the mixture foams, about 5 minutes. The foam means your yeast is alive and ready to go. Stir in 1 tablespoon of the olive oil.

3. In a separate large bowl, combine the flour, xanthan gum, and salt.

4. Add the wet ingredients to the dry ingredients and mix to form a dough ball that is soft and slightly sticky to the touch.

5. Drizzle 1 tablespoon of the olive oil into the mixing bowl and roll the dough ball in it to evenly coat.

6. Drizzle a liberal amount of olive oil onto a 9 × 13-inch baking pan. Use your hand to spread the oil and evenly coat the bottom and sides of the pan.

7. Transfer the dough ball to the pan and use your hands to spread the dough to the edges of the pan. Form a ½-inch lip around the edge of the crust. Cover with a kitchen towel and let rise in a warm location for 30 minutes.

8. Parbake the naked dough for 10 minutes.

9. Add the topping: Top with the sliced mozzarella and then the tomatoes, then sprinkle with the dried oregano and basil. (If using shredded mozzarella, add the tomatoes first, *then* the cheese.)

10. Bake for 10 or more additional minutes, until the edges of the crust are golden brown. Remove from the oven and let rest for 5 minutes. Slice and serve.

PER SERVING (1 slice): 305 calories; 11 g fat; 43 g carbohydrate; 14 g protein; 7 g fiber

—Adapted from *Artisanal Gluten-Free Cooking,* 2nd Ed.

Quinoa–Sweet Potato Veggie Burgers

MAKES 8 PATTIES

This is a launching pad recipe. Eat these as traditional burgers, or branch out and try them on a bed of wilted spinach topped with a poached egg. Skip the carrots and add shredded golden beets or chopped mushrooms. Be creative!

30 gluten-free flax crackers (such as Mary's Gone Crackers original seed crackers), plus more if needed
2 tablespoons olive oil
1 onion, chopped (about ½ cup)
2 stalks celery, diced
4 garlic cloves, minced
½ cup canned chickpeas, drained and rinsed, plus more if needed
1 cup cooked quinoa
1 medium sweet potato, baked, flesh scooped out (about 1 cup cooked)
½ cup shredded carrots
2 teaspoons all-purpose herb seasoning, such as Simply Organic All-Purpose Seasoning
½ teaspoon sea salt
Freshly ground black pepper

1. Preheat the oven to 375°F. Grease a baking sheet.

2. Place the crackers in a food processor and pulse until coarsely ground (not a powder, but not chunky). Set aside.

3. Heat the oil in a large skillet over medium heat. Add the onion, celery, and garlic. Cook, stirring often, until the onion and celery have softened, about 5 minutes.

4. Remove from the heat, add the chickpeas, and stir. Lightly mash the chickpeas with a fork until they are semicrushed.

5. Transfer to a large bowl, add the remaining ingredients, and mix well. The mixture should be moist but firm enough to shape into patties. If the mixture is too moist, add more ground crackers. If too dry, add more mashed chickpeas.

6. Form into burger-shaped patties and place on the prepared baking sheet. Bake for 20 to 25 minutes, until golden brown.

PER SERVING (1 patty): 211 calories; 6 g fat; 34 g carbohydrate; 6 g protein; 4 g fiber

Roasted Brussels Sprouts and Cipollini Onions

MAKES 4 SERVINGS

Cipollini onions are a little tricky to peel, but they're delicious and blend nicely with Brussels sprouts, giving you a double dose of powerful nutrients.

> 1 pound Brussels sprouts (14 to 16 sprouts; about 3 cups), trimmed
>   and quartered
> 4 to 6 cipollini onions, peeled and quartered
> 2 tablespoons olive oil
> Sea salt and freshly ground black pepper

1. Preheat the oven to 400°F.

2. Place the Brussels sprouts and onions in a medium bowl. Drizzle with 1 tablespoon of the olive oil, sprinkle with salt and pepper, and stir to coat the vegetables.

3. Pour the remaining 1 tablespoon of olive oil into a large cast-iron or other ovenproof skillet to cover the bottom of the skillet.

4. Spread the vegetables in a single layer in the skillet. Place the skillet on the center rack of the oven and roast for 15 minutes. Stir to ensure even browning, then roast for another 10 minutes.

PER SERVING: 120 calories; 5 g fat; 16 g carbohydrate; 5 g protein; 5 g fiber

▶ **NUTRITION BONUS:** good source of vitamin C

Roasted Salmon and Asparagus

MAKES 4 SERVINGS

Whether you make this dish as a pre- or postrace dinner, the high omega-3s in the salmon and the mix of antioxidant nutrients and B vitamins in the asparagus make for a perfect performance or recovery meal. Serve with a side of wild rice or quinoa and a green salad.

> Olive oil cooking spray
> 1 pound, 5 ounces wild-caught salmon fillet
> Olive oil
> Sea salt and freshly ground black pepper
> 1½ pounds fresh asparagus
> 2 garlic cloves, minced

1. Preheat the oven to 425°F. Cover a large baking sheet with tinfoil. Mist with olive oil.

2. Carefully rinse and pat dry the salmon fillet. Pour a little olive oil onto your hands and run them over the entire fillet until evenly coated.

3. Place the fillet skin-side down on the prepared baking sheet and sprinkle with salt and pepper.

4. Wash and trim the asparagus. Pat dry and place in a medium bowl. Drizzle 1 tablespoon of olive oil over the asparagus and toss gently until evenly coated. Place the asparagus in a single layer next to the salmon on the same baking sheet. Sprinkle the asparagus with the garlic and season with salt and pepper.

5. Place on the center rack of the oven and bake for 10 to 20 minutes, depending on the thickness of the salmon. Remove when the fish flakes easily with a fork. Using tongs, turn the asparagus once while baking to ensure even roasting.

PER SERVING: 300 calories; 15 g fat; 6 g carbohydrate; 35 g protein; 3 g fiber

▶ **NUTRITION BONUS:** very high in vitamin B$_{12}$, good source of selenium

Spinach and Chickpeas

MAKES 2 LARGE SERVINGS

Tasty, nutritious, and easy—what more could you ask for in a meal!

4 slices uncooked bacon, diced
½ small onion, diced
One 15-ounce can chickpeas, drained and rinsed
1 garlic clove, minced
6 cups spinach leaves
1 cup cooked brown rice

1. Sauté the bacon in a skillet over medium-high heat. When it is crispy, add the onion and chickpeas and sauté until the onion is soft and the chickpeas are golden, about 5 minutes.

2. Add the garlic, mix, then add the spinach and sauté until the spinach is wilted. Serve over the rice.

PER SERVING: 497 calories; 10 g fat; 81 g carbohydrate; 22 g protein; 14 g fiber

▶ **NUTRITION BONUS:** good source of vitamin A and iron

Spinach Pesto

MAKES ½ TO ⅔ CUP (4 SERVINGS)

Drizzle this pesto over roasted chicken, serve it with veggies and crackers, use it on pizza, substitute it as a condiment on wraps or sandwiches, or serve it with pasta. It's healthy and delicious, and the taste is a bit of a surprise.

⅓ cup chopped walnuts
2 cups baby spinach
¼ cup chopped fresh parsley
¼ cup shredded Parmesan
1 garlic clove, chopped
¼ teaspoon sea salt
3 tablespoons olive oil

1. Place the walnuts in a food processor and pulse until finely ground.

2. Add the spinach, parsley, Parmesan, garlic, and salt.

3. Slowly pour the olive oil into the top spout while pulsing. Pulse until the ingredients become a fine paste.

4. Store in the refrigerator.

PER SERVING: 219 calories; 21 g fat; 3 g carbohydrate; 7 g protein; 1 g fiber

Stuffed Peppers

MAKES 4 SERVINGS

These fragrant stuffed bell peppers make for a substantial all-in-one dish with perfectly balanced flavors.

4 bell peppers (green, yellow, orange, or red)
Olive oil
½ medium onion, diced
1 garlic clove, minced
1 pound ground turkey (see note)
One 14.5-ounce can no-salt-added diced tomatoes, with juice
3 cups cooked jasmine rice
1 teaspoon gluten-free Worcestershire sauce
1 teaspoon dried oregano
½ teaspoon dried basil
Salt and freshly ground black pepper
½ cup shredded Cheddar or mozzarella

1. Preheat the oven to 350°F.

2. Cut the tops off the peppers and remove the stems, seeds, and membranes. Dice the tops and set aside.

3. Drizzle a bit of olive oil in the bottom of a baking pan. (Choose a pan in which the peppers will fit fairly snugly so they will remain upright while baking in step 6.) Place the peppers cut-side down in the baking pan and rub with olive oil. Bake for 25 minutes, or until the flesh is tender and the skin starts to brown.

4. Meanwhile, heat a small amount of olive oil in a skillet over medium-high heat. Add the onion, reserved diced pepper, and garlic and sauté until the onion is translucent. Add the ground turkey and cook, stirring occasionally, until browned. Stir in the tomatoes (including the liquid from the can), rice, Worcestershire sauce, oregano, and basil and season with salt and pepper.

5. Remove the peppers from the oven and turn them over so the cut sides are facing upward (like a bowl). Fill each pepper with the filling. Sprinkle the cheese on top.

6. Bake for an additional 20 to 25 minutes, until the cheese is melted and browned.

NOTE: To make vegetarian stuffed peppers, substitute 2 cups (one 15-ounce can) rinsed chickpeas for the ground turkey.

PER SERVING: 465 calories; 23 g fat; 27 g carbohydrate; 37 g protein; 5 g fiber

▶ **NUTRITION BONUS**: good source of vitamin C, iron, and selenium

—Adapted from *Artisanal Gluten-Free Cooking*, 2nd Ed.

Sweet and Spicy Moroccan Stew

MAKES 6 SERVINGS

The sweet and spicy smells of garam masala, curry, and cayenne make this nourishing stew hard to resist. Eat alone as a stew or pour over brown rice.

2 tablespoons olive oil
1 large onion, chopped (about 1 cup)
4 garlic cloves, minced
1 pound grass-fed beef stew meat
Sea salt and freshly ground black pepper
4 cups gluten-free chicken stock
1 large sweet potato, cut into 1-inch cubes (about 3 cups)
One 15-ounce can chickpeas, drained and rinsed
1 cup diced tomatoes, fresh or canned
¼ cup coconut milk
6 Medjool dates, pitted and chopped into small chunks
2 teaspoons curry powder
1 teaspoon garam masala
¼ teaspoon cayenne pepper
¼ teaspoon salt
¼ cup chopped fresh cilantro

1. Heat the oil over medium-low heat in large stockpot. Add the onion and cook for about 5 minutes, stirring often. Add the garlic and sauté for another 2 to 3 minutes. Using a slotted spoon, remove the onion and garlic and set aside.

2. Turn up the heat to medium, add the meat, and season with salt and pepper. Cook, stirring occasionally, until browned on all sides. Return the onion and garlic to the pot and add the chicken stock and sweet potato. Simmer for 20 minutes.

3. Add the chickpeas, tomatoes, coconut milk, dates, curry powder, garam masala, cayenne, and salt. Simmer for 45 to 60 minutes.

4. Add the cilantro, stir well, and simmer for another 5 minutes. Ladle into soup bowls or large mugs.

PER SERVING: 456 calories; 17 g fat; 47 g carbohydrate; 31 g protein; 8 g fiber

▶ **NUTRITION BONUS:** good source of B vitamins, vitamin A and C, iron, and zinc

Turkey Burgers and Sweet Potato Fries

MAKES 4 SERVINGS

Yes, it's true—a burger and fries can be delicious and over-the-top healthy too. This satisfying combination is packed with beneficial nutrients and rich in antioxidants. It makes for a perfect recovery meal. On second thought, it's perfect anytime.

TURKEY BURGERS
1 pound ground turkey
2 garlic cloves, minced
¼ cup finely diced onion
1 tablespoon gluten-free Worcestershire sauce
1 teaspoon olive oil
1 teaspoon all-purpose herb seasoning, preferably Simply Organic
    All-Purpose Seasoning
½ teaspoon sea salt
Freshly ground black pepper
4 gluten-free hamburger buns
Optional garnishes: gluten-free ketchup, mayonnaise, or mustard,
    lettuce, tomato slices, onion slices, pickle slices

SWEET POTATO FRIES
4 sweet potatoes, peeled if not organic
1½ tablespoons olive oil
Sea salt and freshly ground black pepper

1. Preheat the oven to 425°F. Lightly grease a baking sheet.

2. Prepare the burgers: Combine all the burger ingredients in a medium bowl and mix well. Shape into four patties.

3. Prepare the sweet potato fries: Cut the sweet potatoes into ½-inch wedges. Try to cut each piece into a similar-size wedge for uniform baking.

4. Place the sweet potatoes in a large bowl and drizzle with the oil. Mix well to coat. Sprinkle with salt and pepper.

5. Arrange the sweet potatoes in a single layer on the prepared baking sheet. You can also arrange them on a wire cooling rack on the baking sheet for uniform baking and less turning.

6. Place on the center rack of the oven and bake for about 30 minutes, turning once or twice.

7. Grill or panfry the patties until thoroughly cooked. Serve on gluten-free buns with the desired garnishes.

PER SERVING (1 burger with bun, without garnishes): 475 calories; 24 g fat; 33 g carbohydrate; 33 g protein; 2 g fiber

PER SERVING (sweet potato fries): 157 calories; 5 g fat; 26 g carbohydrate; 2 g protein; 4 g fiber

Turkey Meatballs and Spaghetti

MAKES 6 SERVINGS

Lean ground turkey and gluten-free, whole-grain spaghetti pasta make this a great prerace or pregame meal the night before a big event.

ITALIAN MEATBALLS
1 pound ground turkey
2 eggs
1⅓ cups gluten-free bread crumbs
½ medium onion, chopped (reserving the rest for sauce)
2 teaspoons dried basil
1½ teaspoons dried oregano
1 teaspoon garlic powder
1½ teaspoons salt
1 teaspoon freshly ground black pepper
1 tablespoon olive oil

MARINARA SAUCE
1 tablespoon olive oil
½ medium onion, chopped
2 garlic cloves, minced
1 teaspoon dried basil
1 teaspoon dried oregano
One 14.5-ounce can no-salt-added diced tomatoes
Salt and freshly ground black pepper

One 12-ounce package gluten-free spaghetti or other gluten-free pasta

1. Preheat the oven (or toaster oven) to 350°F.

2. Make the meatballs: Combine the turkey, eggs, bread crumbs, onion, basil, oregano, garlic powder, salt, and pepper in a large mixing bowl. Mix thoroughly with your hands. Form into about thirty meatballs, using a heaping tablespoon of the mixture for each.

3. Heat the olive oil in a large skillet over medium-high heat. Add the meatballs and cook (in batches, if needed), turning occasionally, until browned on all sides.

4. Transfer the meatballs to an ungreased, rimmed baking sheet and bake for about 15 minutes, until cooked through.

5. Make the sauce: Heat the olive oil in a medium saucepan over medium heat. Add the onion and garlic and sauté until soft. Add the basil and oregano and sauté for another minute or so. Add the tomatoes and season with salt and pepper. Simmer over medium heat to let the flavors meld, at least 5 minutes.

6. Blend the sauce using a handheld immersion blender and simmer for 5 to 10 minutes longer. Add additional salt and pepper to taste.

7. Cook the pasta in a large pot of boiling salted water until al dente. Drain and return to the pot.

8. Add the marinara sauce to the pasta and mix well. Add the meatballs. Mix and serve.

PER SERVING: 537 calories; 19 g fat; 64 g carbohydrate; 30 g protein; 4 g fiber

—Adapted from *Artisanal Gluten-Free Cooking*, 2nd Ed.

Turkey-Quinoa Meatloaf

MAKES 4 SERVINGS

Nutrient-dense quinoa makes a nice stand-in for bread crumbs in this comforting meatloaf. If you have leftovers, the meatloaf makes for good sandwiches the next day.

MEATLOAF
¼ cup uncooked quinoa, rinsed well
½ cup gluten-free chicken stock
1 small onion, quartered
½ red bell pepper, quartered and seeded
1 carrot, cut into a few pieces
2 garlic cloves
1 pound ground turkey
1 large egg
1½ tablespoons ketchup (preferably unsweetened)
10 dashes gluten-free hot sauce (such as Frank's)
2 tablespoon gluten-free Worcestershire sauce
1 teaspoon salt
1 teaspoon freshly ground black pepper

GLAZE
2 tablespoons light brown sugar
2 teaspoons gluten-free Worcestershire sauce

1. Make the meatloaf: Combine the quinoa and chicken stock in a pot and bring to a boil. Turn down the heat, cover, and simmer for about 12 minutes, until all the liquid is absorbed and the quinoa is translucent. Stir, turn out into a large bowl, and let cool.

2. Meanwhile, put the onion, bell pepper, carrot, and garlic in the bowl of a food processor and pulse to chop finely. Preheat the oven to 350°F.

3. In the large bowl, combine the cooked quinoa and all other the meatloaf ingredients and "knead" with your hands until well mixed.

4. Form the mixture into a loaf shape on a large pan.

5. Make the glaze: Whisk together the brown sugar and Worcestershire sauce to make a glaze, then brush it over the meatloaf to coat evenly.

6. Bake for 45 minutes, or until the internal temperature measures at least 150°F in the center with a meat thermometer. (The meatloaf will continue cooking for a little while after it's removed from the oven, raising the temperature to the safe range of at least 160°F).

7. Remove from the oven and let rest for 10 minutes before slicing.

PER SERVING: 393 calories; 17 g fat; 25 g carbohydrate; 35 g protein; 2 g fiber

Twice-Baked Potatoes

MAKES 8 SERVINGS

Twice-baked potatoes don't need detailed instructions. They're made for creative add-ins depending on what you have on hand. Serve with grilled chicken or steak and a side salad for a perfect pre- or postrace dinner.

> 5 large russet potatoes, scrubbed and pierced with a fork
> 4 to 6 tablespoons unsalted butter
> ¼ cup whole milk
> ¾ cup Colby-Jack cheese, shredded
> One 4-ounce can diced green chiles, hot or mild, drained
> 1 teaspoon crushed red pepper flakes, optional
> Sea salt and freshly ground black pepper

1. Preheat the oven to 400°F. Place the potatoes directly on the center rack of the oven. Bake for 1 hour. Pierce with a knife to make sure they are thoroughly cooked. If the potatoes are extra large, you may need to bake them for 10 or 15 minutes longer.

2. Remove the potatoes and turn the oven down to 350°F.

3. Cut the potatoes in half lengthwise. Hold each half potato with an oven mitt or dish towel, scoop out the flesh, and put it in a medium bowl. Leave enough flesh in the skin that the skin doesn't tear.

4. Add the butter, milk, ½ cup of the cheese, the chiles, and the pepper flakes, if using. Using a potato masher, mash the mixture until the butter has melted and the other ingredients are incorporated. Chunks are good, so don't overmash it. Season with salt and pepper to taste.

5. Place eight potato skins (resembling boats) side by side on a baking sheet; set the remaining two potato skins aside to cool. Using a large spoon, scoop the mixture into the eight skins. As you had baked one additional potato, they should be abundantly filled.

6. Sprinkle the potatoes with the remaining ¼ cup of cheese and place the baking sheet on the center rack of the oven. Bake for 20 to 30 minutes, until the cheese is lightly browned and the potatoes are hot.

7. Serve immediately, and give the dog the extra empty potato skins after they have sufficiently cooled.

PER SERVING: 281 calories; 9 g fat; 43 g carbohydrate; 8 g protein; 3 g fiber

▶ **NUTRITION BONUS:** good source of vitamin B_6 and vitamin C

IIIIIIIIIIIIIIIIIIIIIIIIIIIIIIIIIII **DESSERTS** IIIIIIIIIIIIIIIIIIIIIIIIIIIIIIIIIIII

Apple-Pecan Crumble

MAKES 8 SERVINGS

This juicy crumble beats any traditional apple pie. It's good with a combination of tart and sweet apples, but use any apple available. You can't go wrong with this dessert, especially if you serve it with vanilla ice cream.

APPLE FILLING
6 to 8 apples, cored and sliced (about 6 cups apple slices; see note)
½ cup packed light brown sugar
2 tablespoons all-purpose gluten-free flour mix (see page 252)
1 teaspoon ground cinnamon
¼ teaspoon freshly grated nutmeg
Pinch of salt

CRUMBLE TOPPING
¾ cup all-purpose gluten-free flour mix (see page 252)
⅓ cup packed light brown sugar
½ teaspoon ground cinnamon
⅓ cup unsalted butter
1 cup pecans, coarsely chopped

1. Preheat the oven to 400°F.

2. Make the apple filling: Place the apples in a large bowl. Place the brown sugar, flour, cinnamon, nutmeg, and salt in a small bowl and whisk well. Pour over the apple slices and mix to coat.

3. Arrange the apple slices in a 9-inch pie plate.

4. Make the crumble topping: Whisk together the flour, brown sugar, and cinnamon in a medium bowl. Add the butter and pecans. Using your hands, mix all the ingredients so the butter is well incorporated. Sprinkle the mixture on top of the apples and pat down to cover all the apples.

5. Place the pan on the center rack of the oven. Bake for 30 minutes, then cover with a piece of tinfoil to prevent overbrowning. Bake for another 15 minutes.

6. Serve hot out of the oven.

NOTE: Apple peels are loaded with antioxidants and fiber. They also contain pesticides if the apples are not organic, so choose organic and don't bother peeling.

PER SERVING: 371 calories; 19 g fat; 51 g carbohydrate; 3 g protein; 5 g fiber

Cacao Fondue Dip

MAKES 2 CUPS

Warning: This healthy version of chocolate dipping sauce is addicting. Simple, rich, creamy, and satisfying, it's a perfect balance of healthy ingredients and chocolate perfection. Serve this sauce with fresh strawberries, sliced apples, pears, jicama, and even celery.

10 Medjool dates, pitted and chopped
¾ cup water, plus more if needed
¾ cup unsweetened cacao powder
½ cup almond butter
⅓ cup coconut milk

1. Place the chopped dates in a wide, shallow bowl. Cover the dates with the water and let soak for at least 30 minutes.

2. Place the dates and soaking water in a food processor. Pulse until well blended.

3. Add the remaining ingredients and pulse until a thick sauce forms. If it is too thick, slowly add water, 1 tablespoon at a time, until it reaches the desired consistency.

4. Serve, or cover and store in the refrigerator. This sauce tastes just as good chilled and served again later.

PER SERVING (¼ cup): 213 calories; 10 g fat; 34 g carbohydrate; 3 g protein; 6 g fiber

Sweet Potato–Walnut Cupcakes

MAKES 24 CUPCAKES

Sweet potato—a favorite carbohydrate of many athletes—and walnuts make these cupcakes a healthier indulgent treat. They are a cake, and they do have some sugar, so they're not for every day. But if you abide by the 80/20 rule (page 159), these are a great choice for the 20 percent!

WALNUT TOPPING
1 cup packed brown sugar
½ cup (1 stick) butter
2 teaspoons ground cinnamon
1 cup chopped walnuts

CUPCAKES
½ cup (1 stick) butter, at room temperature
1 cup packed brown sugar
1 cup granulated sugar
2 teaspoons gluten-free pure vanilla extract
4 large eggs, at room temperature
¾ cup sour cream
1 cup mashed, cooked sweet potato (steamed or boiled)
2½ cups all-purpose gluten-free flour mix (see page 252)
2 teaspoons xanthan gum
1 tablespoon gluten-free baking powder
1 teaspoon baking soda
½ teaspoon salt
2 teaspoons ground cinnamon
½ teaspoon ground ginger
½ teaspoon ground allspice

1. Make the topping: Combine the brown sugar, butter, cinnamon, and walnuts in a medium saucepan over medium-high heat and cook, stirring occasionally, until the mixture boils and the sugar dissolves. Remove from the heat and set aside.

2. Make the cupcakes: Preheat the oven to 350°F. Place paper liners in 24 muffin tin cups.

3. With an electric mixer, cream together the butter and sugars until light and fluffy. Add the vanilla.

4. Add the eggs one at a time, mixing to incorporate after each addition.

5. Add the sour cream and sweet potato. Mix well.

6. In a separate bowl, combine the flour, xanthan gum, baking powder, baking soda, salt, cinnamon, ginger, and allspice. Mix with a whisk.

7. Add the dry ingredients to the wet ingredients and mix for about 10 seconds at medium-low speed to incorporate. Scrape down the sides of the bowl and mix at high speed for about 5 seconds, just until the batter is completely mixed and smooth.

8. Divide the batter among the prepared muffin cups. When the walnut topping is cool enough to touch, break into pieces, then sprinkle over the cupcakes.

9. Bake for 25 minutes, until a toothpick inserted in the center of a muffin comes out clean. Allow to cool completely in the tins.

PER SERVING (1 cupcake): 285 calories; 14 g fat; 39 g carbohydrate; 4 g protein; 2 g fiber

—Adapted from *Artisanal Gluten-Free Cupcakes*

METRIC CONVERSION CHARTS

FLOUR	
1 cup Artisan Gluten-Free Flour Blend (page 252)	125 g
1 cup commercial all-purpose gluten-free flour blend	115 to 150 g
1/2 cup brown rice flour	62 g

SUGAR	
1 cup white sugar	200 g
1 cup packed brown sugar	230 g
1/3 cup turbinado sugar	80 g

SWEETENERS	
1/3 cup maple syrup	104 g
1/4 cup maple syrup	75 g
1/3 cup honey	112 g

COCOA AND CHOCOLATE	
1/2 cup chocolate chips	110 g
3/4 cup unsweetened cacao powder	62 g

BUTTER		
1/2 cup	1 stick	113 g
1/3 cup	1/2 stick	76 g
1/4 cup		56.5 g

CHEESE	
1/2 cup shredded Cheddar	57 g
3/4 cup shredded Colby-Jack	85 g
1/2 cup shredded mozzarella	56 g
1 cup crumbled feta	150 g
1 cup shredded Parmesan or three-cheese blend	80 g

PRODUCE	
1 cup fresh blueberries	48 g
1/4 cup fresh blueberries	39 g
1/2 cup fresh pitted cherries	77 g
1 cup dried cranberries	120 g
1/2 cup frozen cranberries	51 g
1 cup raisins	145 g
1 cup chopped cucumber	133 g
1 cup canned corn	82 g
1 cup chopped onion	160 g
1 cup leafy greens	35 g
1 cup chopped parsley	60 g
1 cup chopped fresh herbs (e.g., basil, cilantro)	40 to 45 g
1/4 cup coarsely chopped cilantro	10 g
1 cup chopped zucchini	124 g

GRAINS AND LEGUMES	
1 cup cooked basmati or jasmine rice	175 g
1 cup cooked brown rice	195 g
1 cup gluten-free rolled oats	101 g
1 cup uncooked quinoa	170 g
1 cup cooked quinoa	185 g
1/2 cup quinoa flakes	52 g
1/2 cup cooked chickpeas	82 g
1 cup dried red lentils	192 g

NUTS AND SEEDS	
1 cup whole almonds	142 g
1 cup chopped almonds	90 g
1 cup almond butter	250 g
1 cup almond meal	113 g
1 cup pecan halves	108 g
1 cup chopped pecans	114 g
1 cup walnut halves	100 g
1 cup chopped walnuts	119 g
1 cup raw pumpkin seeds	138 g

WEIGHTS		
1 pound	16 ounces	450 g
3/4 pound	12 ounces	340 g
1/2 pound	8 ounces	225 g
1/4 pound	4 ounces	115 g
	1 ounce	30 g
	1/2 ounce	15 g

OTHER	
1 1/3 cups gluten-free bread crumbs	120 g
1 cup unsweetened coconut flakes	60 g
1 cup shredded coconut	93 g

TEMPERATURES	
500°F	260°C
425°F	220°C
400°F	200°C
375°F	190°C
350°F	175°C
325°F	163°C
300°F	150°C
160°F	71°C
155°F	68°C
150°F	66°C
145°F	63°C
115°F	46°C

LENGTHS	
12 inches	30 cm
9 inches	23 cm
8 inches	20 cm
6 inches	15 cm
2 inches	5 cm
1 inch	2.5 cm
1/2 inch	1.25 cm
1/4 inch	5 mm

VOLUMES			
1 gallon	16 cups	128 fl oz	3.8 L
1 quart	4 cups	32 fl oz	950 ml
1 pint	2 cups	16 fl oz	475 ml
	1 cup	8 fl oz	250 ml
	3/4 cup	6 fl oz	185 ml
	1/2 cup	4 fl oz	125 ml
	1/3 cup	2 2/3 fl oz	80 ml
	1/4 cup	2 fl oz	60 ml
	2 tablespoons	1 fl oz	30 ml

GLOSSARY

For additional definitions, see the list "Possible Signs and Symptoms of Gluten Exposure" in chapter 1 on page 33.

ABSORPTION   The uptake of nutrients into the body following digestion

ADENOSINE DIPHOSPHATE (ADP)   A compound converted to adenosine triphosphate (ATP) when the body stores energy, and created from ATP when the body uses its stored energy

ADENOSINE TRIPHOSPHATE (ATP)   The compound in which the body stores energy (in the bond between two phosphate atoms)

ADIPOSE TISSUE   Fat storage tissue

AEROBIC   Occurring with the assistance of oxygen

ALKALOIDS   Naturally occurring protective compounds found in plants, which may impact digestive and joint health in sensitive people when ingested in large enough quantities or concentrations

ALLERGEN   A substance that triggers an inappropriate immune response; a type of antigen

(FOOD) ALLERGY   An adverse reaction that occurs when protein fractions in food cause an immunologic response

AMENORRHEA   Cessation of the menstrual cycle

AMINO ACIDS   The structural components of protein

ANAEROBIC   Occurring in the absence of oxygen

ANAPHYLAXIS   An extreme, sometimes life-threatening reaction to an allergen

ANEMIA   A deficit of healthy, functioning red blood cells, often due to iron deficiency and subsequent low hemoglobin content, which results in decreased oxygen-carrying capacity

ANTIBODY   A protein produced by the body in response to a specific antigen

ANTIGEN   Any substance that provokes an immune response and the formation of antibodies, including allergens, bacteria, and viruses

ANTIOXIDANTS   Beneficial molecules that inhibit the damaging action of free radicals

APPETITE   The body's integrated response to the smell, sight, taste, or thought of food that stimulates eating

AUTOIMMUNE   When the immune system attacks the body's own cells

BODY MASS INDEX (BMI)   An approximate measure, not always accurate for athletes, of whether one's weight is healthy or unhealthy based on the relation between weight and height

BONE DENSITY   The amount of mineral components per section of bone; used to gauge osteoporosis, osteopenia, and osteomalacia

BONKING   The sudden onset of severe muscle fatigue due to extreme glucose and glycogen depletion (also called *hitting the wall*)

CALCIUM   The most abundant mineral in the body; found mainly in the bones and teeth

CALORIE   The unit by which food energy is measured

CARB-LOAD   The act of increasing dietary carbohydrate intake and reducing training load in advance of an event in order to maximize glycogen storage in the muscles (also called *carbo-loading, carbohydrate loading*)

CARBOHYDRATES   Energy-yielding macronutrients that include sugars, starches, and fibers

CARDIOVASCULAR   Pertaining to the heart and blood vessels

CELIAC DISEASE   A genetically predisposed, multisystem autoimmune disease triggered by ingesting gluten which primarily injures the small intestine

CEREAL   An agricultural grain crop used for food, such as wheat, corn, or oats; may or may not contain gluten

CHROMOSOME   A threadlike molecule made of DNA (genetic material) and protein, found in the nucleus of a cell

CLEANSE   A temporary clean-eating plan and health regimen (usually one to three weeks) designed to identify food allergens and remove toxins from the body (contrast *fasting*, which involves severe caloric restriction or total abstinence from food for a certain period of time)

CROHN'S DISEASE An inflammatory bowel disease that impacts the health of the intestines

CROSS-CONTAMINATION When an unintended substance (such as gluten) is found somewhere it shouldn't be (such as in a gluten-free meal)

CROSS-REACTIVITY When one antigen stimulates an immune antibody response originally precipitated by another, similar antigen (such as when corn causes a response normally triggered by wheat)

CYTOKINES Chemical messengers secreted by immune cells that cause an inflammatory response

DEHYDRATION A condition in which the body doesn't have as much water and other fluids as it should, including:

> *hyperosmotic dehydration* When water is lost faster than electrolytes, as through sweating, eventually resulting in fluid loss from both intra- and extracellular spaces
>
> *isosmotic dehydration* An overall reduction in extracellular, but not intracellular, fluid without change in electrolyte concentrations, caused by gastrointestinal fluid loss via diarrhea or vomiting

DENATURING "Unfolding" a protein's quaternary, tertiary, and/or secondary structure

DETOX Ridding the body of toxins

DIABETES A group of metabolic disorders marked by limited or absent production and improper utilization of insulin which negatively impact blood glucose management, including:

> *type 1 diabetes* When the pancreas fails to make insulin
>
> *type 2 diabetes* When the body's cells fail to respond to insulin; more common than type 1

DIGESTION The mechanical and chemical (enzymatic) process of breaking down food into small, absorbable components

DIPLOID Containing two complete sets of chromosomes, such as from a mother and father (in humans); from *di*, meaning two, and *ploid*, meaning the number of sets of chromosomes in a cell

EINKORN An early cultivated form of diploid wheat; an ancestor of modern wheat

ELECTROLYTES Salts that dissolve in water and dissociate into positive and negative ions, making them electrically conductive

EMMER A tetraploid wheat resulting from the hybridization of two wild forms of diploid grasses; an ancestor of modern wheat

EMPTY CARBS   Carbohydrates that provide basic caloric energy but lack additional nutrients

ENDOGENOUS   Formed within the body

ENDURANCE   The ability to sustain activity for a long period of time (also called *stamina*)

ENZYMES   Proteins that facilitate chemical reactions without being changed themselves in the process

ESSENTIAL AMINO ACIDS   Amino acids that the body cannot synthesize in the amounts needed and must obtain through diet

EXOGENOUS   From outside the body

(GLUTEN) EXORPHINS   Opiate-like peptides formed during the breakdown of gluten during peptic digestion in the stomach

EXTRACELLULAR FLUID   Body fluid located outside the cells

FATS   Lipids in foods or the body, composed mostly of triglycerides

FEMALE ATHLETE TRIAD   A syndrome marked by a trio of challenges: disordered eating, amenorrhea, and osteoporosis

FIBER   The component of plants that is not broken down by human digestive enzymes (but some forms are digested by bacteria in the GI tract)

FLEXIBILITY   The ability to bend and twist without injury; usually applies to muscles, ligaments, tendons, and joints

FOOD-DEPENDENT, EXERCISE-INDUCED GASTROINTESTINAL DISTRESS   A unique disorder brought on by strenuous exercise after the ingestion of trigger foods, causing allergic gastrointestinal problems

FORTIFICATION   The artificial addition of nutrients that were either removed from a food or not sufficiently present in the first place, such as calcium-fortified orange juice

(GLUTEN OR PROTEIN) FRACTION   A component segment or amino acid subset of a larger protein

FREE RADICAL   An unstable or highly reactive atom or molecule that contains at least one unpaired electron; can cause oxidative damage to cells

FRUCTOSE   A monosaccharide, also known as *fruit sugar*, naturally found in fruits, honey, saps, some vegetables, agave nectar, and corn syrup

FUNCTIONAL TRAINING   Uses large-scale, everyday, whole-body motions that call upon multiple muscle groups for balance, coordination, strength, and endurance

GASTROENTEROLOGIST   A doctor specializing in the branch of medicine that focuses on disorders of the stomach and intestines

GASTROINTESTINAL   Pertaining to the gastrointestinal (GI) tract of the body, which handles the digestion of food and absorption of nutrients

GELATINIZATION (OF STARCHES)   The process in which starch is broken down in the presence of water and heat

GENOME   An organism's total hereditary information; encoded in DNA and divided into components called *genes*

GLIADIN   The fraction of gluten found in wheat that causes a toxic reaction in susceptible people (although not the only toxic fraction in grains); most closely studied in celiac disease

GLUCOSE   A monosaccharide also known as *blood sugar*

GLUCOSE TOLERANCE   The body's appropriate metabolic response to sugar (how efficiently glucose is cleared from the blood)

GLUTAMINE   An amino acid commonly found in proteins; plays a role in gut health and immune function

GLUTAMINE PEPTIDE   A protein compound commonly used as a sports supplement, especially among bodybuilders, that may be derived from wheat gluten (and thus, not gluten-free)

GLUTEN   Common term for a group of storage proteins found in wheat, barley, and rye that cause problems for people with gluten intolerance

GLUTEN-FREE   Containing no gluten

GLUTEN INTOLERANCE   An umbrella term used to describe all conditions in which someone reacts negatively to gluten and which respond positively to a gluten-free diet, especially celiac disease, wheat allergy, and gluten sensitivity

GLUTEN SENSITIVITY   A condition that affects the largest branch of gluten sufferers and is the result of a different immune response than is the case with celiac disease or wheat allergy

(BEING) "GLUTENED"   Having unintentionally ingested gluten and experienced negative side effects as a result

GLUTENIN   A protein component of wheat gluten (together with gliadin)

GLYCEMIC INDEX (GI)   A method to classify the increase in blood glucose and insulin in response to ingesting a specific food

GLYCEMIC LOAD (GL)   Measures a food's impact on blood glucose and insulin levels, accounting for its glycemic index, its typical serving size, and the portion of that serving that contributes to the food's glycemic index value; potentially a more accurate measure than the glycemic index, since it prorates the GI value according to the food

GLYCEROL   A three-carbon molecule that serves as the "backbone" of a triglyceride

GLYCOGEN   The form in which carbohydrate (glucose) is stored in the liver and muscles

GLYCOLYSIS   The series of chemical reactions that produce ATP

GRAIN   The seed or fruit of a cereal grass; used as a food source

HEME   The iron-holding part of hemoglobin and myoglobin; the source of the iron in animal-based foods

HEMOGLOBIN   The protein in red blood cells that carries oxygen throughout the body

HEXAPLOID   Containing six complete sets of chromosomes

HISTAMINE   A substance produced by immune cells in response to an antigen, causing inflammation

HITTING THE WALL   *see* Bonking

HORMONE   A chemical messenger secreted by a gland in a regulatory response to altered conditions in the body

HYDRATION   The state of appropriate water/fluid content in the body

HYDROGENATION   To combine with hydrogen; in unsaturated fats, the addition of hydrogen to fill bonds, increase shelf life, and make otherwise liquid fats solid at room temperature—a process that produces trans fats in partially hydrogenated fats

HYPERSENSITIVITY   An abnormal response; excessively sensitive

HYPONATREMIA   A potentially deadly condition also known as *water intoxication* or *water poisoning*; typically brought on by excessive water intake coupled with high electrolyte loss

IMPACT   The degree to which an exercise jolts the body (both high- and low-impact exercises may be either high or low *intensity*)

    high-impact exercise   Activities and exercises in which both feet leave the ground simultaneously, such as running; can help strengthen bones and yield other athletic benefits *low-impact exercise*   Walking, cycling, swimming, and other exercises that do not involve both feet leaving the ground simultaneously

INFLAMMATION   The body's response to injury; includes redness and swelling

INSULIN   A hormone secreted by the pancreas involved in the control of blood glucose; shuttles glucose (and amino acids) from the blood into cells, including muscles

INSULIN RESISTANCE   When the body's cells have a reduced ability to respond to insulin, thus preventing normal glucose metabolism

INSULIN SENSITIVITY   Cells' responsiveness to insulin

INTENSITY   The amount of physical output as compared to an athlete's maximum possible effort; can be expressed as a percentage of VO_2 max, maximum heart rate, and other measures

INTERVAL TRAINING   Training that involves alternating periods of high- and low-intensity exercise, toggling above and below the lactate threshold (also known as *polarized training*)

INTRACELLULAR FLUID   Body fluid located inside the cells

IRON   An essential nutrient; in the body, mostly present in hemoglobin and myoglobin

IRRITABLE BOWEL SYNDROME   A condition characterized by abdominal pain, constipation, and/or diarrhea

ISOLATION TRAINING   The stereotypical gym experience; utilizing free weights and machines to focus on one muscle group at the exclusion of others

JUICING   Extracting nutrient-rich liquid, but not fiber, from vegetables and fruits; in the context of this book, not to be confused with the euphemism for using illegal steroids

KETOGENIC DIET   A very low-carbohydrate, modest protein, high-fat diet that induces a state of nutritional ketosis

KETONES   Organic compounds, some of which are by-products of fat breakdown, that can provide energy for the brain, especially during fasting and other times when glucose levels plummet

(NUTRITIONAL) KETOSIS   An intentionally induced state of elevated ketone levels through careful dietary manipulation

LACTATE THRESHOLD   The level of exertion at which lactic acid begins to build up in the muscles and blood faster than it can be broken down or converted to other compounds; about 85 percent output (also called the *anaerobic threshold* or *aerobic threshold*)

LACTIC ACID A compound produced during anaerobic metabolism

LACTOSE A disaccharide composed of galactose and glucose; also known as *milk sugar*

LACTOSE INTOLERANCE The inability to digest lactose (milk sugar), which causes digestive distress; different from *milk allergy*, which is an immune response to the protein in milk (casein)

LEAKY GUT A breach of the gut lining that separates the contents of the intestine from systemic circulation, usually due to damage; can be exacerbated by gluten and intense exercise (also known as *increased intestinal permeability*)

LEUCINE A branched-chain essential amino acid that is thought to improve muscle regeneration after strenuous exercise

LIPIDS A family of compounds that includes fats (triglycerides), cholesterol, and waxes

LONG SLOW DISTANCE TRAINING Exercising at a reduced intensity (50 to 70 percent output) for a greater duration of time and distance

MACRONUTRIENTS Energy-yielding nutrients, including carbohydrates, protein, and fat

MALNUTRITION A condition that occurs when the body doesn't get enough nutrients, either from deficient nutrient intake or nutrient malabsorption

MAX HEART RATE The fastest the heart can safely beat with exercise

METABOLISM The chemical reactions that occur within living cells; *energy metabolism* is the process by which the body obtains and utilizes the energy from food

MICRONUTRIENTS Nutrients, including vitamins and minerals, that are required in small quantities for normal growth and development and must be obtained from food or supplements

MINERALS Organic substances needed by the body that must be obtained through food or supplements

MORPHINE A narcotic drug obtained from opium; both an alkaloid and an opiate

NALOXONE A drug that blocks opiate receptors in the nervous system, turning off the effects of morphine and other opioids

NATURAL KILLER (NK) CELLS   Defensive cells that are part of the innate (nonspecific) immune system and act by releasing chemicals that destroy the disease-causing organism's cell membrane and nucleus

NEURONS   Cells of the nervous system specialized to transmit messages throughout the body

NIGHTSHADES   A diverse group of plants that contain alkaloids; the most common being potatoes, tomatoes, eggplants, and peppers

NONESSENTIAL AMINO ACIDS   Amino acids that can be synthesized in the body

OILS   Fats that are liquid at room temperature

OPIATES   Substances that resemble or contain the narcotic compounds found in opium

OPIOIDS   Opium-like compounds that bind to opiate receptors in the body

OSTEOMALACIA   A condition in which the bones are soft and decalcified

OSTEOPENIA   A reduction of bone mass; less severe than osteoporosis

OSTEOPOROSIS   A condition in which the bones lose tissue, become weak, and are at greater risk of fracture

OXALATES   Naturally occurring compounds found in plants that can inhibit calcium absorption

OXIDATIVE SYSTEM   Aerobic energy pathways that involve carbohydrate and fat oxidation

PEPSIN   A protein-digesting enzyme in the stomach

PEPTIDES   Two or more amino acids linked in a chain

PERIODIZATION   Breaking into segments, specifically:
> *fitness periodization*   Breaking down training into smaller, more achievable components, and tailoring training into various phases that support peaking for major competitions
> *dietary periodization*   Changing one's diet to support different phases of training and competing

PHOSPHOCREATINE (PCR)   An intracellular high-energy phosphate compound important during intense exercise; part of the anaerobic energy pathway system

PHYTOCHEMICAL   Describes the health-promoting nutrients found in plants, which are also known as *phytonutrients*

PLASMA   The colorless, extracellular fluid found in blood vessels

POISSON BINOMIAL DISTRIBUTION   A mathematical way to measure the likelihood of multiple true or false events taking place when the probability of each individual event is different

POLYPLOIDY   A condition in which an organism's cells contain more than two sets of chromosomes

PROLAMINS   Storage proteins found in grains and rich in the amino acid proline: gliadin and glutenin in wheat, hordein in barley, secalin in rye, avenin in oats

PROTEIN   A macronutrient composed of a chain of linked amino acids

RECOVERY   Return to a normal state of health

RHEUMATOID ARTHRITIS   An autoimmune disease involving painful inflammation of the joints and related structures

SACCHARIDES   Sugar units (carbohydrates) classified according to size: *mono-* (one sugar unit), *di-* (two sugar units), *poly-* (many sugar units)

SATIETY   The state of hunger satisfaction after a meal; inhibits eating

SMALL INTESTINE   The principal organ for the digestion of food and absorption of nutrients

SMOOTHIE   A blended drink made from vegetables, fruit, and other ingredients; includes the pulp and fiber

SODIUM-POTASSIUM PUMP   The most common of the transporter proteins that actively pump substances across cell membranes

STARCH   A complex carbohydrate (plant polysaccharide) composed of multiple units of glucose

STEATORRHEA   The presence of excess fat in feces, which may float or be loose, oily, or unusually foul smelling; often the result of poor fat absorption in the intestine

STOMACH   The muscular, saclike portion of the digestive tract between the esophagus and the small intestine, which churns swallowed food with enzymes and acid

STRENGTH TRAINING   An activity that progressively taxes muscles to improve power and strength

STRESSOR   A condition, substance, or stimulus that triggers the stress response

SUCROSE   Table sugar; a disaccharide

SUGAR   A simple carbohydrate (as opposed to starch)

SYMPTOM   A subjective mental or physical feature indicating a disease or disorder, noticed by the person experiencing the symptom (as opposed to a sign, noticed by a doctor or other third-party observer)

TEMPO TRAINING   Training at or near the lactate threshold (also called the *anaerobic threshold*), about 75 to 85 percent output

TETRAPLOID   Containing four complete sets of chromosomes

TONICITY   A measure of the osmotic pressure gradient across cell membranes; in sports drinks, refers to carbohydrate concentration in relation to blood:

> *hypertonic*   Describes drinks that have a higher carbohydrate concentration than blood and cause cell shrinkage
>
> *hypotonic*   Describes drinks such as water that have a lower carbohydrate concentration than blood and cause cell swelling
>
> *isotonic*   Describes drinks that match the carbohydrate concentration of blood and have the best rates of fluid, carbohydrate, and electrolyte transport

TOXICITY   The degree of toxic effect or damage on an organism

TRIGGER   A stressor that can turn on gluten intolerance, such as excessive dietary gluten, pregnancy and childbirth, sickness, intense physical exertion, or lifestyle stress

TRIGLYCERIDE   A molecule of glycerol with three fatty acids attached; the main form of fat in the diet

TWIGS, STICKS, AND LOGS   A dietary strategy and framework for fueling activity, consisting of:

> *twigs*   Fast-acting, high–glycemic index simple carbohydrates
>
> *sticks*   Longer-lasting, low–glycemic index complex carbohydrates
>
> *logs*   Slow-burning, long-lasting fats

VITAMIN D   Can be synthesized by the body with the help of sunlight; important in bone growth and maintenance

VITAMINS   Organic (carbon-containing) essential nutrients necessary for normal biological function that must be obtained from the diet

VO$_2$ MAX   An individual's maximum capacity to transport and use oxygen during exercise; an important predictor of peak physical performance

WHEAT   A gluten-containing cereal grain from the genus *Triticum*; includes modern bread wheat, durum, einkorn, emmer, and spelt

WHEAT ALLERGY   A rapid allergic response to wheat that triggers the release of histamine

WHEAT-DEPENDENT, EXERCISE-INDUCED ANAPHYLAXIS   A potentially life-threatening response to gluten that occurs when wheat is ingested in conjunction with exercise

NOTES

NOTE: Any direct quotation not attributed in these endnotes is taken from an interview with the speaker.

INTRODUCTION

1. F. Fidanza, "Diets and Dietary Recommendations in Ancient Greece and Rome and the School of Salerno," *Progress in Food and Nutrition Science* 3, no. 3 (1979): 79–99.
    A. P. Simopoulos, "The Mediterranean Diets: What Is So Special About the Diet of Greece? The Scientific Evidence," *Journal of Nutrition* 131, no. 11 (November 2001): 3065S–73S.
    W. E. Sweet, *Sport and Recreation in Ancient Greece* (New York: Oxford University Press, 1987), 200.
    A. Trichopoulou, "Mediterranean Diet: The Past and the Present," *Nutrition, Metabolism & Cardiovascular Diseases* 11, no. 4 (August 2001): 1S–4S.
    J. C. Waterlow, "Diet of the Classical Period of Greece and Rome," *European Journal of Clinical Nutrition* 43, no. 2 (1989): 3S–12S.

2. A. C. Grandjean, "Diets of Elite Athletes: Has the Discipline of Sports Nutrition Made an Impact?" *Journal of Nutrition* 127, no. 5 (May 1, 1997): 874S–77S.
    L. E. Grivetti and E. A. Applegate, "From Olympia to Atlanta: A Cultural-Historical Perspective on Diet and Athletic Training," *Journal of Nutrition* 127, no. 5 (May 1997): 860S–68S.
    S. Sell, "Eating Was No Idle Game in Ancient Greece," USA Today (August 12, 2004): www.usatoday.com/travel/destinations/2004-08-12-greek-food-main_x.htm (accessed November 28, 2011).
    C. Walker, "Ancient Olympians Followed Atkins Diet, Scholar Says," National Geographic News (August 10, 2004): http://news.nationalgeographic.com/news/2004/08/0810_040810_olympic_food.html (accessed November 29, 2011).

3. H. B. Falls, ed., *Exercise Physiology* (New York: Academic Press, 1968), 157.
    H. A. Harris, "Nutrition and Physical Performance: The Diet of Greek Athletes," *Proceedings of the Nutrition Society* 25, no. 2 (March 12, 1966): 90.
    T. Perrottet, *The Naked Olympics: The True Story of the Ancient Games* (New York: Random House, 2004), 35.
    W. J. Raschke, ed., *The Archaeology of the Olympics* (Madison, WI: University of Wisconsin Press, 1988), 176.
    Xenophon, *Memorabilia*, 3.14.3.

4. P. K. Skiadas and J. G. Lascaratos, "Dietetics in Ancient Greek Philosophy: Plato's Concepts of Healthy Diet," *European Journal of Clinical Nutrition* 55, no. 7 (July 2001): 532–37.

5. B. Dowd and J. Walker-Smith, "Samuel Gee, Aretaeus, and the Coeliac Affection," *British Medical Journal* 2, no. 5909 (April 6, 1974), 46.

G. Kristjansson, "Food Antigen Sensitivity in Coeliac Disease Assessed by the Mucosal Patch Technique," *Digital Comprehensive Summaries of Uppsala Dissertations from the Faculty of Medicine 80,* Uppsala Universitet, Sweden, 16.

P. E. Makovicky et al., "From Historical Data and Opinions to Present Challenges in the Field of Celiac Disease," *Epidemiologie, Mikrobiologie, Imunologie* 57, no. 3 (August 2008): 90–96.

W. F. Paveley, "From Aretaeus to Crosby: A History of Coeliac Disease," *British Medical Journal* 297, no. 6664 (December 24, 1988): 1646.

6. G. Gasbarrini et al., "When Was Celiac Disease Born?: The Italian Case from the Archaeologic Site of Cosa," *Journal of Clinical Gastroenterology* 44, no. 7 (August 2010): 502–3.

7. A. D. Georgoulis et al., "Herodicus, the Father of Sports Medicine," *Knee Surgery, Sports Traumatology, Arthroscopy* 15, no. 3 (March 2007): 315–18.

8. J. A. Murray et al., "Increased Prevalence and Mortality in Undiagnosed Celiac Disease," *Gastroenterology* 137, no. 1 (July 2009): 88–93.

9. S. Cambers, "Is Novak Djokovic's Year the Best Ever in Men's Tennis?" *The Guardian* (November 17, 2011): www.guardian.co.uk/sport/blog/2011/nov/17/novak-djokovic-guardian-sport-network (accessed November 30, 2011).
    C. McHardy, "Sampras Hails Djokovic's 'Best Year Ever,'" *Sport 360* (October 1, 2011): www.sport360.com/article/sampras-hails-djokovics-best-year-ever (accessed November 30, 2011).
    S. Tignor, "Is Djokovic Having Best Men's Tennis Year Ever?" *NBC Sports* (September 13, 2011): http://nbcsports.msnbc.com/id/44500220/ns/sports-tennis/ (accessed November 30, 2011).
    J. Wertheim, "Effect of Djokovic's Fall Slump on 'Best Year Ever' Talks," *Sports Illustrated* (November 30, 2011): sportsillustrated.cnn.com/2011/writers/jon_wertheim/11/30/djokovic-mailbag/index.html (accessed November 30, 2011).
    K. Wilkinson, "US Open Champion Novak Djokovic on Brink of Best-Ever Year," *BBC Sport* (September 13, 2011): http://news.bbc.co.uk/sport2/hi/tennis/14896786.stm (accessed November 30, 2011).

10. C. M. Cerqueira et al., "The Food and Nutrient Intakes of the Tarahumara Indians of Mexico," *American Journal of Clinical Nutrition* 43, no. 4 (April 1979): 905–15.
    C. McDougall, *Born to Run: A Hidden Tribe, Superathletes, and the Greatest Race the World Has Never Seen* (New York: Alfred A. Knopf, 2010), 15–16, 44.

11. V. O. Onywera et al., "Demographic Characteristics of Elite Kenyan Distance Runners," *Journal of Sports Science* 24, no. 4 (April 2006): 415–22.

12. D. L. Christensen et al., "Food and Macronutrient Intake of Male Adolescent Kalenjin Runners in Kenya," *British Journal of Nutrition* 88, no. 6 (December 2002): 711–17.

13. M. P. McMurry et al., "Changes in Lipid and Lipoprotein Levels and Body Weight in Tarahumara Indians After Consumption of an Affluent Diet," *New England Journal of Medicine* 325, no. 24 (December 12, 1991): 1704–8.

14. K. Barada et al., "Celiac Disease in Middle Eastern and North African Countries: A New Burden?" *World Journal of Gastroenterology* 16, no. 12 (March 28, 2010): 1449–57.
    C. Catass et al., "Why Is Coeliac Disease Endemic in the People of the Sahara?" *Lancet* 354, no. 9179 (August 21, 1999): 647–48.

A. G. Cummins and I. C. Roberts-Thomson, "Prevalence of Celiac Disease in the Asia-Pacific Region," *Journal of Gastroenterology and Hepatology* 24, no. 8 (August 2009): 1347–51.

B. S. Ramakrishna, "Celiac Disease: Can We Avert the Impending Epidemic in India?" *Indian Journal of Medical Research,* no. 133 (January 2011): 5–8.

J. M. Remes-Troche et al., "Celiac Disease Could Be a Frequent Disease in Mexico: Prevalence of Tissue Transglutaminase Antibody in Healthy Blood Donors," *Journal of Clinical Gastroenterology* 40, no. 8 (September 2006), 697–700.

CHAPTER 1

1. E. J. Helmerhort et al., "Discovery of a Novel and Rich Source of Gluten-Degrading Microbial Enzymes in the Oral Cavity," *PLoS ONE* 5, no. 10:e13264.

2. P. Masson et al., "Peptic Hydrolysis of Gluten, Glutenin and Gliadin from Wheat Grain: Kinetics and Characterisation of Peptides," *Journal of the Science of Food and Agriculture* 37, no. 12 (December 1986): 1223–35.

3. D. Stepniak et al., "Highly Efficient Gluten Degradation with a Newly Identified Prolyl Endoprotease: Implications for Celiac Disease," *American Journal of Physiology—Gastrointestinal and Liver Physiology* 291, no. 4 (October 2006): G621–29.

4. M. K. Kagnoff, "Celiac Disease: Pathogenesis of a Model Immunogenetic Disease," *Journal of Clinical Investigation* 117, no. 1 (January 2, 2007): 41–49.

5. C. Storrs, "Will a Gluten-Free Diet Improve Your Health?" *Health.com* (April 5, 2011): www.health.com/health/article/0,,20479423,00.html (accessed December 21, 2011).

6. P. R. Shewry, "Wheat," *Journal of Experimental Botany* 60, no. 6 (2009): 1537–53.

7. J. Diamond, *Guns, Germs, and Steel* (New York: W. W. Norton & Co., 2005).

8. M. Feldman, "Wheats," *Evolution of Crop Plants* (Essex, UK: Longman Scientific and Technical, 1995), 185–192.

9. B. C. Curtis, "Wheat in the World," *FAO Plant Production and Protection Series: Bread Wheat,* Food and Agriculture Organization of the United Nations, Italy (2002): www.fao.org/docrep/006/y4011e/y4011e04.htm#bm04 (accessed December 10, 2011).

10. E.-S.M. Abdel-Aal, "Einkorn: Functional Wheat for Health Promotion," AACC International Cereal Science Knowledge Database (April 2009): www.aaccnet.org/CerScienceKnowledgedb/Summary/EAbdelaal.asp (accessed December 10, 2011).

11. *International Wheat Genome Sequencing Consortium,* www.wheatgenome.org (accessed January 25, 2012).

12. Y. Qiang Gu et al., "Rapid Genome Evolution Revealed by Comparative Sequence Analysis of Orthologous Regions from Four Triticeae Genomes," *Plant Physiology* 135, no. 1 (April 2004): 459–70.

13. B. C. Curtis, "Wheat in the World," *FAO Plant Production and Protection Series: Bread Wheat,* Food and Agriculture Organization of the United Nations, Italy (2002): www.fao.org/docrep/006/y4011e/y4011e04.htm#bm04 (accessed December 10, 2011).

14. B. Dowd and J. Walker-Smith, "Samuel Gee, Aretaeus, and the Coeliac Affection," *British Medical Journal* 2, no. 5909 (April 6, 1974): 46.
Gudjon Kristjansson, "Food Antigen Sensitivity in Coeliac Disease Assessed by the Mucosal Patch Technique," *Digital Comprehensive Summaries of Uppsala Dissertations from the Faculty of Medicine 80,* Uppsala Universitet, Sweden, 16.
P. E. Makovick et al., "From Historical Data and Opinions to Present Challenges in the Field of Celiac Disease," *Epidemiologie, Mikrobiologie, Imunologie,* 57, no. 3 (August 2008): 90–96.
W. F. Paveley, "From Aretaeus to Crosby: A History of Coeliac Disease," *British Medical Journal* 297, no. 6664 (December 24, 1988): 1646.

15. A. Fasano et al., "Prevalence of Celiac Disease in At-Risk and Not-At-Risk Groups in the United States: A Large Multicenter Study," *Archives of Internal Medicine* 163, no. 3 (February 10, 2003): 286–92.

16. J. A. Murray et al., "Increased Prevalence and Mortality in Undiagnosed Celiac Disease," *Gastroenterology* 137, no. 1 (July 2009), 88–93.

17. "Wheat's Role in the U.S. Diet Has Changed over the Decades," *United States Department of Agriculture Economic Research Service Briefing Room,* www.ers.usda.gov/briefing/wheat/consumption.htm (accessed December 10, 2011).

18. O. Molberg et al., "Mapping of Gluten T-cell Epitopes in the Bread Wheat Ancestors: Implications for Celiac Disease," *Gastroenterology* 128, no. 2 (February 2005): 393–401.

19. H. C. van den Broeck et al., "Presence of Celiac Disease Epitopes in Modern and Old Hexaploid Wheat Varieties: Wheat Breeding May Have Contributed to Increased Prevalence of Celiac Disease," *Theoretical and Applied Genetics* 121, no. 8 (November 2010): 1527–39.

20. P-F. Qi et al., "The γ-gliadin Multigene Family in Common Wheat (*Triticum aestivum*) and Its Closely Related Species," *BMC Genomics,* no. 10 (April 21, 2009): 168.
E. Salentijn et al., "Tetraploid and Hexaploid Wheat Varieties Reveal Large Differences in Expression of Alpha-gliadins from Homoeologous Gli-2 Loci," *BMC Genomics,* no. 10 (January 26, 2009): 48.
T. W. Van Herpen et al., "Alpha-gliadin Genes from the A, B, and D Genomes of Wheat Contain Different Sets of Celiac Disease Epitopes," *BMC Genomics,* no. 7 (January 10, 2006): 1.

21. D. Pizzuti et al., "Lack of Intestinal Mucosal Toxicity of *Triticum monococcum* in Celiac Disease Patients," *Scandinavian Journal of Gastroenterology* 41, no. 11 (2006): 1305–11.
H. C. van den Broeck et al., "Presence of Celiac Disease Epitopes in Modern and Old Hexaploid Wheat Varieties: Wheat Breeding May Have Contributed to Increased Prevalence of Celiac Eisease," *Theoretical and Applied Genetics* 121, no. 8 (November 2010): 1527–39.

22. A. Gregorini e. al., "Immunogenicity Characterization of Two Ancient Wheat α-gliadin Peptides Related to Coeliac Disease," *Nutrients* 1, no. 2 (February 2009): 276–90.

D. Kasarda and R. D'Ovidio, "Deduced Amino Acid Sequence of an Ð-gliadin Gene from Spelt Wheat (Spelta) Includes Sequences Active in Celiac Disease," *Cereal Chemistry* 76, no. 4 (July/August 1999): 548–51.

23. J. Gil-Humanes et al., "Effective Shutdown in the Expression of Celiac Disease–Related Wheat Gliadin T-cell Epitopes by RNA Interference," *Proceedings of the National Academy of Sciences of the United States of America* 107, no. 39 (September 28, 2010): 17023–28.

L. Spaenij-Dekking et al., "Natural Variation in Toxicity of Wheat: Potential for Selection of Nontoxic Varieties for Celiac Disease Patients," *Gastroenterology* 129, no. 3 (2005): 797–806.

Z. Xie et al., "Molecular Characterization of the Celiac Disease Epitope Domains in α-gliadin Genes in *Aegilops tauschii* and Hexaploid Wheats (*Triticum aestivum* L.)," *Theoretical and Applied Genetics* 121, no. 7 (November 2010): 1239–51.

24. O. Molberg et al., "Mapping of Gluten T-cell Epitopes in the Bread Wheat Ancestors: Implications for Celiac Disease," *Gastroenterology* 128, no. 2 (February 2005): 393–401.

25. L. Greco, "From the Neolithic Revolution to Gluten Intolerance: Benefits and Problems Associated with the Cultivation of Wheat," *Journal of Pediatric Gastroenterology and Nutrition* 24, no. 5 (May 1997): 14S–16S.

P. F. Qi et al., "The Gamma-Gliadin Multigene Family in Common Wheat (*Triticum aetsivum*) and Its Closely Related Species," *BMC Genomics*, no. 10 (April 21, 2009): 168.

26. "Wheat's Role in the U.S. Diet Has Changed over the Decades," *United States Department of Agriculture Economic Research Service Briefing Room*, www.ers.usda.gov/briefing/wheat/consumption.htm (accessed December 10, 2011).

27. C. Frangou, "Gluten Sensitivity Baffles Celiac Disease Specialists," *Gastroenterology & Endoscopy News* 61, no. 10 (October 2010): 28, www.gastroendonews.com/ViewArticle.aspx?d=In%2Bthe%2BNews&d_id=187&i=October%2B2010&i_id=672&a_id=16015 (accessed December 11, 2011).

28. "Celiac Disease," *National Digestive Diseases Information Clearing House*, U.S. Department of Health and Human Services (September 2008), NIH Publication No. 08-4269, http://digestive.niddk.nih.gov/ddiseases/pubs/celiac (accessed December 11, 2011).

"Celiac Disease," National Foundation for Celiac Awareness, www.celiaccentral.org/Celiac-Disease/21 (accessed December 11, 2011).

Celiac Disease Center at Columbia University, www.celiacdiseasecenter.columbia.edu/CF-HOME.htm (accessed December 11, 2011).

University of Chicago Celiac Disease Center, www.cureceliacdisease.org/ (accessed December 11, 2011).

University of Maryland Center for Celiac Research, http://medschool.umaryland.edu/celiac (accessed December 11, 2011).

29. "Wheat Allergy," *Mayo Clinic Diseases and Conditions*, www.mayoclinic.com/health/wheat-allergy/DS01002 (accessed December 11, 2011).

30. E. Morita et al., "Food-Dependent Exercise-Induced Anaphylaxis," *Journal of Dermatological Science* 47, no. 2 (August 2007): 109–17.
E. Morita et al.," Food-Dependent Exercise-Induced Anaphylaxis—Importance of Omega-5 Gliadin and HMW-Glutenin as Causative Antigens for Wheat-Dependent Exercise-Induced Anaphylaxis," *Allergology International* 58, no. 4 (December 2009): 493–98.

31. E. F. Verdu et al., "Between Celiac Disease and Irritable Bowel Syndrome: The 'No Man's Land' of Gluten Sensitivity and IBS," *American Journal of Gastroenterology* 104, no. 6 (June 2009): 1587–94.

32. A. Fasano et al., "Divergence of Gut Permeability and Mucosal Immune Gene Expression in Two Gluten-Associated Conditions: Celiac Disease and Gluten Sensitivity," *BMC Medicine,* no. 9 (2011): 23, www.biomedcentral.com/1741-7015/9/23 (accessed December 11, 2011).

CHAPTER 2

1. F. Brouns and E. Beckers, "Is the Gut an Athletic Organ? Digestion, Absorption and Exercise," *Sports Medicine* 15, no. 4 (1993): 2242–57.

2. I. H. Anderson et al., "Incomplete Absorption of the Carbohydrate in All-Purpose Wheat Flour," *New England Journal of Medicine* 304, no. 15 (1981): 891–92.
J. Holm and I. Bjorck, "Bioavailability of Starch in Various Wheat-Based Bread Products: Evaluation of Metabolic Responses in Healthy Subjects and Rate and Extent of In Vitro Starch Digestion," *American Journal of Clinical Nutrition* 55, no. 2 (February 1992): 420–29.
M. Olesen and E. Gudmand-Hoyer, "Maldigestion and Colonic Fermentation of Wheat Bread in Humans and the Influence of Dietary Fat," *American Journal of Clinical Nutrition* 66, no. 1 (1997): 62–66.

3. C. Berti et al., "In Vitro Starch Digestibility and In Vivo Glucose Response of Gluten-Free Foods and Their Gluten Counterparts," *European Journal of Nutrition* 43, no. 4 (August 2004): 198–204.
D. J. Jenkins et al., "The Effect of Starch-Protein Interaction in Wheat on the Glycemic Response and Rate of In Vitro Digestion," *American Journal of Clinical Nutrition* 45, no. 5 (1987): 946–51.

4. *Jay Beagle—Washington Capitals,* http://capitals.nhl.com/club/player.htm?id=8474291 (accessed January 4, 2012).

5. C. V. Gisolfi, "Is the GI System Built for Exercise?" *News in Physiological Sciences* 15, no. 3 (June 2000): 114–19.
G. P. Lambert et al., "Gastrointestinal Permeability During Exercise: Effects of Aspirin and Energy-Containing Beverages," *Journal of Applied Physiology* 90, no. 6 (June 2001): 2075–80.
T. Marchbank et al., "The Nutriceutical Bovine Colostrum Truncates the Increase in Gut Permeability Caused by Heavy Exercise in Athletes," *American Journal of Physiology—Gastrointestinal and Liver Physiology* 300, no. 3 (March 2011): G477–84.
M. A. Nieuwenhoven et al., "Gastrointestinal Profile of Symptomatic Athletes at Rest and During Physical Exercise," *European Journal of Applied Physiology* 91 no. 4 (April 2004): 429–34.

6. M. G. Clemente et al., "Early Effects of Gliadin on Enterocyte Intracellular Signaling Involved in Intestinal Barrier Function," *Gut* 52, no. 2 (February 1, 2003): 218–23.

S. Drago et al., "Gliadin, Zonulin and Gut Permeability: Effects on Celiac and Non-Celiac Intestinal Mucosa and Intestinal Cell Lines," *Scandinavian Journal of Gastroenterology* 41, no. 4 (April 2006): 408–19.

L. Elli et al., "Imaging Analysis of the Gliadin Direct Effect on Tight Junctions in an In Vitro Three-Dimensional Lovo Cell Line Culture System," *Toxicology In Vitro* 25 no. 1 (February 2011): 45–50.

A. Fasano, "Zonulin and Its Regulation of Intestinal Barrier Function: The Biological Door to Inflammation, Autoimmunity, and Cancer," *Physiological Reviews* 91, no. 1 (January 2011): 151–75.

S. Friis et al., "Gliadin Uptake in Human Enterocytes: Differences Between Coeliac Patients in Remission and Control Individuals," *Gut* 33, no. 11 (1992): 1487–92.

G. R. Sandler et al., "Rapid Disruption of Intestinal Barrier Function by Gliadin Involves Altered Expression of Apical Junctional Proteins," *FEBS Letters* 579, no. 21 (August 29, 2005): 4851–55.

J. Visser et al., "Tight Junctions, Intestinal Permeability, and Autoimmunity," *Annals of the New York Academy of Sciences* 1165 (May 2009): 195–205.

7. L. M. Sollid, "Coeliac Disease: Dissecting a Complex Inflammatory Disorder," *Nature Reviews Immunology* 2, no. 9 (September 2002): 647–55.

8. C. Giovannini et al., "Induction of Apoptosis in Caco-2 Cells by Wheat Gliadin Peptides," *Toxicology* 145, no. 1 (April 7, 2000): 63–71.

C. Giovannini et al., "Wheat Gliadin Induces Apoptosis of Intestinal Cells via an Autocrine Mechanism Involving Fas-Fas Ligand Pathway," *FEBS Letters* 540, nos. 1–3 (April 10, 2003): 117–24.

9. D. A. Hudson et al., "Non-Specific Cytotoxicity of Wheat Gliadin Components Towards Cultured Human Cells," *Lancet* 307, no. 7955 (February 14, 1976): 339–41.

10. D. D. Kitts and K. Weiler, "Bioactive Proteins and Peptides from Food Sources: Applications of Bioprocesses Used in Isolation and Recovery," *Current Pharmaceutical Design* 9, no. 16 (June 2003): 1309–23.

11. S. Fukudome and M. Yoshikawa, "Opioid Peptides Derived from Wheat Gluten: Their Isolation and Characterization," *FEBS Letters* 296, no. 1 (January 13, 1992): 107–11.

12. P. Holzer, "Treatment of Opioid-Induced Gut Dysfunction," *Expert Opinion on Investigational Drugs* 16, no. 2 (February 2007): 181–94.

13. A. E. Kalaydjian et al., "The Gluten Connection: The Association Between Schizophrenia and Celiac Disease," *Acta Psychiatrica Scandinavica* 113, no. 2 (February 2006): 82–90.

14. H. P. F. Peters and W. R. de Vries, "Potential Benefits and Hazards of Physical Activity and Exercise on the Gastrointestinal Tract," *Gut* 48, no. 3 (2001): 435–39.

15. G. Gremion, "Lower Intestinal Distress During Sports Activities," *Revue médicale de la Suisse romande* 7, no. 304 (August 10, 2011): 1525–28.

G. W. K. Ho, "Lower Gastrointestinal Distress in Endurance Athletes," *Current Sports Medicine Reports* 8, no. 2 (March/April 2009): 85–91.

S. J. Karageanes, "Gastrointestinal Infections in the Athlete," *Clinical Journal of Sports Medicine* 26, no. 3 (July 2007): 433–48.

M. A. Nieuwenhoven et al., "Gastrointestinal Profile of Symptomatic Athletes at Rest and During Physical Exercise," *European Journal of Applied Physiology* 91, no. 4 (April 2004): 429–34.

S. A. Paluska, "Current Concepts: Recognition and Management of Common Activity-Related Gastrointestinal Disorders," *Physician and Sports Medicine* 37, no. 1 (April 2009): 54–63.

16. E. P. de Oliveira and R. C. Burini, "The Impact of Physical Exercise on the Gastrointestinal Tract," *Current Opinion in Clinical Nutrition & Metabolic Care* 12, no. 5 (September 2009): 533–38.

17. R. W. F. Ter Steege et al., "Abdominal Symptoms During Physical Exercise and the Role of Gastrointestinal Ischaemia: A Study in 12 Symptomatic Athletes," *British Journal of Sports Medicine* (October 20, 2011) published online first, http://bjsm.bmj.com/content/early/2011/10/20/bjsports-2011-090277.short?rss=1 (accessed December 13, 2011).

R. W. F. Ter Steege et al., "Prevalence of Gastrointestinal Complaints in Runners Competing a Long-Distance Run: An Internet-Based Observational Study in 1281 subjects," *Scandinavian Journal of Gastroenterology* 43, no. 12 (2008): 1477–82.

18. E. H. Alsheik et al., "Division I College Athletes of the Highest Intensity Sports Have More Functional GI Disorders," Digestive Disease Week 2011, poster #SU1346.

19. A. Carroccio et al., "Fecal Assays Detect Hypersensitivity to Cow's Milk Protein and Gluten in Adults with Irritable Bowel Syndrome," *Clinical Gastroenterology and Hepatology,* 9, no. 11 (November 2011): 965–71.

20. J. R. Biesiekierski et al., "Gluten Causes Gastrointestinal Symptoms in Subjects Without Celiac Disease: A Double-Blind Randomized Placebo-Controlled Trial," *American Journal of Gastroenterology* 106, no. 3 (March 2011): 508–14.

E. D. Newnham, "Does Gluten Cause Gastrointestinal Symptoms in Subjects Without Celiac Disease?" *Journal of Gastroenterology and Hepatology* 26, no. 3 (April 2011): S132–34.

21. E. P. de Oliveira and R. C. Burini, "Food-Dependent, Exercise-Induced Gastrointestinal Distress," *Journal of the International Society of Sports Nutrition* 8 (September 28, 2011): 12.

22. J. F. Ludvigsson et al., "Small-Intestinal Histopathology and Mortality Risk in Celiac Disease," *Journal of the American Medical Association* 302, no. 11 (2009): 1171–78.

23. C. G. Beckett et al., "Gluten-Induced Nitric Oxide and Pro-Inflammatory Cytokine Release by Cultured Coeliac Small Intestine Biopsies," *European Journal of Gastroenterology & Hepatology* 11, no. 5 (May 1999): 529–36.

T. T. MacDonald and G. Monteleone, "Immunity, Inflammation, and Allergy in the Gut," *Science* 307, no. 5717 (March 25, 2005): 1920–25.

R. T. Przemioslo et al., "Raised Pro-Inflammatory Cytokines Interleukin 6 and Tumor Necrosis Factor Alpha in Coeliac Disease Mucosa Detected by Immunochemistry," *Gut* 35, no. 10 (1994): 1398–1403.

24. *Kyle Korver,* www.kylekorver.com (accessed January 4, 2012).

25. G. De Palma et al., "Effects of a Gluten-Free Diet on Gut Microbiota and Immune Function in Healthy Adult Human Subjects," *British Journal of Nutrition* 102, no. 8 (2009): 1154–60.

26. "2012 Annual 'Best of' Poll Results," *Austin Fit Magazine* (January 2012): www .austinfitmagazine.com/Lifestyle/Reviews/2012/January/best-of-2012.html (accessed January 3, 2012).
    Mauro Pilates, www.mauropilates.com (accessed January 3, 2012).

27. "Burkina Faso," *FAO Initiative on Soaring Food Prices,* Food and Agriculture Organization of the United Nations, www.fao.org/isfp/country-information/ burkina-faso/en (accessed December 14, 2011).
    C. De Filippo et al., "Impact of Diet in Shaping Gut Microbiota Revealed by a Comparative Study in Children from Europe and Rural Africa," *Proceedings of the National Academy of Sciences* 107, no. 33 (August 17, 2010): 14691–96.
    T. Reardon and P. Matlon, "Seasonal Food Insecurity and Vulnerability in Drought-Affected Regions of Burkina Faso," *Seasonal Variability in Third World Agriculture,* International National Food Policy Research Institute, 1989, 118–36.

28. S. K. Anderson, "Biology of Natural Killer Cells: What Is the Relationship Between Natural Killer Cells and Cancer? Will an Increased Number and/or Function of Natural Killer Cells Result in Lower Cancer Incidence?" *Journal of Nutrition* 135, no. 12 (December 1, 2005): 2910S.

29. N. M. Moyna et al., "Exercise-Induced Alterations in Natural Killer Cell Number and Function," *European Journal of Applied Physiology and Occupational Physiology* 74, no. 3 (1996): 227–33.
    D. C. Nieman et al., "Effects of High- vs Moderate-Intensity Exercise on Natural Killer Cell Activity," *Medicine & Science in Sports & Exercise* 25, no. 10 (October 1993): 1126–34.
    N. P. Walsh et al., "Position Statement, Part One: Immune Function and Exercise," *Exercise Immunology Review* 17 (2011) 6–63.
    N. P. Walsh et al., "Position Statement, Part Two: Maintaining Immune Health," *Exercise Immunology Review* 17 (2011): 64–103.

30. B. K. Pederson and H. Ullum, "NK Cell Response to Physical Activity: Possible Mechanisms of Action," *Medicine & Science in Sports & Exercise* 26, no. 2 (1994): 140–46.

31. M. Gleeson and N. C. Bishop, "The T Cell and NK Cell Immune Response to Exercise," *Annals of Transplantation* 10, no. 4 (2005): 43–48.
    M. W. Kakanis et al., "The Open Window of Susceptibility to Infection After Acute Exercise in Healthy Young Male Elite Athletes," *Exercise Immunology Review* 16 (2010): 119–37.
    B. K. Pederson and A. D. Toft, "Effects of Exercise on Lymphocytes and Cytokines," *British Journal of Sports Medicine* 34, no. 4 (2000): 246–51.
    R. J. Shephard and P. N. Shek, "Effects of Exercise and Training on Natural Killer Cell Counts and Cytolytic Activity: A Meta-analysis," *Sports Medicine* 28, no. 3 (September 1999): 177–95.

32. T. D. Noakes, "Food Allergy in Runners," *Journal of the American Medical Association* 247, no. 10 (1982): 1406.

33. "Celiac Marathoner Eyes World Championships and Beyond," *The Savvy Celiac* (January 28, 2011): http://thesavvyceliac.com/2011/01/28/celiac-marathoner-eyes-world-championships-and-beyond (accessed January 3, 2012).

34. "Insights," *Kate Smyth Official Website*, www.katesmyth.com.au (accessed January 3, 2012).

35. "Interview: Elite 2011 Chicago Marathon Runner Ryan Hall," *Time Out Chicago* (September 26, 2011): http://timeoutchicago.com/shopping-style/the-rundown-blog/14961417/interview-elite-2011-chicago-marathon-runner-ryan-hall (accessed January 3, 2012).

36. E. Strout, "Stephanie Rothstein Is Running Free," *ESPN W.* (May 20, 2011): http://espn.go.com/espnw/features-profiles/6566470/stephanie-rothstein-running-free (accessed January 3, 2012).

37. J. W. Barber, "Serious Fuel: Picky Bars—Created by Pros, These Bars Meet a Range of Dietary Needs," *Lava Magazine* (July 19, 2011): http://lavamagazine.com/training/serious-fuel-picky-bars/#axzz1iSBoT2RN (accessed January 3, 2012).

38. "Gluten-Free Athlete Profile: John Forberger, AKA Gluten Free Triathlete," *Gluten Free Fitness* (November 24, 2010): www.glutenfreefitness.com/gluten-free-athlete-profile-jon-forberger-aka-gluten-free-triathlete (accessed January 3, 2012).

39. "Team Gluten Free—Experts," *Celiac Disease Foundation Team Gluten-Free*, www.teamglutenfree.org/experts.html (accessed January 3, 2012).

40. I. Dille, "Gluten-Free Diets: The Word on Wheat—Is a Voluntary Gluten-Free Diet a Good Choice for Cyclists?" *Bicycling*, www.bicycling.com/training-nutrition/nutrition-weight-loss/word-wheat (accessed January 3, 2012).
V. Gregory, "Winning Without Wheat," *Men's Journal* (February 18, 2010): www.mensjournal.com/winning-without-wheat (accessed January 3, 2012).
S. Staber, "Christian Vande Velde's Secret?" *Velo News* (May 11, 2009): http://velonews.competitor.com/2009/05/nutrition/christian-vande-veldes-secret_91925 (accessed January 3, 2012).

41. *Xterra Jenny*, www.xterrajenny.com (accessed January 4, 2012).

42. A. Fasano, "Systemic Autoimmune Disorders in Celiac Disease," *Current Opinion in Gastroenterology* 22, no. 6 (November 2006): 674–79.

43. *Brian Lopes*, www.brianlopes.com/bio.html (accessed January 4, 2012).

44. M. Kieffer et al., "Wheat Gliadin Fractions and Other Cereal Antigens Reactive with Antibodies in the Sera of Coeliac Patients," *Clinical & Experimental Immunology* 50, no. 3 (December 1982): 651–60.

45. M. A. Castany et al., "Natural Killer Cell Activity in Coeliac Disease: Effect of In Vitro Treatment on Effector Lymphocytes and/or Target Lymphoblastoid, Myeloid and Epithelial Cell lines with Gliadin," *Folia Microbiologica* 40, no. 6 (1995): 615–20.

R. Hoggan, "Considering Wheat, Rye, and Barley Proteins as Aids to Carcinogens," *Medical Hypotheses* 49, no. 3 (September 1997): 285–88.

S. Hue et al., "A Direct Role for NKG2D/MICA Interaction in Villous Atrophy During Celiac Disease," *Immunity* 21, no. 3 (September 2004): 367–77.

B. Meresse et al., "Reprogramming of CTLs into Natural Killer–like Cells in Celiac Disease" *Journal of Experimental Medicine* 203, no. 5 (May 15, 2006): 1343–55.

E. M. Nilsen et al., "Gluten Induces an Intestinal Cytokine Response Strongly Dominated by Interferon Gamma in Patients with Celiac Disease" *Gastroenterology* 115, no. 3 (September 1998): 551–63.

46. M. Hadjivassiliou et al., "Gluten Sensitivity: From Gut to Brain," *Lancet Neurology* 9, no. 3 (2010): 318–30.

47. K. K. Adom et al., "Phytochemicals and Antioxidant Activity of Milled Fractions of Different Wheat Varieties," *Journal of Agricultural and Food Chemistry* 53, no. 6 (2005): 2297–2306.

M. M. Belovic et al., "Potential of Bioactive Proteins and Peptides for Prevention and Treatment of Mass Non-Communicable Diseases," *Food and Feed Research* 38, no. 2 (2011): 51–61.

D. J. J. Carr and M. Serou, "Exogenous and Endogenous Opioids as Biological Response Modifiers," *Immunopharmacology* 31, no. 1 (1995): 59–71.

E. G. Fischer, "Opioid Peptides Modulate Immune Functions: A Review," *Immunopharmacology and Immunotoxicology* 10, no. 3 (1988): 265–326.

A. R. French and W. M. Yokoyama, "Natural Killer Cells and Autoimmunity," *Arthritis Research & Therapy* 6, no. 1 (2004): 8–14.

S. Fukudome and M. Yoshikawa "Opioid Peptides Derived from Wheat Gluten: Their Isolation and Characterization," *FEBS Letters* 296, no. 1 (January 13, 1992): 107–11.

R. Hartmann and H. Meisel, "Food-Derived Peptides with Biological Activity: From Research to Food Applications," *Current Opinion in Biotechnology* 18, no. 2 (April 2007): 163–69.

W. A. Hemmings, "The Entry into the Brain of Large Molecules Derived from Dietary Protein," *Proceedings B* 200, no. 1139 (February 23, 1978): 175–92.

N. Horiguchi et al., "Effect of Wheat Gluten Hydrolysate on the Immune System in Healthy Subjects," *Bioscience, Biotechnology, and Biochemistry* 69, no. 12 (December 2005): 2445–49.

J. E. Morley et al., "Neuropeptides: Conductors of the Immune Orchestra," *Life Sciences* 41, no. 5 (August 3, 1987): 527–44.

N. E. S. Sibinga and A. Goldstein, "Opioid Peptides and Opioid Receptors in Cells of the Immune System," *Annual Review of Immunology* 6 (April 1988): 219–49.

L. R. Watkins et al., "Immune Activation: The Role of Pro-inflammatory Cytokines in Inflammation, Illness Responses and Pathological Pain States," *Pain* 63, no. 3 (December 1995): 289–302.

C. Zioudrou et al., "Opioid Peptides Derived from Food Proteins: The Exorphins," *Journal of Biological Chemistry* 254, no. 7 (April 10, 1979): 2446–49.

48. E. Broad, "Allergies and Intolerances in a Flatwater Kayaker," *Medicine & Science in Sports & Exercise* 42, no. 5 (May 2010): 194S–95S.

49. N. Mitchell, "Coeliac Disease Olympic Track Cyclist," *Medicine & Science in Sports & Exercise* 42, no. 5 (May 2010): 195S.

50. L. E. Eberman, and M. A. Cleary, "Celiac Disease in an Elite Female Collegiate Volleyball Athlete: A Case Report," *Journal of Athletic Training* 40, no. 4 (October–December 2005): 360–64.

51. P. Latimer, "Through Illness and Injury, UNC's Taylor Endures," *Lacrosse Magazine* (April 19, 2010): http://laxmagazine.com/college_women/DI/2009-10/news/041910_through_illness_injury_uncs_taylor_prevails (accessed October 29, 2011).
    "Player Bio: Kristen Taylor," *University of North Carolina Tar Heels Official Athletic Site*, www.tarheelblue.com/sports/w-lacros/mtt/taylor_kristen00.html (accessed October 29, 2011).
    Winning Without Gluten, www.winningwithoutgluten.com/about-wwg.html (accessed October 29, 2011).

52. J. E. Leone et al., "Celiac Disease Symptoms in a Female Collegiate Tennis Player: A Case Report," *Journal of Athletic Training* 40, no. 4 (October–December 2005): 365–69.

53. L. A. Mancini et al., "Celiac Disease and the Athlete," *Current Sports Medicine Reports* 10, no. 2 (March–April 2011): 105–8.

54. "About," *Christie Sym*, www.christiesym.com/ChristieSym.com/About.html (accessed January 6, 2012).

55. C. Scott-Thomas, "Gaining Loyalty in the Gluten-Free Market," *Food Navigator USA*, www.foodnavigator-usa.com/Business/Gaining-loyalty-in-the-gluten-free-market (accessed January 4, 2012).

56. "Celiac Disease: Facts and Figures," *National Foundation for Celiac Awareness*, www.celiaccentral.org/Celiac-Disease/Facts-Figures/35 (accessed January 4, 2012).

57. "Making Sense of the Gluten-Free Trend," *The Hartman Group* (September 2, 2009): www.hartman-group.com/hartbeat/making-sense-of-the-gluten-free-trend (accessed January 4, 2012).
    C. Scott-Thomas, "Celiac Disease May Have Little Influence on Soaring Gluten-Free Market," *Food Navigator USA* (February 4, 2011): www.foodnavigator-usa.com/Business/Celiac-disease-may-have-little-influence-on-soaring-gluten-free-market (accessed January 4, 2012).

58. J. Hjelle, "The Weekend I Fed Olympians," *Jen & Company* (July 27, 2011): www.jenandcoblog.com/the-weekend-i-fed-olympians (accessed January 4, 2012).
    S. Stenzel, "Pro Triathlete Interviews before Mpls Triathlon," *St. Paul Examiner* (July 8, 2011): www.examiner.com/triathlon-in-st-paul/pro-triathlete-interviews-before-the-mpls-triathlon (accessed January 4, 2012).

CHAPTER 3

1. V. Mougios, *Exercise Biochemistry* (Champaign, IL: Human Kinetics Publishers, 2006).

2. J. H. Wilmore et al., *Physiology of Sport and Exercise*, 4th Ed. (Champaign, IL: Human Kinetics Publishers, 2007), 50–59.
    V. Gregory, "Winning Without Wheat," *Men's Journal* (February 18, 2010): www.mensjournal.com/winning-without-wheat (accessed January 6, 2012).
    "Our Special 'Anti-inflammatory Diet,'" *Slipstream Sports* (July 25, 2008): www.slipstreamsports.com/2008/07/25/our-special-anti-inflammatory-diet (accessed January 6, 2012).

"Overall Standings," *USA Pro Cycling Challenge,* www.usaprocyclingchallenge.com/standings (accessed January 6, 2012).

S. Staber, "Christian Vande Velde's Secret?" *VeloNews* (May 11, 2009): http://velonews.competitor.com/2009/05/nutrition/christian-vande-veldes-secret_91925 (accessed January 6, 2012).

"The Gluten-Free Bistro to Supply Products to Team Garmin-Cervelo for the USA Pro Cycling Challenge," *The Gluten Free Bistro Blog* (August 15, 2011): www.theglutenfreebistro.com/blog/the-gluten-free-bistro-to-supply-products-to-team-garmin-cervelo-for-the-usa-pro-cycling-challenge (accessed January 6, 2012).

"The Lounge—Athlete—Tejay Van Garderen," *Smith Optics,* www.smithoptics.com/lounge/Team/Bike/Tejay-van-Garderen (accessed January 6, 2012).

3. M. Vogt et al., "Effects of Dietary Fat on Muscle Substrates, Metabolism, and Performance in Athletes," *Medicine & Science in Sports & Exercise* 35, no. 6 (June 2003): 952–60.

4. *Ibid.*

5. *Natalie Jill Fitness,* http://nataliejillfitness.com/about/being-celiac (accessed January 4, 2012).

CHAPTER 4

1. "Jenn Suhr," *USA Track & Field,* www.usatf.org/Athlete-Bios/Jenn-%28Stuczynksi%29-Suhr.aspx (accessed January 6, 2012).

D. Leon Moore, "Jenn Suhr Seeks World Title After Battling Illness," *USA Today* (August 25, 2011): www.usatoday.com/sports/olympics/story/2011-08-25/Jenn-Suhr-seeks-world-title-after-battling-illness/50138128/1 (accessed January 6, 2012).

"Pole Vault Champion Hurdles Celiac Disease," *Athletes for Awareness Blog—National Foundation for Celiac Awareness* (August 11, 2011): www.celiaccentral.org/News/NFCA-Blogs/Athletes-For-Awareness/Celiac-Disease-Athletes-For-Awareness/158/vobid--5877 (accessed January 6, 2012).

P. Shinn, "Jenn Suhr: Going Up Again in Pole Vaulting," *Team USA News* (August 29, 2011): www.teamusa.org/news/2011/08/29/jenn-suhr-going-up-again-in-pole-vaulting/44393 (accessed January 6, 2012).

J. Sullivan, "Suhr Feeling Free and Clear," *Buffalo News* (August 7, 2011): www.buffalonews.com/sports/other/article514628.ece (accessed January 6, 2012).

C. Vito, "Jenn Suhr Grabs No. 1 Spot in Women's Pole Vault Rankings," *Rochester Democrat & Chronicle* (January 2, 2012).

2. W. McArdle et al., *Exercise Physiology: Energy, Nutrition, and Human Performance* (Baltimore, MD: Lippincott Williams & Wilkins, 2007), 31.

3. *Ibid.* 31.

4. P. J. Horvath et al., "The Effects of Varying Dietary Fat on the Nutrient Intake in Male and Female Runners," *Journal of the American College of Nutrition* 19, no. 1 (February 2000): 42–51.

5. W. McArdle et al., *Exercise Physiology: Energy, Nutrition, and Human Performance* (Baltimore, MD: Lippincott Williams & Wilkins, 2007), 28.

6. P. Bronski, "I'm Deficient, You're Deficient, We're All Deficient?" *No Gluten, No Problem* (November 2009): http://noglutennoproblem.blogspot.com/2009/11/im-

deficient-youre-deficient-were-all_04.html (accessed December 19, 2011).

L. Kinsey et al., "A Dietary Survey to Determine If Patients with Coeliac Disease Are Meeting Current Healthy Eating Guidelines and How Their Diet Compares to That of the British General Population," *European Journal of Clinical Nutrition* 62, no. 11 (November 2008): 1333–42.

K. Ohlund et al., "Dietary Shortcoming in Children on a Gluten-Free Diet," *Journal of Human Nutrition and Dietetics* 23, no. 3 (June 2010): 294–300.

T. Thompson et al., "Gluten-Free Diet Survey: Are Americans with Coeliac Disease Consuming Recommended Amounts of Fibre, Iron, Calcium and Grain Foods?" *Journal of Human Nutrition and Dietetics* 18, no. 3 (June 2005): 163–69.

7. "Player Bio: Diana Rolniak," *The Official Athletic Site of the University of Utah,* http:// utahutes.cstv.com/sports/w-baskbl/mtt/rolniak_diana00.html (accessed January 4, 2012).

8. S. O. Fetissov et al., "Autoantibodies Against Appetite-Regulating Peptide Hormones and Neuropeptides: Putative Modulation by Gut Microflora," *Nutrition* 24, no. 4 (April 2008): 348–59.

9. M. R. Cohen et al., "Naloxone Reduces Food Intake in Humans," *Psychosomatic Medicine* 47, no. 2 (March–April 1985): 132–38.
    E. Trenchard and T. Silverstone, "Naloxone Reduces the Food Intake of Normal Human Volunteers," *Appetite* 4, no. 1 (March 1983): 43–50.

10. A. Drewnowski et al., "Naloxone, an Opiate Blocker, Reduces the Consumption of High-Fat Foods in Obese and Lean Female Binge Eaters," *American Journal of Clinical Nutrition* 61, no. 6 (June 1995): 1206–12.

11. J. E. Morley et al., "Effect of Exorphins on Gastrointestinal Function, Hormonal Release, and Appetite," *Gastroenterology* 84, no. 6 (1983): 1517–23.

12. C. Berti et al., "Effect on Appetite Control of Minor Cereal and Pseudocereal Products," *British Journal of Nutrition* 94, no. 5 (November 2005): 850–58.

13. A. Bensaid et al., "Protein Is More Potent than Carbohydrate for Reducing Appetite in Rats," *Physiology & Behavior* 75, no. 4 (April 1, 2002): 577–82.
    J. Bowen et al., "Appetite Regulatory Hormone Responses to Various Dietary Proteins Differ by Body Mass Index Status Despite Similar Reductions in *ad Libitum* Energy Intake," *Journal of Clinical Endocrinology & Metabolism* 91, no. 8 (August 2006): 2913.
    V. Lang et al., "Satiating Effect of Proteins in Healthy Subjects: A Comparison of Egg Albumin, Casein, Gelatin, Soy Protein, Pea Protein, and Wheat Gluten," *American Journal of Clinical Nutrition* 67, no. 6 (June 1998): 1197–1204.

14. M. T. Bardella et al., "Body Composition and Dietary Intakes in Adult Celiac Disease Patients Consuming a Strict Gluten-Free Diet," *American Journal of Clinical Nutrition* 72, no. 4 (October 2000): 937–39.

15. J. A. Murray et al., "Effect of a Gluten-Free Diet on Gastrointestinal Symptoms in Celiac Disease," *American Journal of Clinical Nutrition* 79, no. 4 (April 2004): 669–73.

16. J. Cheng et al., "Body Mass Index in Celiac Disease: Beneficial Effect of a Gluten-Free Diet," *Journal of Clinical Gastroenterology* 44, no. 4 (April 2010): 267–71.

17. N. R. Reilly et al., "Celiac Disease in Normal-Weight and Overweight Children: Clinical Features and Growth Outcomes Following a Gluten-Free Diet," *Journal of Pediatric Gastroenterology and Nutrition* 53, no. 5 (November 2011): 528–31.

18. W. Dickey and N. Kearney, "Overweight in Celiac Disease: Prevalence, Clinical Characteristics, and Effect of a Gluten-Free Diet," *American Journal of Gastroenterology* 101, no. 10 (October 2006): 2356–59.

19. *Kicking 4 Celiac Foundation*, www.kicking4celiac.org/?page_id=5 (accessed January 4, 2012).

CHAPTER 5

1. L. A. Mancini et al., "Celiac Disease and the Athlete," *Current Sports Medicine Reports,* American College of Sports Medicine 10, no. 2 (March–April 2011): 105–8.

2. G. Tortora and S. Grabowski, *Principles of Anatomy and Physiology* (New York: John Wiley & Sons, Inc., 2003), 639–40.

3. M. Waller and E. Haymes, "The Effects of Heat and Exercise on Sweat Iron Loss," *Medicine & Science in Sports & Exercise* 28, no. 2 (1996): 197–203.

4. M. Buckman, "Gastrointestinal Bleeding in Long Distance Runners," *Annals of Internal Medicine* 101, no. 1 (1984): 127–28.

5. A. Ahmadi et al., "Iron Status in Female Athletes Participating in Team Ball-Sports," *Pakistan Journal of Biological Sciences* 13, no. 2 (January 15, 2010): 93–96.
   P. Bartsch et al., "Pseudo-anemia Caused by Sports," *Therapeutische Umschau* 55, no. 4 (April 1998): 251–55.
   S. Reinke et al., "Absolute and Functional Iron Deficiency in Professional Athletes During Training and Recovery," *International Journal of Cardiology,* epub ahead of print, www.sciencedirect.com/science/article/pii/S0167527310010028 (accessed December 19, 2011).

6. J. Brumitt et al., "Comprehensive Sports Medicine Treatment of an Athlete Who Runs Cross-Country and Is Iron Deficient," *North American Journal of Sports Physical Therapy* 4, no. 1 (February 2009): 13–20.

7. L. M. Sinclair and P. S. Hinton, "Prevalence of Iron Deficiency With and Without Anemia in Recreationally Active Men and Women," *Journal of the American Dietetic Association* 105, no. 6 (June 2005): 975–78.

8. D. M. Dellavalle and J. D. Haas, "Impact of Iron Depletion Without Anemia on Performance in Trained Endurance Athletes at the Beginning of a Training Season: A Study of Female Collegiate Rowers," *International Journal of Sport Nutrition and Exercise Metabolism* 21, no. 6 (December 2011): 501–6.

9. J. E. Botero-Lopez et al., "Micronutrient Deficiencies in Patients with Typical and Atypical Celiac Disease," *Journal of Pediatric Gastroenterology and Nutrition* 53, no. 3 (September 2011): 265–70.
   A. Carroccio et al., "Sideropenic Anemia and Celiac Disease: One Study, Two Points of View," *Digestive Disease and Sciences* 43, no. 3 (March 1998): 673–78.

A. Parfenov, "Hematological Disorders in Celiac Disease," *Terapevticheskii Arkhiv* 83, no. 7 (2011): 68–73.

10. *USDA National Nutrient Database for Standard Reference*, www.nal.usda.gov/fnic/foodcomp/search (accessed December 27, 2011).

11. "All-Purpose GF Baking Flour," www.glutino.com/our-products/gluten-free-pantry/beths-all-purpose-gf-baking-flour-us (accessed December 27, 2011).

12. "Bifera FAQ," www.bifera.com/bifera-supplement-faq/how-much-iron-does-bifera-contain (accessed December 27, 2011).
    "Iron," www.naturemade.com/Products/Minerals/Iron (accessed December 27, 2011).

13. "GF All Purpose Baking Flour," www.bobsredmill.com/gf-all_purpose-baking-flour.html?&cat=15 (accessed December 27, 2011).

14. A. Kiskini et al., "Sensory Characteristics and Iron Dialyzability of Gluten-Free Bread Fortified with Iron," *Food Chemistry* 102, no. 1 (2007): 309–16.

15. J. McGinnis, "Enriching Gluten-Free Products Doesn't Make Them 'Healthy,'" *Bartlett's Integrated Health Journal* (December 20, 2011): www.bartlettshealth.com/enriching-gluten-free-products-doesn't-make-them-healthy (accessed December 21, 2011).

16. B. Annibale et al., "Efficacy of Gluten-Free Diet Alone on Recovery from Iron Deficiency Anemia in Adult Celiac Patients," *American Journal of Gastroenterology* 96, no. 1 (January 2001): 132–37.
    L. R. Saez et al., "Refractory Iron-Deficiency Anemia and Gluten Intolerance—Response to Gluten-Free Diet," *Revista Española de Enfermedades Digestivas* 103, no. 7 (July 2011): 349–54.

17. T. Thompson et al., "Gluten-Free Diet Survey: Are Americans with Coeliac Disease Consuming Recommended Amounts of Fibre, Iron, Calcium and Grain Foods?" *Journal of Human Nutrition and Dietetics* 18, no. 3 (June 2005): 163–69.
    D. Wild et al., "Evidence of High Sugar Intake, and Low Fibre and Mineral Intake, in the Gluten-Free Diet," *Alimentary Pharmacology & Therapeutics* 32, no. 4 (August 2010): 573–81.

18. L. A. Garvican et al., "Haemoglobin Mass in an Anaemic Female Endurance Runner Before and After Iron Supplementation," *International Journal of Sports Physiology and Performance* 6, no. 1 (March 2011): 137–40.
    P. Nielsen and D. Nachtigall, "Iron Supplementation in Athletes: Current Recommendations," *Sports Medicine* 26, no. 4 (October 1998): 207–16.
    S. Radjen et al., "Effect of Iron Supplementation on Maximal Oxygen Uptake in Female Athletes," *Vojnosanitetski Pregled* 68, no. 2 (February 2011): 130–35.
    E. P. Zaitseva, "Efficiency of Using Vitamin-Mineral Complexes in the Prevention of Iron-Deficiency States in Athletes," *Gig Sanit*, no. 4 (July–August 2010), 66–69.

19. S. Mettler and M. B. Zimmermann, "Iron Excess in Recreational Marathon Runners," *European Journal of Clinical Nutrition* 64, no. 5 (May 2010): 490–94.
    H. Zoller and W. Vogel, "Iron Supplementation in Athletes—First Do No Harm," *Nutrition* 20, no. 7–8 (July–August 2004): 615–19.

20. *Ibid.*

21. E. Whitney et al., *Understanding Normal and Clinical Nutrition* (Belmont, CA: Wadsworth/Thomson Learning, 2002), 404.

22. A. Cranney et al., "Effectiveness and Safety of Vitamin D in Relation to Bone Health," *Evidence Report—Technology Assessment,* no. 158 (August 2007) 1–235.

23. W. McArdle et al., *Exercise Physiology: Energy, Nutrition, and Human Performance* (Philadelphia, PA: Lea & Febiger, 1986), 297.

24. E. Whitney et al., *Understanding Normal and Clinical Nutrition* (Belmont, CA: Wadsworth/Thomson Learning, 2002), 404–5.

25. *Amy Yoder Begley,* www.yoderbegley.com (accessed January 5, 2012).

26. R. Bescos Garcia and F. A. Rodriguez Guisado, "Low Levels of Vitamin D in Professional Basketball Players After Wintertime: Relationship with Dietary Intake of Vitamin D and Calcium," *Nutricion Hospitalaria* 26, no. 5 (October 2011): 945–51.

27. A. Zittermann et al., "Evidence for an Acute Rise of Intestinal Calcium Absorption in Response to Aerobic Exercise," *European Journal of Nutrition* 41, no. 5 (2002): 189–96.

28. C. Blanchet et al., "Leisure Physical Activity Is Associated with Quantitative Ultrasound Measurements Independently of Bone Mineral Density in Postmenopausal Women," *Calcified Tissue International* 73, no. 4 (October 2003): 339–49.

29. A. Arasheben et al., "A Meta-analysis of Bone Mineral Density in Collegiate Female Athletes," *Journal of the American Board of Family Medicine* 24, no. 6 (November 2011): 728–34.
    E. Babaroutsi et al., "Body Mass Index, Calcium Intake, and Physical Activity Affect Calcaneal Ultrasound in Healthy Greek Males in an Age-Dependent and Parameter-Specific Manner," *Journal of Bone and Mineral Metabolism* 23, no. 2 (2005): 157–66.
    K. T. Borer, "Physical Activity in the Prevention and Amelioration of Osteoporosis in Women: Interaction of Mechanical, Hormonal and Dietary Factors," *Sports Medicine* 35, no. 9 (2005): 779–830.
    A. L. Dias Quiterio et al., "Skeletal Mass in Adolescent Male Athletes and Nonathletes: Relationships with High-Impact Sports," *Journal of Strength & Conditioning Research* 25, no. 12 (December 2011): 3439–47.
    Y. Dionyssiotis et al., "Association of Physical Exercise and Calcium Intake with Bone Mass Measured by Quantitative Ultrasound," *BMC Women's Health* 10 (April 7, 2010): 12.
    E. W. Gregg et al., "Correlates of Quantitative Ultrasound in the Women's Healthy Lifestyle Project," *Osteoporosis International* 10, no. 5 (1999): 416–24.
    G. Guillaume et al., "Evaluation of the Bone Status in High-Level Cyclists," *Journal of Clinical Densitometry,* November 8, 2011, epub ahead of print, www.ncbi.nlm.nih .gov/pubmed/22071023 (accessed December 21, 2011).

30. P. Brukner, "Shin Pain—Running," *Medicine and Science in Sports and Exercise: Proceedings of the 52nd American College of Sports Medicine (ACSM) Annual Meeting,* June 2005, 457S.

31. C. Greenhill, "Celiac Disease: Lack of Vitamins D and K Affects Bone Health in Celiac Disease," *Nature Reviews Gastroenterology & Hepatology* 8, no. 12 (November 8, 2011): 660.

D. Margoni et al., "Bone Health in Children with Celiac Disease Assessed by Dual X-Ray Absorptiometry: Effect of Gluten-Free Diet and Predictive Value of Serum Biochemical Indices," *Journal of Pediatric Gastroenterology and Nutrition* (November 15, 2011), epub ahead of print, www.ncbi.nlm.nih.gov/pubmed/22094895 (accessed December 21, 2011).

S. Mora et al., "Reversal of Low Bone Density with a Gluten-Free Diet in Children and Adolescents with Celiac Disease," *American Journal of Clinical Nutrition* 67, no. 3 (March 1998): 477–81.

C. J. Mulder et al., "Celiac Disease Presenting as Severe Osteopenia," *Hawaii Medical Journal* 70, no. 11 (November 2011): 242–44.

32.   L. Matsuoka et al., "Chronic Sunscreen Use Decreases Circulating Concentrations of 25-hydroxyvitamin D: A Preliminary Study," *Archives of Dermatology* 124, no. 12 (December 1988): 1802–4.

CHAPTER 6

1.   C. M. Donaldson et al., "Glycemic Index and Endurance Performance," *International Journal of Sport Nutrition and Exercise Metabolism* 20, no. 2 (April 2010): 154–65.

J. P. Little et al., "The Effects of Low- and High-Glycemic Index Foods on High-Intensity Intermittent Exercise," *International Journal of Sports Physiology and Performance* 4, no. 3 (September 2009): 367–80.

M. J. Sparks et al., "Pre-exercise Carbohydrate Ingestion: Effect of the Glycemic Index on Endurance Exercise Performance," *Medicine & Science in Sports & Exercise* 30, no. 6 (June 1998): 844–49.

C. L. Wu and C. Williams, "A Low Glycemic Index Meal Before Exercise Improves Endurance Running Capacity in Men," *International Journal of Sport Nutrition and Exercise Metabolism* 16, no. 5 (October 2006): 510–27.

2.   Y. J. Chen et al., "Effects of Glycemic Index Meal and CHO-Electrolyte Drink on Cytokine Response and Run Performance in Endurance Athletes," *Journal of Science and Medicine in Sport* 12, no. 6 (November 2009): 697–703.

3.   C. M. Donaldson et al., "Glycemic Index and Endurance Performance," *International Journal of Sport Nutrition and Exercise Metabolism* 20, no. 2 (April 2010): 154–65.

J. Oreilly et al., "Glycaemic Index, Glycaemic Load and Exercise Performance," *Sports Medicine* 40, no. 1 (January 1, 2010): 27–39.

4.   "Insulin Resistance and Pre-diabetes," *National Diabetes Information Clearinghouse,* http://diabetes.niddk.nih.gov/dm/pubs/insulinresistance/#what (accessed December 28, 2011).

5.   K. M. Behall and J. Hallfrisch, "Plasma Glucose and Insulin Reduction After Consumption of Breads Varying in Amylose Content," *European Journal of Clinical Nutrition* 56, no. 9 (2002): 913–20.

6.   L. A. Grant et al., "Determination of Amylose and Amylopectin of Wheat Starch Using High Performance Size-Exclusion Chromatography (HPSEC)," *Cereal Chemistry* 79, no. 6 (2002): 771–73.

"Starch," *International Starch Institute,* www.starch.dk/isi/starch/starch.asp (accessed January 29, 2012).

7.   K. S. Juntunen et al., "Postprandial Glucose, Insulin, and Incretin Responses to Grain Products in Healthy Subjects," *American Journal of Clinical Nutrition* 75, no. 2 (February 2002): 254–62.

8. J. Bao et al., "Food Insulin Index: Physiologic Basis for Predicting Insulin Demand Evoked by Composite Meals," *American Journal of Clinical Nutrition* 90, no. 4 (October 2009): 986–92.

    M. Gannon et al., "An Increase in Dietary Protein Improves the Blood Glucose Response in Persons with Type 2 Diabetes," *American Journal of Clinical Nutrition.* 78, no. 4 (October 2003): 734–41.

    L. Mortensen et al., "Differential Effects of Protein Quality on Postprandial Lipemia in Response to a Fat-Rich Meal in Type 2 Diabetes: Comparison of Whey, Casein, Gluten, and Cod Protein," *American Journal of Clinical Nutrition* 90, no. 1 (July 2009): 41–48.

    M. Nilsson et al., "Glycemia and Insulinemia in Healthy Subjects After Lactose-Equivalent Meals of Milk and Other Food Proteins: The Role of Plasma Amino Acids and Incretins," *American Journal of Clinical Nutrition* 80, no. 5 (November 2004): 1246–53.

    F. Q. Nuttall et al., "Effect of Protein Ingestion on the Glucose and Insulin Response to a Standardized Oral Glucose Load," *Diabetes Care* 7, no. 5 (September–October 1984): 465–70.

    G. A. Spiller et al., "Effect of Protein Dose on Serum Glucose and Insulin Response to Sugars," *American Journal of Clinical Nutrition* 46, no. 3 (September 1987): 474–80.

9. S. C. Packer et al., "The Glycaemic Index of a Range of Gluten-Free Foods," *Diabetic Medicine* 17, no. 9 (September 2000): 657–60.

    M. E. Segura and C. M. Rosell, "Chemical Composition and Starch Digestibility of Different Gluten-Free Breads," *Plant Foods for Human Nutrition* 66, no. 3 (September 2011): 224–30.

10. P. A. Crapo et al., "Postprandial Plasma-Glucose and -Insulin Responses to Different Complex Carbohydrates," *Diabetes* 26, no. 12 (December 1977): 1178–83.

    J. Holm and I. Bjorck, "Bioavailability of Starch in Various Wheat-Based Bread Products: Evaluation of Metabolic Responses in Healthy Subjects and Rate and Extent of In Vitro Starch Digestion," *American Journal of Clinical Nutrition* 55, no. 2 (February 1992): 420–29.

    D. J. Jenkins et al., "The Effect of Starch-Protein Interaction in Wheat on the Glycemic Response and Rate of In Vitro Digestion," *American Journal of Clinical Nutrition* 45, no. 5 (May 1987): 946–51.

11. S. Fukudome et al., "Effect of Gluten Exorphins a5 and b5 on the Postprandial Plasma Insulin Level in Conscious Rats," *Life Sciences* 57, no. 7 (July 1995): 729–34.

12. R. Amin et al., "A Longitudinal Study of the Effects of a Gluten-Free Diet on Glycemic Control and Weight Gain in Subjects with Type 1 Diabetes and Celiac Disease," *Diabetes Care* 25, no. 7 (July 2002): 1117–22.

    E. Bosi et al., "Gluten-Free Diet in Subjects at Risk for Type 1 Diabetes: A Tool for Delaying Progression to Clinical Disease?" *Advances in Experimental Medicine and Biology* 569 (2005): 157–58.

    M. Donath et al., "Inflammatory Mediators and Islet β-cell Failure: A Link Between Type 1 and Type 2 Diabetes," *Journal of Molecular Medicine* 81, no. 8 (2003): 455–70.

    G. Frisk et al., "A Unifying Hypothesis on the Development of Type 1 Diabetes and Celiac Disease: Gluten Consumption May Be a Shared Causative Factor," *Medical Hypotheses* 70, no. 6 (2008): 1207–9.

    M. Fuchtenbusch et al., "Elimination of Dietary Gluten and Development of Type 1 Diabetes in High Risk Subjects," *Review of Diabetic Studies* 1, no. 1 (Spring 2004): 39–41.

    D. P. Funda et al., "Gluten-Free but Also Gluten-Enriched (Gluten+) Diet Prevent Diabes in NOD Mice; the Gluten Enigma in Type 1 Diabetes," *Diabetes/Metabolism Research and Reviews* 24, no. 1 (January–February 2008): 59–63.

D. P. Funda et al., "Gluten-Free Diet Prevents Diabetes in NOD Mice," *Diabetes/Metabolism Research and Reviews* 15, no. 5 (September–October 1999): 323–27.

A. Giongo et al., "Microbiology of Type 1 Diabetes: Possible Implications for Management of the Disease," *Diabetes Management* 1, no. 3 (May 2011): 325–31.

A. Hansen et al., "Diabetes Preventive Gluten-Free Diet Decreases the Number of Caecal Bacteria in Non-obese Diabetic Mice," *Diabetes/Metabolism Research and Reviews* 22, no. 3 (2006): 220–25.

D. Hansen et al., "Clinical Benefit of a Gluten-Free Diet in Type 1 Diabetic Children with Screening-Detected Celiac Disease: A Population-Based Screening Study with 2 Years' Follow-up," *Diabetes Care* 29, no. 11 (November 2006): 2452–56.

S. Hummel and A. Ziegler, "Early Determinants of Type 1 Diabetes: Experience from the BABYDIAB and BABYDIET Studies," *American Journal of Clinical Nutrition* 94, no. 6 (December 2011): 1821S–23S.

D. Lefebvre et al., "Dietary Proteins as Environmental Modifiers of Type 1 Diabetes Mellitus," *Annual Review of Nutrition*, no. 26 (August 2006): 175–202.

V. Malalasekera et al., "Potential Reno-Protective Effects of a Gluten-Free Diet in Type 1 Diabetes," *Diabetologia* 52, no. 5 (2009): 798–800.

M. R. Pastore et al., "Six Months of Gluten-Free Diet Do Not Influence Autoantibody Titers, but Improve Insulin Secretion in Subjects at High Risk for Type 1 Diabetes," *Journal of Clinical Endocrinology & Metabolism* 88, no. 1 (January 2003): 162–65.

O. Saadah et al., "Effect of Gluten-Free Diet and Adherence on Growth and Diabetic Control in Diabetics with Coeliac Disease," *Archives of Disease in Childhood* 89, no. 9 (September 2004): 871–76.

I. Sanchez-Albisua et al., "Coeliac Disease in Children with Type 1 Diabetes Mellitus: The Effect of the Gluten-Free Diet," *Diabetic Medicine* 22, no. 8 (August 2005): 1079–82.

13. *Ibid.*

14. A. Bonen et al., "Glucose Tolerance Is Improved After Low- and High-Intensity Exercise in Middle-Age Men and Women," *Canadian Journal of Applied Physiology* 23, no. 6 (December 1988): 583–93.

J. Eriksson et al., "Aerobic Endurance Exercise or Circuit-Type Resistance Training for Individuals with Impaired Glucose Tolerance?" *Hormone and Metabolic Research* 30, no. 1 (1998): 37–41.

G. H. Goodpaster et al., "Skeletal Muscle Lipid Content and Insulin Resistance: Evidence for a Paradox in Endurance-Trained Athletes," *Journal of Clinical Endocrinology & Metabolism* 86, no. 12 (December 1, 2001): 5755–61.

G. W. Heath et al., "Effects of Exercise and Lack of Exercise on Glucose Tolerance and Insulin Sensitivity," *Journal of Applied Physiology* 55, no. 2 (August 1983): 512–17.

J. O. Holloszy et al., "Effects of Exercise on Glucose Tolerance and Insulin Resistance," *Acta Medica Scandinavica* 220, no. S711 (December–January 1986): 55–65.

J. L. Ivy, "Role of Exercise Training in the Prevention and Treatment of Insulin Resistance and Non-Insulin-Dependent Diabetes Mellitus," *Sports Medicine* 24, no. 5 (1997): 321–26.

D. S. King et al., "Time Course for Exercise-Induced Alterations in Insulin Action and Glucose Tolerance in Middle-Aged People," *Journal of Applied Physiology* 78, no. 1 (January 1995): 17–22.

V. A. Koivisto et al., "Insulin Binding to Monocytes in Trained Athletes: Changes in the Resting State and After Exercise," *Journal of Clinical Investigation* 64, no. 4 (October 1979): 1011–15.

X-R. Pan et al., "Effects of Diet and Exercise in Preventing NIDDM in People with Impaired Glucose Tolerance: The Da Qing IGT and Diabetes Study," *Diabetes Care* 20, no. 4 (April 1997): 537–44.

M. E. Reed et al., "The Effects of Two Bouts of High- and Low-Volume Resistance Exercise on Glucose Tolerance in Normoglycemic Women," *Journal of Strength & Conditioning Research* (December 8, 2011), epub ahead of print, www.ncbi.nlm.nih.gov/pubmed/22158138 (accessed December 20, 2011).

M. A. Rogers et al., "Improvement in Glucose Tolerance After 1 Wk of Exercise in Patients with Mild NIDDM," *Diabetes Care* 11, no. 8 (September 1988): 613–18.

D. R. Seals et al., "Glucose Tolerance in Young and Older Athletes and Sedentary Men," *Journal of Applied Physiology* 56, no. 6 (June 1984): 1521–25.

M. A. Smutok et al., "Effects of Exercise Training Modality on Glucose Tolerance in Men with Abnormal Glucose Regulation," *International Journal of Sports Medicine* 15, no. 6 (1994): 283–89.

S. L. Wee et al., "Influence of High and Low Glycemic Index Meals on Endurance Running Capacity," *Medicine & Science in Sports & Exercise* 31, no. 3 (March 1999): 393–99.

J. C. Young et al., "Exercise Intensity and Glucose Tolerance in Trained and Nontrained Subjects," *Journal of Applied Physiology* 67, no. 1 (1989): 39–43.

15. "Ginger Vieira," *Living in Progress*, http://living-in-progress.com/2010/12/ginger-vieira (accessed January 5, 2012).

16. J. Wahlberg et al., "Dietary Risk Factors for the Emergence of Type 1 Diabetes-Related Autoantibodies in 2½-Year-Old Swedish Children," *British Journal of Nutrition* 95, no. 3 (2006): 603–8.

A-G. Ziegler et al., "Early Infant Feeding and Risk of Developing Type 1 Diabetes–Associated Autoantibodies," *Journal of the American Medical Association* 290, no. 13 (2003): 1721–28.

17. R. Kawamori, "Diabetes Trends in Japan," *Diabetes/Metabolism Research and Reviews* 18, no. 3 (September–October 2002): S9–S13.

S. E. Neville et al., "Diabetes in Japan: A Review of Disease Burden and Approaches to Treatment," *Diabetes/Metabolism Research and Reviews* 25, no. 8 (November 2009): 705–16.

W. Yang et al., "Prevalence of Diabetes Among Men and Women in China," *New England Journal of Medicine* 362, no. 12 (2010): 1090–1101.

18. H. Lijeberg et al., "Metabolic Responses to Starch in Bread Containing Intact Kernels Versus Milled Flour," *European Journal of Clinical Nutrition* 46, no. 8 (August 1992): 561–75.

A. Nanri et al., "Rice Intake and Type 2 Diabetes in Japanese Men and Women: The Japan Public Health Center–Based Prospective Study," *American Journal of Clinical Nutrition* 92, no. 6 (December 2010): 1468–77.

Q. Sun et al., "White Rice, Brown Rice, and Risk of Type 2 Diabetes in US Men and Women," *Archives of Internal Medicine* 170, no. 11 (June 14, 2010): 961–69.

19. A. M. Najjar et al., "The Acute Impact of Ingestion of Breads of Varying Composition on Blood Glucose, Insulin and Incretins Following First and Second Meals," *British Journal of Nutrition* 101, no. 3 (February 2009): 391–98.

20. M. Maki et al., "Increased Prevalence of Coeliac Disease in Diabetes," *Archives of Disease in Childhood* 59, no. 8 (1984): 739–42.

R. Troncone et al., "Gluten Sensitivity in a Subset of Children with Insulin Dependent Diabetes Mellitus," *American Journal of Gastroenterology* 98, no. 3 (March 2003): 590–95.

21. C. Berti et al., "In Vitro Starch Digestibility and In Vivo Glucose Response of Gluten-Free Foods and Their Gluten Counterparts," *European Journal of Nutrition* 43, no. 4 (August 2004): 198–204.

22. H. M. DeMarco et al., "Pre-exercise Carbohydrate Meals: Application of Glycemic Index," *Medicine & Science in Sports & Exercise* 31, no. 1 (January 1999): 164–70.

M. A. Febbraio et al., "Preexercise Carbohydrate Ingestion, Glucose Kinetics, and Muscle Glycogen Use: Effect of the Glycemic Index," *Journal of Applied Physiology* 89, no. 5 (November 2000): 1845–51.

M. Hargreaves et al., "Pre-exercise Carbohydrate and Fat Ingestion: Effects on Metabolism and Performance," *Journal of Sports Sciences* 22, no. 1 (2004): 31–38.

J. F. Horowitz et al., "Lipolytic Suppression Following Carbohydrate Ingestion Limits Fat Oxidation During Exercise," *American Journal of Physiology—Endocrinology and Metabolism* 273, no. 4 (October 1997): E768–75.

J. P. Kirwan et al., "A Moderate Glycemic Meal Before Endurance Exercise Can Enhance Performance," *Journal of Applied Physiology* 84, no. 1 (January 1998): 53–59.

W. Shiou-Liang et al., "Influence of High and Low Glycemic Index Meals on Endurance Running Capacity," *Medicine & Science in Sports & Exercise* 31, no. 3 (March 1999): 393–99.

M. J. Sparks et al., "Pre-exercise Carbohydrate Ingestion: Effect of the Glycemic Index on Endurance Exercise Performance," *Medicine & Science in Sports & Exercise* 30, no. 6 (June 1998): 844–49.

S. H. S. Wong et al., "Effect of the Glycaemic Index of Pre-exercise Carbohydrate Meals on Running Performance," *European Journal of Sport Science* 8, no. 1 (2008): 23–33.

C-L. Wu et al., "The Influence of High-Carbohydrate Meals with Different Glycaemic Indices on Substrate Utilisation During Subsequent Exercise," *British Journal of Nutrition* 90, no. 6 (2003): 1049–56.

23. L. M. Burke et al., "Carbohydrate Intake During Prolonged Cycling Minimizes Effect of Glycemic Index of Preexercise Meal," *Journal of Applied Physiology* 85, no. 6 (December 1998): 2220–26.

M. A. Febbraio et al., "Effects of Carbohydrate Ingestion Before and During Exercise on Glucose Kinetics and Performance," *Journal of Applied Physiology* 89, no. 6 (December 2000): 2220–26.

M. C. Riddell et al., "Substrate Utilization During Exercise Performed With and Without Glucose Ingestion in Female and Male Endurance Trained Athletes," *International Journal of Sport Nutrition and Exercise Metabolism* 13, no. 4 (December 2003): 407–21.

J. A. Romijn et al., "Regulation of Endogenous Fat and Carbohydrate Metabolism in Relation to Exercise Intensity and Duration," *American Journal of Physiology—Endocrinology and Metabolism* 265, no. 3 (September 1993): E380–91.

24. L. B. Borghouts and H. A. Keizer, "Exercise and Insulin Sensitivity: A Review," *International Journal of Sports Medicine* 21, no. 1 (January 2000): 1–12.

"What You Eat After Exercise Matters," *Science Daily* (January 28, 2010): www .sciencedaily.com/releases/2010/01/100128122142.htm (accessed January 26, 2012).

J. F. Wojtaszewski et al., "Insulin Signaling and Insulin Sensitivity After Exercise in Human Skeletal Muscle," *Diabetes* 49, no. 3 (March 2000): 325–31.

25. C. Frosig and E. Richter, "Improved Insulin Sensitivity After Exercise: Focus on Insulin Signaling," *Obesity* 17, Suppl. 3 (2009): S15–20.

L. Goodyear and B. Kahn, "Exercise, Glucose Transport, and Insulin Sensitivity," *Annual Review of Medicine* 49 (February 1998): 235–61.

P. Hansen et al., "Increased GLUT-4 Translocation Mediates Enhanced Insulin Sensitivity of Muscle Glucose Transport After Exercise," *Journal of Applied Physiology* 85, no. 4 (October 1998): 1218–22.

26. G. Perseghin et al., "Increased Glucose Transport–Phosphorylation and Muscle Glycogen Synthesis After Exercise Training in Insulin-Resistant Subjects," *New England Journal of Medicine* 335, no. 18 (October 1996): 1357–62.

27. M. Beelen et al., "Impact of Caffeine and Protein on Post-Exercise Muscle Glycogen Synthesis," *Medicine & Science in Sports & Exercise* (October 7, 2011), epub ahead of print, www.ncbi.nlm.nih.gov/pubmed/21986807 (accessed December 17, 2011).
L. M. Burke et al., "Carbohydrates and Fat for Training and Recovery," *Journal of Sports Sciences* 22, no. 1 (2004): 15–30.
W. R. Lunn et al., "Chocolate Milk and Endurance Exercise Recovery: Protein Balance, Glycogen and Performance," *Medicine & Science in Sports & Exercise* (September 7, 2011), epub ahead of print, www.ncbi.nlm.nih.gov/pubmed/21904247 (accessed December 17, 2011).
E. J. Stevenson et al., "The Metabolic Responses to High Carbohydrate Meals with Different Glycemic Indices Consumed During Recovery from Prolonged Strenuous Exercise," *International Journal of Sport Nutrition and Exercise Metabolism* 15, no. 3 (June 2005): 291–307.

28. S. H. Wong et al., "Effect of Glycemic Index Meals on Recovery and Subsequent Endurance Capacity," *International Journal of Sports Medicine* 30, no. 12 (December 2009): 898–905.

29. P. M. Siu et al., "Effect of Frequency of Carbohydrate Feedings on Recovery and Subsequent Endurance Run," *Medicine & Science in Sports & Exercise* 36, no. 2 (February 2004): 315–23.

30. J. W. Coburn et al., "Effects of Leucine and Whey Protein Supplementation During Eight Weeks of Unilateral Resistance Training," *Journal of Strength & Conditioning Research* 20, no. 2 (2006): 284–91.
M. Negro et al., "Branched-Chain Amino Acid Supplementation Does Not Enhance Athletic Performance but Affects Muscle Recovery and the Immune System," *Journal of Sports Medicine and Physical Fitness* 48, no. 3 (September 2008): 347–51.
I. Rieu et al., "Increased Availability of Leucine with Leucine-Rich Whey Proteins Improves Postprandial Muscle Protein Synthesis in Aging Rats," *Nutrition* 23, no. 4 (April 2007): 323–31.
J. E. Tang et al., "Ingestion of Whey Hydrolysate, Casein, or Soy Protein Isolate: Effects on Mixed Muscle Protein Synthesis at Rest and Following Resistance Exercise in Young Men," *Journal of Applied Physiology* 107, no. 3 (September 2009) 987–92.
K. D. Tipton et al., "Ingestion of Casein and Whey Proteins Result in Muscle Anabolism After Resistance Exercise," *Medicine & Science in Sports & Exercise* 36, no. 12 (December 2004): 2073–81.

31. M. Gleeson, "Dosing and Efficacy of Glutamine Supplementation in Human Exercise and Sport Training," *Journal of Nutrition* 138, no. 10 (October 2008): 2045S–49S.

32. N. Koikawa et al., "Delayed-Onset Muscle Injury and Its Modification by Wheat Gluten Hydrolysate," *Nutrition* 25, no. 5 (May 2009): 493–98.

33. M. Holecek. "Relation Between Glutamine, Branched-Chain Amino Acids, and Protein Metabolism," *Nutrition* 18, no. 2 (February 2002): 130–33.
K. Sawaki et al., "Effects of Distance Running and Subsequent Intake of Glutamine Rich Peptide on Biomedical Parameters of Male Japanese Athletes," *Nutrition Research* 24, no. 1 (January 2004): 59–71.

34. J. Antonio and C. Street, "Glutamine: A Potentially Useful Supplement for Athletes," *Canadian Journal of Applied Physiology* 24, no. 1 (1999): 1–14.

L. M. Castell and E. A. Newsholm, "The Effects of Oral Glutamine Supplementation on Athletes After Prolonged Exhaustive Exercise," *Nutrition* 13, nos. 7–8 (July–August 1997): 738–42.

L. M. Castell et al., "Does Glutamine Have a Role in Reducing Infections in Athletes?" *European Journal of Applied Physiology* 73, no. 5 (November 1992): 488–90.

E. E. Lyon, "Supplements for the Gluten Free Athlete—Glutamine Edition," *Gluten Free Fitness* (January 31, 2010): www.glutenfreefitness.com/supplements-for-the-gluten-free-athlete-glutamine-edition (accessed December 17, 2011).

35. L. M. Burke et al., "Effect of Coingestion of Fat and Protein with Carbohydrate Feedings on Muscle Glycogen Storage," *Journal of Applied Physiology* 78, no. 6 (June 1995): 2187–92.

A. H. Manninen, "Hyperinsulinaemia, Hyperaminoacidaemia and Post-exercise Muscle Anabolism: The Search for the Optimal Recovery Drink," *British Journal of Sports Medicine* 40, no. 10 (2006): 900–905.

G. J. Wilson et al., "Leucine or Carbohydrate Supplementation Reduces AMPK and eEF2 Phosphorylation and Extends Postprandial Muscle Protein Synthesis in Rats," *American Journal of Physiology—Endocrinology and Metabolism* 301, no. 6 (December 2011): E1236–42.

36. G. D. Cartee et al., "Prolonged Increase in Insulin-Stimulated Glucose Transport in Muscle After Exercise," *American Journal of Physiology—Endocrinology and Metabolism* 256, no. 4 (April 1989): E494–99.

37. "Position of the American Dietetic Association, Dietitians of Canada, and the American College of Sports Medicine: Nutrition and Athletic Performance," *Journal of the American Dietetic Association* 109, no. 3 (March 2009): 509–27.

38. A. C. Grandjean, "Diets of Elite Athletes: Has the Discipline of Sports Nutrition Made an Impact?" *Journal of Nutrition* 127, no. 5 (May 1, 1997): 874S–77S.

39. D. R. Pendergrast et al., "Influence of Exercise on Nutritional Requirements," *European Journal of Applied Physiology* 111, no. 3 (March 2011): 379–90.

40. M. T. Cerquiera et al., "The Food and Nutrient Intakes of the Tarahumara Indians of Mexico," *American Journal of Clinical Nutrition* 32, no. 4 (April 1979): 905–15.

D. L. Christensen et al., "Food and Macronutrient Intake of Male Adolescent Kalenjin Runners in Kenya," *British Journal of Nutrition* 88, no. 6 (December 2002): 711–17.

W. E. Connor et al., "The Plasma Lipids, Lipoproteins, and Diet of the Tarahumara Indians of Mexico," *American Journal of Clinical Nutrition* 31, no. 7 (July 1978): 1131–42.

41. J. A. Hawley et al., "Carbohydrate-Loading and Exercise Performance: An Update," *Sports Medicine* 24, no. 2 (1997): 73–81.

42. F. X. Pizza et al., "A Carbohydrate Loading Regimen Improves High Intensity, Short Duration Exercise Performance," *International Journal of Sport Nutrition* 5, no. 2 (June 1995): 110–16.

L. H. Rauch et al., "The Effects of Carbohydrate Loading on Muscle Glycogen Content and Cycling Performance," *International Journal of Sport Nutrition* 5, no. 1: 25–36.

M. A. Tarnopolsky et al., "Carbohydrate Loading and Metabolism During Exercise in Men and Women," *Journal of Applied Physiology* 78, no. 4 (April 1995): 1360–68.

43. V. A. Bussau et al., "Carbohydrate Loading in Human Muscle: An Improved 1 Day Protocol," *European Journal of Applied Physiology* 87, no. 3 (September 1999): 290–95.

44. L. M. Burke et al., "Eating Patterns and Meal Frequency of Elite Australian Athletes," *International Journal of Sport Nutrition and Exercise Metabolism* 13, no. 4 (December 2003): 521–38.

J. A. Hawley and L. M. Burke, "Effect of Meal Frequency and Timing on Physical Performance," *British Journal of Nutrition* 77, Suppl. 1 (April 1997): S91–103.

D. Jenkins et al., "Nibbling Versus Gorging: Metabolic Advantages of Increased Meal Frequency," *New England Journal of Medicine* 321, no. 14 (October 5, 1989): 929–34.

K. A. Kirsch and H. von Ameln, "Feeding Patterns of Endurance Athletes," *European Journal of Applied Physiology and Occupational Physiology* 47, no. 2 (1981): 197–208.

P. M. La Bounty et al., "International Society of Sports Nutrition Position Stand: Meal Frequency," *Journal of the International Society of Sports Nutrition* 8 (March 16, 2011): 4.

W. P. Verboeket-van de Venne and K. R. Westerterp, "Influence of the Feeding Frequency on Nutrient Utilization in Man: Consequences for Energy Metabolism," *European Journal of Clinical Nutrition* 45, no. 3 (991): 161–69.

45. B. S. Anand, et al., "The Role of Various Cereals on Coeliac Disease," *QJM: An International Journal of Medicine* 47, no. 185 (January 1978): 101–10.

S. U. Friis, "Enzyme-Linked Immunosorbent Assay for Quantitation of Cereal Proteins Toxic in Coeliac Disease," *Clinica Chimica Acta* 178, no. 3 (December 30, 1988): 261–70.

M. Kieffer, et al., "Wheat Gliadin Fractions and Other Cereal Antigens Reactive with Antibodies in the Sera of Coeliac Patients," *Clinical & Experimental Immunology* 50, no. 3 (December 1982): 651–60.

B. Moron, et al., "Sensitive Detection of Cereal Fractions That Are Toxic to Celiac Disease Patients by Using Monoclonal Antibodies to a Main Immunogenic Wheat Peptide," *American Journal of Clinical Nutrition* 87, no. 2 (February 2008): 405–14.

D. J. Unsworth and E. J. Holborow, "Does the Reticulin Binding Property of Cereal Proteins Demonstrable In Vitro Have Pathogenetic Significance for Coeliac Disease?" *Gut* 26, no. 11 (November 1985): 1204–9.

46. F. Cabrera-Chavez et al., "Transglutaminase Treatment of Wheat and Maize Prolamins of Bread Increases the Serum IgA Reactivity of Celiac Disease Patients," *Journal of Agricultural and Food Chemistry* 56, no. 4 (February 27, 2008): 1387–91.

F. Kluge et al., "Gluten-Sensitive Enteropathy—in the Light of New Clinical and Pathogenetic Aspects," *Klinische Wochenschrift* 61, no. 14 (July 15, 1983): 669–79.

G. Kristjansson et al., "Gut Mucosal Granulocyte Activation Precedes Nitric Oxide Production: Studies in Coeliac Patients Challenged with Gluten and Corn," *Gut* 54, no. 6 (June 2005): 769–74.

E. Vainio and E. Varjonen, "Antibody Response Against Wheat, Rye, Barley, Oats and Corn: Comparison Between Gluten-Sensitive Patients and Monoclonal Antigliadin Antibodies," *International Archives of Allergy and Immunology* 106, no. 2 (February 1995): 134–38.

47. J. Kolberg et al., "Immunoblotting Detection of Lectins in Gluten and White Rice Flour," *Biochemical and Biophysical Research Communications* 142, no. 3 (February 13, 1987): 717–23.
    R. Troncone et al., "An Analysis of Cereals That React with Serum Antibodies in Patients with Coeliac Disease," *Journal of Pediatric Gastroenterology and Nutrition* 6, no. 3 (May–June 1987): 346–50.

48. E. K. Janatuinen et al., "A Comparison of Diets With and Without Oats in Adults with Celiac Disease," *New England Journal of Medicine* 333, no. 16 (October 19, 1995): 1033–37.
    M. Silano et al., "In Vitro Tests Indicate That Certain Varieties of Oats May Be Harmful to Patients with Coeliac Disease," *Journal of Gastroenterology and Hepatology* 22, no. 4 (April 2007): 528–31.

49. "About," *The Official Website of Dana Vollmer,* www.danavollmer.com/#!about (accessed January 6, 2012).
    K. Anderson, "Vollmer Achieves Individual Glory, Wins U.S.' First Gold at Swim Worlds," *Sports Illustrated* (July 25, 2011): http://sportsillustrated.cnn.com/2011/writers/kelli_anderson/07/25/Vollmer-wins-first-US-gold/index.html#ixzz1TKsMOmyd (accessed January 6, 2012).
    J. Devaney, "U.S. Swimmer Dana Vollmer 'Lives on Pizza,'" *Universal Sports,* November 30, 2011, www.universalsports.com/news-blogs/blogs/blog=splashed/postid=569394.html (accessed January 6, 2012).
    K. Egan, "GF Swimmer Aims for 2nd Olympic Gold," *Gluten-Free Living,* Winter 2011, 62–63.
    "Swimmer Dana Vollmer Wins Gold after Going Gluten-Free," *Gluten Freeville* (July 27, 2011): http://glutenfreeville.com/research/volmer (accessed January 6, 2012).

50. F. G. Chirdo et al., "Presence of High Levels of Non-degraded Gliadin in Breast Milk from Healthy Mothers," *Scandinavian Journal of Gastroenterology* 33, no. 11 (November 1988): 1186–92.
    E. Hopman et al., "Presence of Gluten Proteins in Breast Milk: Implications for the Development of Celiac Disease," thesis, https://openaccess.leidenuniv.nl/bitstream/handle/1887/13118/02.pdf?sequence=6 (accessed January 25, 2012).
    T. Thompson "Gluten Peptides in Human Breast Milk: Implications for Cow's Milk?" *Gluten Free Dietitian* (January 24, 2012): www.glutenfreedietitian.com/newsletter/2012/01/24/gluten-peptides-in-human-breast-milk-implications-for-cow's-milk (accessed January 25, 2012).
    R. Troncone et al., "Passage of Gliadin into Human Breast Milk," *Acta Paediatrica Scandinavica* 76, no. 3 (May 1987): 453–56.

51. R. Ford, "Gluten in Cow's Milk?" *Gluten-Free Planet,* http://gluten-freeplanet.blogspot.com/2011/04/gluten-in-cows-milk.html (accessed December 18, 2011).

52. L. Dekking et al., "Intolerance of Celiac Disease Patients to Bovine Milk Is Not Due to the Presence of T-cell Stimulatory Epitopes of Gluten," *Nutrition* 25, no. 1 (January 2009): 122–23.

53. W. Daniewski et al., "Gluten Content in Special Dietary Use Gluten-Free Products and Other Food Products," *Roczniki Panstwowego Zakladu Higieny* 61, no. 1 (2010): 51–55.
    T. Thompson and E. Mendez, "Commercial Assays to Assess Gluten Content of Gluten-Free Foods: Why They Are Not Created Equal," *Journal of the American Dietetic Association* 108, no. 10 (October 2008): 1682–87.

54. "About," *The Adventures of Pip,* www.adventuresofpip.com/about/ (accessed January 5, 2012).
"Snowbird Athlete: Pip Hunt," *Snowbird Ski and Summer Resort,* www.snowbird.com/athletes/athletes/piphunt.html (accessed January 5, 2012).

55. T. Thompson et al., "Gluten Contamination of Grains, Seeds, and Flours in the United States: A Pilot Study," *Journal of the American Dietetic Association* 110, no. 6 (June 2010): 937–40.

CHAPTER 7

1. W. McArdle et al., *Exercise Physiology: Energy, Nutrition, and Human Performance* (Baltimore, MD: Lippincott Williams & Wilkins, 2007), 74–77.

2. W. McArdle et al., *Exercise Physiology: Energy, Nutrition, and Human Performance* (Philadelphia, PA: Lea & Debiger, 1986), 45–46.

3. "Dehydration," *Mayo Clinic,* www.mayoclinic.com/health/dehydration/DS00561/DSECTION=symptoms (accessed December 29, 2011).
R. Murray, "Dehydration, Hyperthermia, and Athletes: Science and Practice," *Journal of Athletic Training* 31, no. 3 (July–September 1996): 248–52.
C. Wright. "Dehydration in Sport: Why It Is Vital an Athlete Maintains Hydration Levels During Exercise," *Peak Performance,* www.pponline.co.uk/encyc/dehydration-in-sport-why-it-is-vital-an-athlete-maintains-hydration-levels-during-exercise-316 (accessed December 29, 2011).

4. G. Reynolds, "Health and Fitness Report 2012," *Outside,* January 2012, 85.

5. R. Dudek, *High-Yield Physiology* (Baltimore, MD: Lippincott Williams & Wilkins, 2008), 77.
M. N. Sawka and S. J. Montain, "Fluid and Electrolyte Supplementation for Exercise Heat Stress," *American Journal of Clinical Nutrition* 72, no. 2 (August 2000): 564S–72S.

6. D. Liska et al., *Clinical Nutrition: A Functional Approach* (Gig Harbor, WA: Institute of Functional Medicine, 2004), 165–67.

7. F. Carswell and R. Lindsay, "Sodium/Potassium ATPase Activity in Coeliac Disease," *Archives of Disease in Childhood* 49, no. 3 (March 1974): 245.

8. "Player Bio: Andie Cozzarelli," *NC State University Official Athletic Site,* www.gopack.com/sports/c-track/mtt/cozzarelli_andie00.html (accessed January 5, 2012).

9. "Hyponatremia," *U.S. National Library of Medicine,* www.ncbi.nlm.nih.gov/pubmedhealth/PMH0001431 (accessed December 29, 2011).

10. B. Knechtle et al., "Do Male 100-km Ultra-Marathoners Overdrink?" *International Journal of Sports Physiology and Performance* 6, no. 2 (June 2011): 195–207.
B. Knechtle et al., "Prevalence of Exercise-Associated Hyponatremia in Male Ultraendurance Athletes," *Clinical Journal of Sports Medicine* 21, no. 3 (May 2011): 226–32.

C. A. Rust et al., "No Case of Exercise-Associated Hyponatraemia in Top Male Ultra-Endurance Cyclists: The 'Swiss Cycling Marathon,'" *European Journal of Applied Physiology* (June 9, 2011), epub ahead of print, www.ncbi.nlm.nih.gov/pubmed/21656229 (accessed December 21, 2011).

R. J. Shephard, "Suppression of Information on the Prevalence and Prevention of Exercise-Associated Hyponatraemia," *British Journal of Sports Medicine* 45, no. 15 (December 2011): 1238–42.

11.   J. Dugas, "Sodium Ingestion and Hyponatraemia: Sports Drinks Do Not Prevent a Fall in Serum Sodium Concentration During Exercise," *British Journal of Sports Medicine* 40, no. 4 (April 2006): 372.

12.   S. Cohen, "Peak Performance: GF Athletes at Top of Their Game," *Gluten-Free Living*, Winter 2011, 43–46, 62–63.
"Jeff Spear," *Go Columbia Lions—Official Website of Columbia University Athletics*, www.gocolumbialions.com/ViewArticle.dbml?SPSID=45280&SPID=4049&DB_LANG=C&DB_OEM_ID=9600&ATCLID=691245&Q_SEASON=2009 (accessed January 5, 2012).
"Jeff Spear," *USA Fencing*, http://usfencing.org/athletes/jeff-spear (accessed January 5, 2012).
A. Richard and J. Spear, "College Without Pizza: Life at Columbia with Celiac Disease," *Columbia College Today*, November/December 2010, www.college.columbia.edu/cct/nov_dec10/alumni_corner (accessed January 5, 2012).

13.   D. S. Rowlands et al., "Unilateral Fluid Absorption and Effects on Peak Power After Ingestion of Commercially Available Hypotonic, Isotonic, and Hypertonic Sports Drinks," *International Journal of Sport Nutrition and Exercise Metabolism* 21, no. 6 (December 2011): 480–91.

14.   K. J. Spaccarotella and W. D. Andzel, "Building a Beverage for Recovery from Endurance Activity: A Review," *Journal of Strength & Conditioning Research* 25, no. 11 (November 2011): 3198–3204.

15.   V. A. Convertino et al., "American College of Sports Medicine Position Stand: Exercise and Fluid Replacement," *Medicine & Science in Sports & Exercise* 28, no. 1 (January 1996): i–vii.

16.   "Results," *Tyler Stewart: Hard Riding, Dog-Walking Ironman Champion Triathlete*, www.tyler-stewart.com/?page_id=25 (accessed January 5, 2012).

CHAPTER 8

1.   E. Rejc et al., "Energy Expenditure and Dietary Intake of Athletes During an Ultraendurance Event Developed by Hiking, Cycling and Mountain Climbing," *Journal of Sports Medicine and Physical Fitness* 50, no. 3 (September 2010): 296–302.

2.   L. M. Burke, "'Fat Adaptation' for Athletic Performance: The Nail in the Coffin?" *Journal of Applied Physiology* 100, no. 1 (January 2006): 7–8.
L. M. Burke et al., "Adaptations to Short-Term High-Fat Diet Persist During Exercise Despite High Carbohydrate Availability," *Medicine & Science in Sports & Exercise* 34, no. 1 (January 2002): 83–91.
L. M. Burke et al., "Effect of Fat Adaptation and Carbohydrate Restoration on Metabolism and Performance During Prolonged Cycling," *Journal of Applied Physiology* 89, no. 6 (December 2000): 2413–21.

A. L. Carey et al., "Effects of Fat Adaptation and Carbohydrate Restoration on Prolonged Endurance Exercise," *Journal of Applied Physiology* 91, no. 1 (July 2001): 115–22.
W. K. Yeo et al., "Fat Adaptation in Well-Trained Athletes: Effects on Cell Metabolism," *Applied Physiology, Nutrition, and Metabolism* 36, no. 1 (February 2011): 12–22.

3. S. Phinney, "Ketogenic Diets and Physical Performance," *Nutrition & Metabolism* 1, no. 1 (August 2004): 2.

4. B. Pfeiffer et al., "Nutritional Intake and Gastrointestinal Problems During Competitive Endurance Events," *Medicine & Science in Sports & Exercise* (July 19, 2011), epub ahead of print, www.mendeley.com/research/nutritional-intake-gastrointestinal-problems-during-competitive-endurance-events (accessed December 17, 2011).

5. "Player Profile: Sarah-Jane Smith," *ALPG*, www.alpg.com.au/index.php?page_id=player&id=1223 (accessed January 6, 2012).
G. Roberts-Grey, "Sarah Jane Smith: Taking a Swing at Celiac Disease," *Celebrity Health Minute* (November 2, 2010): http://celebrityhealthminute.com/2010/11/02/sarah-jane-smith-taking-a-swing-at-celiac-disease (accessed January 6, 2012).
"Sarah-Jane Kenyon Points Aim at Five LPGA Cards," *LPGA Futures Tour,* www.lpga.com/content_1.aspx?pid=16916&mid=2 (accessed January 6, 2012).
"Sarah-Jane Smith Eyes LPGA Major," *Athletes for Awareness Blog—National Foundation for Celiac Awareness* (June 22, 2011): www.celiaccentral.org/News/NFCA-Blogs/Athletes-For-Awareness/Celiac-Disease-Athletes-For-Awareness/158/vobid--5621 (accessed January 6, 2012).
"Sarah-Jane Smith—LPGA Tour," *Yahoo! Sports,* http://sports.yahoo.com/golf/lpga/players/Sarah+Jane+Smith/8549 (accessed January 6, 2012).

6. L. Altobelli, "NFL Workout: Strapped In: A System Designed by a Navy SEAL Got the Saints' Drew Brees in Shape to Succeed," *Sports Illustrated* (January 9, 2007): http://sportsillustrated.cnn.com/2007/players/01/09/nfl.workout0115/index.html (accessed December 31, 2011).

7. J. Libonati, "FSU Quarterback Clint Tricket Goes Gluten Free After Celiac Disease Diagnosis," *Gluten Free Works* (October 4, 2011): http://glutenfreeworks.com/blog/2011/10/04/fsu-quaterback-clint-trickett-goes-gluten-free-after-celiac-disease-diagnosis (accessed December 31, 2011).

8. "Phillies Player Goes Gluten-Free," *National Foundation for Celiac Awareness,* www.celiaccentral.org/News/NFCA-Blogs/Athletes-For-Awareness/Celiac-Disease-Athletes-For-Awareness/158/vobid--4948 (accessed December 31, 2011).

9. "Anita's Story," *PhenomeNall Nutrition,* www.phenomenallnutrition.com/about.html (accessed January 6, 2012).
K. Crouse, "The Care and (Healthy) Feeding of the Jaguars," *New York Times* (December 11, 2010): www.nytimes.com/2010/12/12/sports/football/12jaguars.html (accessed January 6, 2012).

10. K. Birch, "Female Athlete Triad," *British Medical Journal* 330 (2005): 244.

11. W. McArdle et al., *Exercise Physiology: Energy, Nutrition, and Human Performance* (Philadelphia, PA: Lea & Febiger, 1986), 179–81.

12. M. Brach et al., "Implementation of Preventive Strength Training in Residential Geriatric Care: A Multi-centre Study Protocol with One Year of Interventions on Multiple Levels," *BMC Geriatrics* 9 (2009): 51.

13. "Diet Mix Up Knocks Greg Henderson," *Road Cycling* (June 13, 2011): www.roadcycling.co.nz/RaceTalk/diet-mix-up-knocks-greg-henderson.html (accessed December 31, 2011).

14. "Kelsey Holbert," *Milwaukee Athletics—Women's Soccer,* http://uwmpanthers.cstv.com/sports/w-soccer/mtt/holbert_kelsey00.html (accessed January 5, 2012).
J. Trost, "Soccer Spotlight's on Kelsey Holbert," *Chicago Tribune* (April 27, 2011): http://articles.chicagotribune.com/2011-04-27/sports/ct-spt-0428-prep-soc-spotlight-20110427_1_lions-advance-pepsi-showdown-breast-cancer-treatment (accessed January 5, 2012).

CHAPTER 9

1. R. J. Maughan, "Fasting and Sport: An Introduction," *British Journal of Sports Medicine* 44, no. 7 (June 2010): 473–75.

2. A. Kelinson, "An Off-Season Cleanse for Triathletes," *Triathlete*, December 12, 2011, http://triathlon.competitor.com/2011/12/nutrition/an-off-season-cleanse-for-triathletes_17306 (accessed December 17, 2011).

CHAPTER 10

1. J. Henderson, *Long Slow Distance: The Human Way to Train* (Mountain View, CA: Tafnews Press, 1969).

2. S. Trappe et al., "Single Muscle Fiber Adaptations with Marathon Training," *Journal of Applied Physiology* 101, no. 3 (September 2006): 721–27.

3. F. A. Dolgener et al., "Long Slow Distance Training in Novice Marathoners," *Research Quarterly for Exercise and Sport* 65, no. 4 (1994): 339–46.

4. J. Majerczak et al., "Endurance Training Decreases the Non-linearity in the VO_2-Power Output Relationship in Humans," *Experimental Physiology* (December 23, 2011), epub ahead of print, www.ncbi.nlm.nih.gov/pubmed/22198015 (accessed January 2, 2012).

5. D. C. Poole and G. A. Gaesser, "Response of Ventilatory and Lactate Thresholds to Continuous and Interval Training," *Journal of Applied Physiology* 58, no. 4 (April 1985): 1115–21.

6. T. Kavanagh and R. J. Shephard, "The Effects of Continued Training on the Aging Process," *Annals of the New York Academy of Sciences* 301 (October 1977): 656–70.

7. W. K. Allen et al., "Lactate Threshold and Distance-Running Performance in Young and Older Endurance Athletes," *Journal of Applied Physiology* 58, no. 4 (April 1985): 1281–84.

8. V. Billat et al., "Effect of Training on the Physiological Factors of Performance in Elite Marathon Runners (Males and Females)," *International Journal of Sports Medicine* 23, no. 5 (2002): 336–41.
    A. M. Stewart and W. G. Hopkins, "Seasonal Training and Performance of Competitive Swimmers," *Journal of Sports Sciences* 18, no. 11 (2000): 873–84.

9. B. Knechtle et al., "Personal Best Marathon Performance Is Associated with Performance in a 24-h Run and Not Anthropometry or Training Volume," *British Journal of Sports Medicine* 43, no. 11 (2009): 836–39.

10. M. C. Elliott et al., "Power Athletes and Distance Training: Physiological and Biomechanical Rationale for Change," *Sports Medicine* 37, no. 11 (November 1, 2007): 47–57.

11. R. Dotan, "'Reverse Lactate Threshold'—A Novel, Single-Session Approach to Reliable, High Resolution Estimation of the Anaerobic Threshold," *International Journal of Sports Physiology and Performance* (December 2, 2011), epub ahead of print, www.ncbi.nlm.nih.gov/pubmed/22180336 (accessed January 2, 2012).
    P. Janssen, *Lactate Threshold Training* (Champaign, IL: Human Kinetics, 2001).
    H. N. Soultanakis et al., "Lactate Threshold and Performance Adaptations to 4 Weeks of Training in Untrained Swimmers: Volume vs. Intensity," *Journal of Strength and Conditioning Research* 26, no. 1 (January 2012): 131–37.

12. V. L. Billat et al., "Very Short (15 s–15 s) Interval-Training Around the Critical Velocity Allows Middle-Aged Runners to Maintain VO_2 Max for 14 Minutes," *International Journal of Sports Medicine* 22, no. 3 (2001): 201–8.

13. H. Yu et al., "A Quasi-Experiment Study of Training Load of Chinese Top-Level Speed Skaters: Threshold vs. Polarized Model," *International Journal of Sports Physiology and Performance* (December 12, 2011), epub ahead of print, www.ncbi.nlm.nih.gov/pubmed/22173214 (accessed January 2, 2012).

14. T. A. Astorino et al., "Effect of High-Intensity Interval Training on Cardiovascular Function, VO_2 Max, and Muscular Force," *Journal of Strength & Conditioning Research* 26, no. 1 (January 2012): 138–45.
    V. L. Billat, "Interval Training for Performance: A Scientific and Empirical Practice: Special Recommendations for Middle- and Long-Distance Running. Part I: Aerobic Interval Training," *Sports Medicine* 31, no. 1 (January 1, 2001): 13–31.

15. K. A. Burgomaster et al., "Six Sessions of Sprint Interval Training Increases Muscle Oxidative Potential and Cycle Endurance Capacity in Humans," *Journal of Applied Physiology* 98, no. 6 (June 2005): 1985–90.

16. J. Helgerud et al., "Aerobic High-Intensity Intervals Improve VO_2max More Than Moderate Training," *Medicine & Science in Sports & Exercise* 39, no. 4 (April 2007): 665–71.

17. P. B. Laursen and D. G. Jenkins, "The Scientific Basis for High-Intensity Interval Training: Optimising Training Programmes and Maximising Performance in Highly Trained Endurance Athletes," *Sports Medicine* 32, no. 21 (November 1, 2002): 53–73.
     A. W. Midgley et al., "Is There an Optimal Training Intensity for Enhancing the Maximal Oxygen Uptake of Distance Runners? Empirical Research Findings, Current Opinions, Physiological Rationale and Practical Recommendations," *Sports Medicine* 36, no. 16 (November 2, 2006): 117–32.

18. M. J. Gibala et al., "Short-Term Sprint Interval Versus Traditional Endurance Training: Similar Initial Adaptations in Human Skeletal Muscle and Exercise Performance," *Journal of Physiology* 575, no. 3 (September 2006): 901–11.

19. J. Achten and A .E. Jeukendrup, "Optimizing Fat Oxidation Through Exercise and Diet," *Nutrition* 20, nos. 7–8 (July–August 2004): 716–27.
     J. Achten et al., "Determination of the Exercise Intensity That Elicits Maximal Fat Oxidation," *Medicine & Science in Sports & Exercise* 34, no. 1 (January 2002): 92–97.
     B. Knechtle et al., "Fat Oxidation in Men and Women Endurance Athletes in Running and Cycling," *International Journal of Sports Medicine* 25, no. 1 (2004): 38–44.

20. "Earning a Unique Kona Tattoo: Ryann Fraser," *Ironman* (March 24, 2010): http://ironman.com/profiles/matthew-dale-profiles-the-youngest-finisher-at-last-years-ford-ironman-world-championship#axzz1ieYwHgsd (accessed January 6, 2012).
     Ryann Fraser, www.ryannfraser.com (accessed January 6, 2012).
     Ryann.Fraser's Blog, http://ryannfraser.wordpress.com (accessed January 6, 2012).

21. N. Hellmich, "Vigorous Exercise Burns Calories 14 Hours After Workout," *USA Today* (September 8, 2011): http://yourlife.usatoday.com/fitness-food/exercise/story/2011-09-01/Bonus-for-exercisers-Calories-burn-long-after-workout/50224116/1 (accessed January 2, 2012).

22. E. J. Marcinik et al., "Effects of Strength Training on Lactate Threshold and Endurance Performance," *Medicine & Science in Sports & Exercise* 23, no. 6 (June 1991): 739–43.

23. J. S. Raglin and G. S. Wilson, "Overtraining in Athletes," *Emotions in Sport* (Champaign, IL: Human Kinetics, 2000).

24. J. Crossman et al., "Responses of Competitive Athletes to Lay-offs in Training: Exercise Addiction or Psychological Relief?" *Journal of Sport Behavior* 10, no. 1 (March 1987): 28–38.
     M. Griffiths, "Exercise Addiction: A Case Study," *Addiction Research & Theory* 5, no. 2 (1997): 61–168.
     M. D. Griffiths et al., "The Exercise Addiction Inventory: A Quick and Easy Screening Tool for Health Practitioners," *British Journal of Sports Medicine* 39, no. 6 (2005).
     V. B. Modol et al., "Negative Addiction to Exercise: Are There Differences Between Genders?" *Clinics* 66, no. 2 (2011): 255–60.
     E .F. Pierce et al., "Scores on Exercise Dependence Among Dancers," *Perceptual and Motor Skills* 72, no. 2 (1993): 531–35.
     L. Thaxton, "Physiological and Psychological Effects of Short-Term Exercise Addiction on Habitual Runners," *Journal of Sport & Excersise Psychology* 4, no. 1 (1982): 73–80.

25. M. Ekstedt and G. Kentta, "Recovery Is a Matter of Course for Elite Athletes . . . but Not for Working Professionals," *Lakartidningen* 108, no. 36 (September 7–13, 2011): 1684–87.

26. K. G. Baron et al., "Role of Sleep Timing in Caloric Intake and BMI," *Obesity* 19, no. 7 (July 2011): 1374–81.

L. Brondel et al., "Acute Partial Sleep Deprivation Increases Food Intake in Healthy Men," *American Journal of Clinical Nutrition* (May 2010): www.ajcn.org/content/early/2010/03/31/ajcn.2009.28523.full.pdf+html (accessed January 2, 2012).

W. Derman et al., "The 'Worn-out Athlete': A Clinical Approach to Chronic Fatigue in Athletes," *Journal of Sports Sciences* 15, no. 3 (1997): 341–51.

D. Erlacher, et al., "Sleep Habits in German Athletes Before Important Games or Competitions," *Journal of Sports Science* 29, no. 8 (May 2011): 859–66.

A. V. Nedeltcheva et al., "Sleep Curtailment Is Accompanied by Increased Intake of Calories from Snacks," *American Journal of Clinical Nutrition* 89, no. 1 (January 2009): 126–33.

S. J. Paxton et al., "Does Aerobic Fitness Affect Sleep?" *Psychophysiology* 20, no. 3 (May 1983): 320–24.

C. Samuels, "Sleep, Recovery, and Performance: The New Frontier in High-Performance Athletics," *Physical Medicine and Rehabilitation Clinics of North America* 20, no. 1 (February 2009): 149–59.

J. Savis, "Sleep and Athletic Performance: Overview and Implications for Sports Psychology," *Sport Psychologist* 8, no. 2 (1994): 111–25.

C. M. Shapiro, "Sleep and the Athlete," *British Journal of Sports Medicine* 15, no. 1 (1981): 51–55.

K. Spiegel et al., "Brief Communication: Sleep Curtailment in Healthy Young Men Is Associated with Decreased Leptin Levels, Elevated Ghrelin Levels, and Increased Hunger and Appetite," *Annals of Internal Medicine* 141, no. 11 (December 7, 2004) 846–50.

J. Trinder et al., "Endurance as Opposed to Power Training: Their Effect on Sleep," *Psychophysiology* 22, no. 6 (November 1985): 668–73.

P. H. Walters, "Sleep, the Athlete, and Performance," *Strength & Conditioning Journal* 24, no. 2 (April 2002): 17–24.

PHOTO ACKNOWLEDGMENTS

Page 21 courtesy Ashley DiVeronica.

Page 37 courtesy Washington Capitals | Getty Images.

Page 42 courtesy Bill Smith | Chicago Bulls.

Page 43 courtesy Liana Mauro.

Page 48 courtesy Jenny Smith.

Page 51 by Rob Trnka, courtesy Brian Lopes.

Page 56 courtesy UNC Athletic Communications.

Page 60 by George Strohl | StrohlPhotography.com.

Page 66 courtesy Heather Wurtele.

Page 72 by Martin Rousselot licensed under Creative Commons BY-SA 3.0.

Page 76 by Rich Wysockey, courtesy Natalie Jill.

Page 98 courtesy University of Utah.

Page 108 by Rich Adams, courtesy Terra Castro | Team Luna Chix.

Page 110 courtesy Michael Danke.

Page 112 courtesy Craig Pinto.

Page 120 by Linden Mallory, courtesy Dave Hahn.

Page 126 courtesy Amy Yoder Begley.

Page 131 courtesy Erin Elberson Lyon.

Page 142 courtesy Ginger Vieira.

Page 156 by Jay Beyer | JayBeyer.com.

Page 160 courtesy Amanda Lovato.

Page 168 by Shawn Coleman, courtesy NC State Athletics.

Page 176 by Larry Rosa, courtesy Tyler Stewart.

Page 181 courtesy Kendra Nielsen.

Page 186 by Re Wikstrom | ReWikstrom.com.

Page 188 courtesy Michelle Smith.

Page 193 courtesy Australian Ladies Professional Golf.

Page 195 by Jim Campbell | OmLightPhotography.com.

Page 197 by Oshi Yuval courtesy Elyse Sparkes.

Page 199 courtesy Anita Nall Richesson.

Page 202 courtesy Alex Borsuk.

Page 214 courtesy University of Wisconsin, Milwaukee.

Page 220 courtesy Clea Shannon.

Page 224 by Steve Zdawczynski courtesy Amy Ippoliti.

Page 230 courtesy Kimberly Bouldin.

Page 236 courtesy Carrie Willoughby.

Page 240 courtesy Ryann Fraser.

Page 372 by Nate Baker | UltraRacePhotos.com.

Page 373 by Kirsten Boyer Photography.

ACKNOWLEDGMENTS

THIS BOOK BEGAN several years ago, circa fall 2008, as a nascent idea discussed over glasses of naturally gluten-free wine in a hotel bar in Golden, Colorado. Like any major endeavor—athletic or otherwise—the effort to bring this book from concept to reality involved determination, perseverance, and heart. It went through its cycles of joy and pain, of stumbles and successes. In the end, it proved akin to sprinting a marathon—full speed ahead for far longer than we ever thought we could maintain the momentum.

Team and solo athletes alike know that their successes are not isolated efforts. They are the by-product of a cast of supporting characters: family, friends, coaches, peers, fans. This book is no different. It would not have happened without the participation, contributions, and support of many people. Each of you has our deepest and sincerest gratitude.

To our publisher, Matthew Lore, and everyone at The Experiment (especially Karen, Jack, and Molly), thank you for believing in this book's potential to positively influence the lives of many in the gluten-free and athletic communities.

To our agent, Jenni Ferrari-Adler at Brick House Literary Agents, thank you for your continued support.

To the athletes we interviewed, this book is about and for you. Thank you for sharing your time and your stories, for your honesty and candor and your sincerity and willingness to be an open book to us. Each of you gives a face and a name and a very real and valuable perspective of personal experience to the science behind the link between gluten intolerance and athletics. You illuminate the book with vibrant color; without you, it would have been a black-and-white silent film. This book's readers are better off because you graciously became a part of it. You are an inspiration. There are many of you, each deserving of mention. We recognize you in the only order that seems fair, borrowed from elementary school seating assignments . . . alphabetical. Thank you, thank you, thank you to Jay Beagle, Amy Yoder Begley, Alex Borsuk, Kimberly Bouldin, Terra Castro, Andie Cozzarelli, Michael Danke, Ashley DiVeronica, Ryann Fraser, Dave Hahn, Kelsey Holbert, Pip Hunt, Amy Ippoliti, Natalie Jill, Kyle Korver, Brian Lopes, Amanda Lovato, Erin Elberson Lyon, Liana Mauro, Taylor Mokate, Kendra Nielsen, Craig Pinto, Anita Nall Richesson, Diana Rolniak, Clea Shannon, Jenny Smith, Michelle Smith, Taro Smith, Elyse Sparkes, Tyler Stewart, Christie Sym, Kristen Taylor, Angeli VanLaanen, Ginger Vieira, Carrie Willoughby, and Heather Wurtele.

To the doctors, sports physiologists, and researchers who patiently answered our questions and clarified several important particulars, thank you for sharing your expertise, especially Rodney Ford, Adam Korzun, Allen Lim, Peter Osborne, David Sands, and Yolanda Sanz.

To the food historians who helped us sift through the wheat and barley of ancient Greece, thank you: Louis Grivetti, Donald Kyle, Stephen Miller, and Francine Segan.

From Pete:
To my coauthor, Melissa: Thank you for being willing to run this three-legged race together as coauthors. I've said from the beginning how much I value our gluten-free perspectives—similar, yet different in subtle but important ways that make our respective viewpoints complementary. I firmly believe that each of this book's chapters, and the book as a whole, is more than the sum of our respective contributions. Through our dynamic back-and-forth that unfolded as we worked on the book, our voices and our perspectives came together and merged, in a sense serving to strengthen and magnify the content. It was a real pleasure, and a greatly rewarding and satisfying experience to see this book come to fruition since first discussing it with you years ago. As ever, I value your friendship, and I'm proud to have done this together.

To Kelli, Marin, and Charlotte: Thank you first and foremost for your unconditional love, and second for the bottomless support you offered me on this project. I know that it was most difficult in the final weeks, as the manuscript deadline loomed and I disappeared for hours upon hours, day after day, week after week. You struck a perfect balance between giving me the space and time and quiet I needed to write this book, and making me still feel like an integral part of our family at a time when I temporarily abandoned seemingly all familial and domestic responsibilities and roles. I love you all from the bottom of my heart, more than mere words can ever express.

From Melissa:

As is often the case, we rarely accomplish anything significant without the help of others. To my amazing family: You encouraged me every step of the way. Thank you for putting up with my long hours, my ups and downs, and my moments of doubt. You kept me laughing.

Special thanks go to my mom for raising me on real food, home-cooked meals, and not TV dinners. I can thank *you* for my love of beets. When it comes to culinary skills, you're a hard act to follow.

To my friends, mentors, and blogging buddies (you know who you are), thank you for your guidance, expertise, and support. I'm lucky to have such friends.

To Pete: I don't have words to express my gratitude and appreciation to you for making this book happen and for doing the heavy lifting. Thank you for your integrity, character, and willingness to take on this challenge. Your insight, writing skills, and organizational magic are unmatched; your enthusiasm and humor, a delightful bonus. I am fortunate to call you a friend and grateful that our paths have crossed.

And finally, to my dad, a man who matched the mountains he so dearly loved: I thank you for being the best dad anyone could ever ask for. I am truly blessed.

INDEX

Note: Page numbers in **bold** indicate an "Athlete Insight."

activities. *See* aerobic activity; anaerobic activity; food as fuel; sports
adenosine diphosphate (ADP), 70, 78, 125
adenosine triphosphate (ATP)
    ATP-PCr energy system, 70, 74, 75, 77
    oxidative stress as by-product, 91–92
adipose tissue, 70, 163. *See also* fat oxidation
ADP (adenosine diphosphate), 70, 78, 125
aerobic activity
    and aging, 206
    LSD training, 232–34, 246
    overview, 229
    recovery from, 149
    See also oxidative system
AG (anaerobic glycolysis), 71, 73–74, 78. *See also* anaerobic activity
aging athletes, 205–7, 233
all-purpose flour blend, 252
Almond-Cranberry Energy Bars, 264
Alzner, Karl, 36–37
amaranth, 86
amenorrhea, 203, 204
American College of Sports Medicine, 59
American Journal of Clinical Nutrition, 137–38
amino acids
    body's process for getting to, 20, 22
    overview, 23, 85–86, 114
    and recovery process, 148–49
    See also specific amino acids
amylopectin, 139
amylose, 139
anaerobic activity
    anaerobic glycolysis, 71, 73–74, 78
    and lactate threshold, 231

overview, 229
    recovery from, 149
    tempo training, 234–35, 246
    See also endurance athletes
anemia or iron deficiency, 54, 118, 119, 122, 124
anti-inflammatory support, 215
antinutrients, 179
antioxidants, 91–92, 215
appetite and gluten, 101–2
Apple-Ginger-Beet Green Smoothie, 261
Apple-Pecan Crumble, 307–8
Artisan Gluten-Free Flour Blend, 252
athletes and gluten
    case study, 61–65, 67
    gastrointestinal problems, 39–40
    glucose tolerance and insulin sensitivity, 138–43
    gluten intolerance trigger, 54–59, 68
    and glycemic index, 134–38
    immune system challenges, 45–49
    impaired digestion, 35–37
    incidence of problems, 50–53
    increased reactivity compared to non-athletes, 53, 54–55, 59, 61, 127
    leaky gut and gluten toxicity, 38–39
    overview, 35, 59–61, 68
    subtle effects, 50
    trying a gluten-free diet, 53–54
    See also inflammation
ATP. *See* adenosine triphosphate

Backcountry Muesli, 253–54
backcountry sports, 183–89, 216
balance vs. overtraining, 244–45
Banana-Buckwheat Pancakes with Pecans, 255–56
Banana-Nut Muffins, 254–55

Beagle, Jay, 36–37, **37**, 159, 203, 210
Beans and Greens, 279
Beef Stew, Hearty, 285–86
beets
  about, 261
  Apple-Ginger-Beet Green Smoothie, 261
  Beet-Chocolate Muffins, 256–57
  Beet Endurance Smoothie, 261–62
  Beet Pizza, 291, 292
  Roasted Beet and Spinach Salad,
    275–76
bioenergetics, 81. *See also* food as fuel
Bison Chili with Beans, 280
Bison Tamari Jerky with a Kick, 271
blood sugar
  and fiber, 83
  glucose tolerance and insulin
    sensitivity, 138–43
  and gluten, 140–41
  and insulin sensitivity, 139
  overview, 69, 78, 82, 161
  replenishing, 147–48
  See also diabetes; glycemic index
body fat, 70, 163. *See also* fat oxidation
bone density, 128
  bonking/hitting the wall, 75, 77, 78
Borsuk, Alex, 106, 110–11, **202–3**
Bouldin, Kim, 210, **230–31**
breakfast recipes, 253–60
breast milk, gluten in, 155
Brees, Drew, 196
Bronski, Peter, 8–12
Brussels Sprouts, Roasted, and Cipollini
  Onions, 295–96
buckwheat, 86, 102, 255
Buckwheat-Banana Pancakes with
  Pecans, 255–56

Cabbage-Cherry Recovery Smoothie, 262
Cacao Fondue Dip, 308
calcium, 125–29, 130
calories, 74, 106–7. *See also* weight
carbohydrates
  blood glucose from, 69
  carb loading, 151, 162
  in energy gels or chews, 185, 191–92
  and energy pathways, 70–74, 145
  and gluten, 36

  natural sources, 175, 177
  overview, 78, 81–85
  percentage in diet, 150–51
  in sports drinks, 172–73
carbohydrate oxidation
  and exertion level, 75
  high-glycemic-index foods for, 145
  overview, 71, 73, 74, 78
  for recovery, 148, 149
Castro, Terra, 46, 62, 105–6, **108**, 109
Celebrity Health Minute, 193
Celiac Attack, 215
celiac disease
  consumption of gluten correlation, 27
  and diabetes risk, 144–45
  and effect of gluten-free diet on
    calorie intake, 102–3
  first diagnoses, 2
  and immune system, 52–53
  incidence of, 3, 26–27, 31
  life stories, 8–17
  onset, 55
  and osteoporosis, 125, 128, 203–4
  overview, 30–31
  and weight, 104–5, 104–7
  See also gluten intolerance
Celiac Disease Foundation (CDF), 241
Center for Celiac Research, University of
  Maryland, 26
Cherry-Cabbage Recovery Smoothie, 262
Chicken Tikka Masala, 281–82
Chickpeas and Spinach, 297
chlorophyll, 90
chocolate
  Cacao Fondue Dip, 308
  Chocolate-Beet Muffins, 256–57
  chocolate milk, 149
  Granola-Style Energy Bars, 267–68
  overview, 161, 162
chocolate milk, 149
chronic joint pain, 16, 43, 44
Cipollini Onions and Roasted Brussels
  Sprouts, 295–96
complex carbohydrates, 82–83
conversion chart, 311–12
Cozzarelli, Andie, **168–69**, 201, 211
Cranberry-Almond Energy Bars, 264
creatine phosphate, 70, 74, 75, 77, 78

cross-contamination issue, 155, 200, 211–12, 213, 217
cross-reactivity issues, 152, 154
Current Good Manufacturing Practices (FDA), 155
cytotoxicity, nonspecific, 38

Danielson, Tom, 73
Danke, Michael, 107, **110**, 111, 211–12
dehydration, 165–67, 182
depression, 109–10
dessert recipes, 307–10
detox. *See* sports detox cleanse
diabetes
   and gluten intolerance, 144–45
   insulin sensitivity and glucose tolerance, 138–43
   overview, 143–44
   powerlifter with, 142–43
diarrhea, water loss from, 167
dietary balance, 150–51
diet periodization, 190
digestive system and gluten
   gastrointestinal problems, 39–40
   gluten intolerance appearing to be some other disease, 31
   leaky gut and gluten toxicity, 38–39
   overview, 35–37
   protein extraction problems, 22–23
   women and, 61–67, 204, 216
   See also small intestine
dinner or lunch recipes, 279–306
dip recipes, 272, 277–78
disaccharides, 81, 82
DiVeronica, Ashley, **19**, 21, 212
Djokovic, Novak, 4
Dupuytren's contracture, 15

ECF (extracellular fluid), 164, 166–67
eggs
   Poached Eggs on a Bed of Chard, 289–90
   Scrambled Omelet, 258–59
   Vegetable Frittata, 290–91
electrolytes, 164–65, 170, 172–74, 175, 182
electron transport chain, 73
empty carbohydrates, 83, 85, 114
endogenous opiates (endorphins), 101, 102

endurance athletes
   during activity nutrition, 146–47, 162, 191
   backcountry athletes, 184–85, 216
   beverage for maximum performance, 173
   and bone density, 127
   bonking, 77
   and carb-loading, 151, 162
   and gastrointestinal issues, 39–40
   gluten-free diet among, 47–49
   and glycemic index, 136
   and hyponatremia, 170, 182
   Ironman triathletes case study, 61–65, 67
   from Mexico and Kenya, 4–5, 150
   overview, 216
   recovery choices, 149
   See also fat oxidation; VO$_2$ max
endurance sports, 189–92
energy
   bonking/hitting the wall, 75, 77, 78
   and carb-loading, 151, 162
   food sources, 69–70
   overview, 70, 78
   pathways, 70–74, 78
   utilization of, 74–75
   See also lactate threshold; oxidative system; VO$_2$ max
Energy Bars, Granola-Style, 267–68
energy gels or chews, 185, 191–92
enzymes, 20, 22
essential amino acids, 23, 85–86, 114
essential fatty acids, 215
exercise
   addiction to, 244
   exercise-induced iron deficiency, 119
   fitness factors, 229, 231
   goals, 228–29
   measuring output, 231–35, 238
   See also training
exertion test, 232
exogenous opioids, 101
exorphins (opioids), 39, 52, 101–2
extracellular fluid (ECF), 164, 166–67

Fasano, Alessio, 30, 32, 205
fat
   for endurance athletes, 189–90
   malabsorption of, 117, 133

overview, 70, 78, 87–89
in recovery mode, 148
sources, 89
fat oxidation
and endurance sports, 189–90, 216, 233
and exertion level, 75
and frequency of meals, 152
low-glycemic-index foods for, 136, 145, 146
overview, 73–74, 78
sustaining, 149
training leading to, 239, 241–42
fatty acids, 88
FDA Current Good Manufacturing Practices, 155
female athletes, 61–65, 67, 203–4, 216
Female Athlete Triad, 203–4
fiber, 83, 85, 179, 180
Ficker, Desirée, 61
fitness, day-to-day diet for, 150–51
fitness factors, 229, 231
flexibility and stretching, 243–44
Flour Blend, Artisan Gluten-Free, 252
flours, 27, 97, 122–23, 248–49, 252
nutritional comparison of starches and, 248–49
Food Allergen Labeling and Consumer Protection Act, 93
food as fuel
after activity, 147–49, 162
before activity, 145, 151, 162
during activity, 146–47, 162, 191
eating right, 108–9
energy gels or chews, 185, 191–92
gluten-free processed foods, 98–100
for hydration, 174–75
juicing, 177, 180
meal size and frequency, 152
nutrient profile of gluten-free grains and wheat, 84
overview, 69–70, 79, 81, 114–15, 133, 161–62
shopping for gluten-free foods, 93–94, 96
smoothies, 177–80, 261–63
twigs, sticks, and logs theory, 146, 185
what not to eat, 92–93, 225–26
what to eat, 94–95, 108–9, 226–27

See also gluten-free diet; macronutrients; micronutrients; nutrient-rich foods; recipes; weight
food-dependent, exercise-induced gastrointestinal distress, 40
food industry and gluten, 23
Ford, Rodney, 155
Fraser, Ryann, **240–41**
free radicals, 91
Fried Rice, 283–84
fruit, dehydrated vs. fresh, 187
Fudge Power Balls, 265
fuel. See food as fuel
functional training, 243

Garderen, Tejay van, 73
Garlic Guacamole, 277–78
gastrointestinal problems, 39–40, 119
genetic changes to wheat, 24–25, 28–29, 34
genetic predisposition
for gluten intolerance, 205
and VO$_2$ max, 229
GI. See gastrointestinal problems; glycemic index
Ginger-Apple-Beet Green Smoothie, 261
glossary, 313–24
glucose, 69, 78, 82. See also blood sugar
glucose tolerance and insulin sensitivity, 138–43. See also diabetes
glutamine, 148–49, 150, 216
glutamine peptide, 148
gluten
and appetite, 101–2
and blood sugar, 140–41
changes over time, 23–26
in cow's milk, 155
and dehydration, 167, 182
diseases related to, 50–51
effect of, 26–30
enzyme resistance of, 22
hidden in diet, 155, 158
myth busting, 101–3
overview, 19–20, 22–23, 34
products containing, 93
reasons for eating, 83
See also athletes and gluten

glutened (accidental exposure to gluten), 11, 158–59, 209–13, 215–16, 225
gluten-free beverages, 174
Gluten Free Certification Organization, 93–94
gluten-free diet
  80/20 rule, 159, 161, 162
  adjusting to, 109–14, 115
  authors' perspective, 3
  bone density recovery, 128–29
  cross-contamination issues, 155, 200, 211–12, 213, 217
  cross-reactivity issues, 152, 154
  decrease in inflammatory response, 41–42, 44
  effect on calorie intake of, 102–3
  female Ironman competitors' results on, 62, 63–65, 66, 67
  flours, 27, 97, 122–23, 248–49, 252
  gluten in gluten-free products, 155
  and glycemic index, 134–38
  isolation as aspect of, 196–98, 200–201
  nutrient profile of gluten-free grains and wheat, 84
  nutritional comparison of flours and starches, 248–49
  Pascal's wager applied to, 53–54
  pitfalls, 96, 98–100
  shopping for gluten-free foods, 93–94, 96
  support for, 201, 203
  and traveling, 207–9, 217
  trying it, 53–54
  variables, 95–96, 122–24
  and weight, 100–103, 105–8
  what to eat, 94–95, 108–9, 226–27
  women and, 204, 216
  See also food as fuel
Gluten-Free Living, 153
gluten-free menus, 208, 217
gluten-free processed foods, 98–100, 185, 191–92
gluten intolerance
  80/20 rule for enjoying food, 159, 161, 162
  in ancient Greece, 2
  athletes with, 59–61
  and diabetes, 144–45
  genetic predisposition, 205
  gluten sensitivity, 32
  incidence of, 62–63
  and iron, 119–22
  overview, 34
  signs and symptoms of, 33
  spectrum, 30–32
  trigger, 54–59, 68
  wheat allergy or sensitivity, 31–32, 43, 196
  widespread nature of, 22–23
  and women, 203–4, 216
  See also celiac disease; Athlete Insights (**bold** page numbers)
gluten sensitivity, 32
glycemic index (GI)
  and carbs as fuel, 145
  factors influencing, 140
  and gluten-free diet, 134–38
  overview, 161
  and replenishing blood sugar, 147–48
  twigs, sticks, and logs theory, 146, 185
glycemic load, 136–38, 161
glycogen
  and anaerobic glycolysis, 71
  and gluten, 36
  and LSD, 233
  maximizing stores, 151
  overview, 78, 82, 162
  and oxidative system, 71, 73–74, 77, 190, 239, 241
  and rehydration, 169, 173, 182
  replenishing stores, 146–49, 191
  running out of, 75, 77
glycogen depletion, 77
glycolysis, 71, 73–74
goals for an exercise routine, 228–29
GORP, 266–67
grain-free diet, 154
Granola-Style Energy Bars, 267–68
Greece, 1–3
Green Salad with Grapefruit and Avocado, 272–73
Greens and Beans, 279
Green Tea-Orange Smoothie, 263
Grilled Cheese Sandwich, 284–85

Hahn, Dave, **120–21**, 211
Hash, High Country, 286–87
heart rate monitors, 231, 232
heme iron, 124
hemoglobin, 118
Henderson, Greg, 209
high-fat diets, 190
histamine, 31
hitting the wall/bonking, 75, 77, 78
Holbert, Kelsey, 201, 213, **214–15**
Hummus, 272
hunger and gluten, 102
Hunt, Pip, **156–57**, 159, 242
hydration
    dehydration, 165–67, 182
    electrolytes, 164–65, 170, 172–74, 175, 182
    food for, 174–75
    juicing, 177, 180
    overview, 163, 182
    rehydration, 169–70
    smoothies, 177–80, 261–63
    sports drinks vs. water, 172–73
    and weather, 174
hydrogenation process, 88
hyperosmotic dehydration, 166
hypertonic beverages, 172, 174
hyponatremia, 170, 182
hypotonic beverages, 172

IBS (irritable bowel syndrome), 39
ICF (intracellular fluid), 164, 166–67
immune system, 90–91, 148, 216
immune system challenges
    and genetics, 76–77
    overview, 52–53
    recovery from meningitis and sports, 57
    sports-related, 45–49, 68
    See also inflammation
impaired digestion, 35–37
individual biology
    and diet, 150–51
    and grain-free diet, 154, 162
    overview, 51–52, 53, 177
    and training, 233–34
    and weight, 100, 103, 104–5
inflammation

anti-inflammatory support, 215
cytokines after exercise, 136
from leaky gut, 38
overview, 40–45
from strenuous sports, 45–47
as sub-symptomatic response to gluten, 72
insulin resistance, 139. *See also* diabetes
insulin sensitivity, 138–43, 147–48
interval training (IT), 235, 238, 246
intestinal permeability, 38–39. *See also* small intestine
intracellular fluid (ICF), 164, 166–67
Ippoliti, Amy, **224–25**
iron
    and athletes, 117, 119
    and gluten-free diet, 122–24
    and gluten-intolerant athletes, 119–22
    overview, 117–18
    sources of, 124–25
iron deficiency or anemia, 54, 118, 119, 122, 124
Ironman triathletes case study, 61–65, 67
irritable bowel syndrome (IBS), 39
isolation training, 243
isosmotic dehydration, 167
isotonic beverages, 172, 173
IT (interval training), 235, 238, 246

Jill, Natalie, **76–77**, 99
Jory, Melissa McLean, 13–17
Journal of the American Medical Association, 41
juicing, 177, 180

Kagnoff, Martin, 22
Kale Chips, 268–69
Kale Salad with Jicama and Cranberries, 274–75
Kalenjin tribe, Kenya, 5, 150
ketosis, 190
Korver, Kyle, **42**, 44–45, 159, 201, 210
Korzun, Adam, 219, 221–22
Krebs cycle, 73

lactate threshold, 75, 231, 232–35, 239, 246
lactic acid, 71, 231

Lasagna, Classic, with a Twist, 282–83
leaky gut and gluten toxicity, 38–39
Leffer, Daniel, 22–23
Leipheimer, Levi, 46, 73, 209
Lentil Dal over Rice, 287–88
leucine and recovery process, 148, 149
lifestyle sports, 194–96
Lim, Allen, 45–46, 114, 200
Lime Tortilla Chips, Spicy, 269
long slow distance (LSD) training, 232–34, 246
Lopes, Brian, **51**
Lovato, Amanda, 61, **160–61**
LSD (long slow distance) training, 232–34, 246
lunch or dinner recipes, 279–306
Lyme disease, 187
Lyon, Erin Elberson, **131–32**
lysine, 86

Macaroni and Cheese, 288–89
macronutrients
    overview, 81–89
    protein, 20, 22, 85–87
    See also entries beginning with carbohydrate; *entries beginning with* fat
malabsorption
    example of, 188
    of fat, 117, 133
    of nutrients, 116, 171, 203–4, 237
    of starch, 36
Mauro, Liana, **43–44**
max heart rate, calculating, 232–35, 238
maximum performance
    beverage of choice for, 173–74
    gluten-free diet and glycemic index, 134–38
    See also VO$_2$ max
Mayo Clinic, 26
McCall, Timothy, 194
McLean, Barney, 13–15
meal size and frequency, 152
metabolic window in recovery mode, 147–48, 161, 162
micronutrients
    antioxidants, 91–92, 215
    overview, 89
    phytochemicals, 90–91

vitamins, 88, 90, 91–92, 130–32
    See also minerals
milk, gluten in, 155
minerals
    antioxidants, 91–92, 215
    calcium, 125–29, 130
    electrolytes, 164–65, 170, 172–74, 175, 182
    overview, 90
    See also iron
Mokate, Taylor, 152
monosaccharides, 81, 82
monounsaturated fats, 88
Moroccan Stew, Sweet and Spicy, 300
Muesli, Backcountry, 253–54
myoglobin, 118

Nall Richesson, Anita, 52, 153, 198, **199–200**
naloxone, 101
Napa cabbage, 262
National Foundation for Celiac Awareness, 12, 93, 194
National Osteoporosis Foundation, 204
natural killer (NK) cells, 45
neurological disorders, 39, 57, 68, 207
Nielsen, Kendra, 99, **181**
nightshades, 179
NK (natural killer) cells, 45
nonheme iron, 124–25
nutrient absorption
    calcium, 125–29, 130
    iron, 117–25
    overview, 116–17, 133
    vitamin D, 130–32
    See also food as fuel
nutrient malabsorption, 116, 171, 203–4, 237
nutrient-rich foods
    calcium, 129
    fats, 89
    fiber, 83, 85, 179, 180
    glutamine, 148–49, 150, 216
    iron, 124–25
    leucine, 149
    overview, 69
    potassium, 164–65
    protein, 86–87
    sodium, 165

vitamin D, 130
See also nutrient absorption
nutritional comparison of flours and
    starches, 248–49

Oatmeal, Old-Fashioned, 257–58
obesity, 103
Olympics, 1–2
opioid effects, 39
opioids (exorphins), 39, 52,
    101–2
Orange–Green Tea Smoothie,
    263
OS. *See* oxidative system
Osborne, Peter, 54, 154, 155, 210
osteomalacia and osteopenia, 128
osteoporosis, 125, 128, 203–4
oxidative stress, 91–92
oxidative system (OS)
    activity and predominate system, 74–75
    and before activity eating, 145
    and bonking, 77
    and interval training, 238, 246
    and iron, 118
    overview, 71, 73–74, 78
    and VO$_2$ max, 118
    See also carbohydrate oxidation; fat ox-
        idation; VO$_2$ max

Paralympics, 236
Pascal's wager, 53–54
PCr (phosphocreatine), 70, 74, 75, 77, 78
Pecan-Apple Crumble, 307–8
Pepitas, Spicy, 270
Peppers, Stuffed, 298–99
pepsin and gluten, 22
perceived exertion measure, 231
periodization, diet, 190
periodization, training, 242, 246
Pesto, Spinach, 297–98
phosphocreatine (PCr), 70, 74, 75, 77, 78
phytochemicals, 90–91
pilates, 243
Pinto, Craig, 111, **112–13**
pizza, 291–94
Poached Eggs on a Bed of Chard, 289–90
polarized training (IT), 235, 238
polyploidy, 25, 28–29

polysaccharides, 81, 82–83
polyunsaturated fats, 88
potassium, 164–65
Potatoes, Twice-Baked, 305–6
Power Pizza, 293–94
processed foods, 83, 85, 98–100
prolamins, 20
protein, 20, 22, 85–87

quinoa, 86
Quinoa Salad with Vinaigrette, 273–74
Quinoa–Sweet Potato Veggie Burgers,
    294–95
Quinoa-Turkey Meatloaf, 303–4

recipes
    about, 247–52
    breakfast, 253–60
    dessert, 307–10
    dips, 272, 277–78
    lunch or dinner, 279–306
    salads, 272–77
    smoothies, 178–80, 261–63
recovery, 147–49, 162, 172, 215–16
refined foods, 83, 85, 98–100
refined grains, 102
rehydration, 169–70
research
    on aging and gluten intolerance, 205
    on athletes with gluten intolerance, 59
    celiac disease patients and weight
        gain/loss, 104–5
    on effect of gluten-free diet on calorie
        intake, 102–3
    on gastrointestinal problems–sports
        relationship, 39
    on global nature of problem, 5–6
    on gluten exorphins, 53, 101–2
    on gluten in gluten-free products, 158
    on incidence of celiac disease, 26–27
    on inflammation and mortality, 41
    on nonhuman enzymes, 22
    on types of wheat and gluten, 27–29
    on wheat flour consumption, 27
resveratrol, 90–91
Roasted Beet and Spinach Salad, 275–76
Rockwell, Michelle, 168
Rolniak, Diana, **98**, 106, 211

salad recipes, 272–77
Salmon, Roasted, and Asparagus, 296–97
Salmon Salad, 276–77
Sands, David, 28, 29
saturated fat, 88
scientific calorie, 74
Scrambled Omelet, 258–59
senior athletes, 205–7, 233
Shannon, Clea, 211, **220–21**
shopping for gluten-free foods, 93–94, 96, 208
silent symptoms, 212–13
simple carbohydrates, 82
Skiing Magazine, 183–84
Slipstream Sports, 72
small intestine
    biopsy for celiac disease diagnosis, 31, 54, 214
    electrolyte absorption, 167
    and fluid intake, 175
    gluten-related damage, 30, 116, 119, 125, 213
    healing, 133
Smith, Jenny, 47, **48–49**, 98, 109, 111
Smith, Michelle, 159, 184, **188–89**
Smith, Sarah-Jane, **193–94**
Smith, Taro, **195**, 195–96
smoothies, 177–80, 261–63
Snacks, Trail Food, On the Go, 264–71
sodium, 164, 165, 166
sodium-potassium pump, 167
soy, 86
Spaghetti, Turkey Meatballs and, 302–3
Sparkes, Elyse, **197**
Spinach and Chickpeas, 297
Spinach and Roasted Beet Salad, 275–76
Spinach Pesto, 297–98
sports
    backcountry recreation, 183–89
    and bone density, 128–29
    duration and intensity factors in energy usage, 74–75
    and gastrointestinal problems, 39–40
    gluten-free endurance athletes, 47–49
    lifestyle sports, 194–96
    matching beverage to, 173–74
    overview, 216–17

team sports, 196–98, 200–201, 203, 216
    See also endurance athletes
sports detox cleanse
    foods to avoid, 225–26
    foods to enjoy, 226–27
    overview, 218–19, 221–22, 227
    process, 222–23
sports drinks, 172–75
Sports Illustrated, 153
starches, 82–83, 139–40
starches, nutritional comparison of flours and, 248–49
Stewart, Tyler, 49, 62, 175, **176**, 177, 211, 244–45
strength training, 149, 206–7, 243
stretching and flexibility, 243–44
Stuffed Peppers, 298–99
subtle effects of gluten, 50
Suhr, Jenn, **80–81**
support for gluten-free diet, 201, 203
Sweet Potato Fries, 301–2
Sweet Potato–Quinoa Veggie Burgers, 294–95
Sweet Potato–Walnut Cupcakes, 309–10
Sym, Christie, **60–61**, 61, 99, 107, 113, 210

Tamari Bison Jerky with a Kick, 271
Tarahumara tribe, Mexico, 4–5, 150
Taylor, Kristen, **56–58**, 99, 198, 201, 211
Team Gluten-Free, 237
team sports, 196–98, 200–201, 203, 216
teff, about, 259
Teff Power Porridge, 259–60
tempo training, 234–35, 246
terminology, 313–24
Toasted Garlic Guacamole, 277–78
training
    balance vs. overtraining, 244–45
    day-to-day diet for, 150–51
    and energy pathways, 75
    event preparation, 151
    interval training, 235, 238, 246
    long slow distance, 232–34, 246
    overview, 238, 245–46
    periodization, 242, 246

strength training, 149, 206–7, 243
stretching and flexibility, 243–44
tempo training, 234–35, 246
See also exercise
training load increase, 58
traveling and gluten-free diet, 207–9, 217
triglycerides, 73–74, 88
Turkey Burgers and Sweet Potato Fries, 301–2
Turkey Meatballs and Spaghetti, 302–3
Turkey-Quinoa Meatloaf, 303–4
Twice-Baked Potatoes, 305–6
twigs, sticks, and logs theory, 146, 185

unsaturated fats, 88
U.S. Census Bureau, 205
U.S. Department of Agriculture (USDA), 27, 93

Vande Velde, Christian, **72–73**
VanLaanen, Angeli, 183–84, **186–87**
Vegetable Frittata, 290–91
Veggie Burgers, Quinoa–Sweet Potato, 294–95
Veggie Pizza, 291–92
Vieira, Ginger, 99, 111, **142–43**
vitamins, 88, 90, 91–92, 130–32
VO₂ max
    and aging, 206
    calculating, 232–35, 238
    and interval training, 235, 246
    and iron, 118, 124
    and LSD training, 233
    overview, 74–75, 229, 231, 245
    and tempo training, 235, 246

Vollmer, Dana, **153–54**

Walnut–Sweet Potato Cupcakes, 309–10
water
    hyponatremia, 170, 182
    percent of body weight, 163
    sipping vs. gulping, 175
    sports drinks vs., 172–73
weather and hydration, 174
weight
    celiac disease examples, 104–5
    elite athlete examples, 105–8
    and gluten-free diet, 100–103, 238–39
    muscle vs. water weight, 163
wheat
    allergic reaction to, 31–32
    history of, 23–26
    nutrient profile of gluten-free grains and, 84
    sensitivity to, 43, 196
wheat-dependent, exercise-induced anaphylaxis, 31–32
whey and whey protein powder, 148
Willoughby, Carrie, **236–37**
wine, 161, 162
"Winning Without Wheat" *(Men's Journal)*, 73
women athletes, 61–65, 67, 203–4, 216
Wurtele, Heather, 62, **66**, 100, 159, 192

Yoder Begley, Amy, 99, 107, **126–27**, 211
yoga, 194–96, 243
Yoga as Medicine (McCall), 194

Zucchini Pizza, 292

ABOUT THE AUTHORS

Peter Bronski

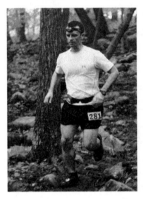

Peter Bronski is an award-winning writer whose work has appeared in more than eighty magazines, including *National Geographic Traveler, Men's Journal, Caribbean Travel & Life, Climbing, Rock & Ice, Snow, Vermont Sports, Elevation Outdoors, Rocky Mountain Sports, Sea Kayaker, AMC Outdoors, Appalachia,* and *Colorado Runner.*

He is the author or coauthor of seven books, including *Artisanal Gluten-Free Cooking,* which *Publishers Weekly* called an "outstanding volume," noting that its "impressive breadth and straightforward instructions make it an essential, horizon-broadening tool for those off gluten."

Pete is also cofounder of the popular and acclaimed blog *No Gluten, No Problem. The Kitchn* included it in a list of "10 Inspiring Blogs for Gluten-Free Food & Cooking," noting Pete's "thorough and lucid writing."

His writing has won numerous awards, including from the North American Travel Journalists Association, Solas Awards for Best Travel Writing, Society of Professional Journalists, and North American Snowsports Journalists Association.

Gluten-free since early 2007, when he was de facto diagnosed with celiac disease, Pete serves as a spokesperson for the National Foundation for Celiac Awareness as one of the organization's Athletes for Awareness. He is passionate about outdoor adventure sports, an endurance athlete currently focused on trail ultramarathons, and a former competitor at the Xterra off-road triathlon U.S. national championship.

He has taught gluten-free cooking demos, educational seminars, and athletic nutrition and training webinars for organizations including the Gluten & Allergen-Free Expo, National Foundation for Celiac Awareness, Gluten-Free Culinary Summit, Whole Foods, and Nourished: A Food Blogger Conference.

Pete and his gluten-free lifestyle have been featured in a variety of online, print, and broadcast media, including *Easy Eats, Gluten-Free Fitness, Edible Front Range,* the *Daily Camera* (Boulder, CO), Denver's NBC television affiliate, and National Public Radio's *The Splendid Table.*

He has been a member of the American Alpine Club, USA Triathlon, North American Travel Journalists Association, and North American Snowsports Journalists Association.

Pete lives in New York's Hudson Valley with his wife, Kelli, and their daughters, Marin and Charlotte.

You can find him at:

www.peterbronski.com
www.artisanglutenfree.com
http://noglutennoproblem.blogspot.com

Melissa McLean Jory

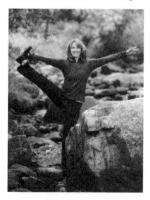

Melissa is a Master Nutrition Therapist and member of the National Association of Nutrition Professionals, a lover of simple food, a fearless cook, and founder in 2007 of the blog *Gluten Free for Good.* She also has a degree in exercise science, a committed yoga practice (she's crazy about inversions), and a passion for the backcountry. In 2007 she completed a two-hundred-hour yoga teacher training program and has followed it up with several additional trainings, including workshops with Matthew Sanford of Mind Body Solutions. Her interest is in bringing yoga to special populations to help transform difficulty into opportunity. She's especially interested in the neurological complications associated with gluten and volunteers in a yoga class for people with Parkinson's disease.

Although she doesn't like the word *disease* attached to it, she has celiac and specializes in gluten-free healing and thriving in her private nutrition practice. She's on a mission to increase awareness and help people navigate the gluten-free lifestyle with confidence, strength, optimal nutrition, and renewed vitality.

Born and raised in Colorado, Melissa grew up skiing, backpacking, hiking, and climbing and has logged hundreds of miles exploring the Rocky Mountain high country. All that time on the trail has fine-tuned her backcountry cooking skills.

She serves on the board of directors of the Colorado Ski & Snowboard Museum & Hall of Fame, is the fitness and nutrition advisor to the Gluten Intolerance Group of Colorado, and is a resource leader for the Celiac Sprue Association of Denver.

Her husband is in the ski business and shares her passion for the great outdoors. They've raised four adventurous kids, and in the process she's packed a zillion school lunches (and has never eaten a Twinkie).

Melissa lives with her family in Golden, Colorado, and finds no limits when it comes to nutritious and tasty gluten-free cooking, whether in the comfort of her kitchen or the wonder of the wilderness.

You can find her at:

www.glutenfreeforgood.com

HILLSBORO PUBLIC LIBRARIES
Hillsboro, OR
Member of Washington County
COOPERATIVE LIBRARY SERVICES